The Medical Profession in Mid-Victorian London

The
Medical Profession
in
Mid-Victorian
London

M. Jeanne Peterson

UNIVERSITY OF CALIFORNIA PRESS

BERKELEY · LOS ANGELES · LONDON

To my parents
Mildred and Clifford Peterson

UNIVERSITY OF CALIFORNIA PRESS

BERKELEY AND LOS ANGELES, CALIFORNIA

UNIVERSITY OF CALIFORNIA PRESS, LTD.

LONDON, ENGLAND

COPYRIGHT © 1978 BY

THE REGENTS OF THE UNIVERSITY OF CALIFORNIA

ISBN 0-520-03343-4

LIBRARY OF CONGRESS CATALOG CARD NUMBER: 76-48362

PRINTED IN THE UNITED STATES OF AMERICA

DESIGNED BY DAVE COMSTOCK

1 2 3 4 5 6 7 8 9

Contents

List of Tables and Appendices   vii

Acknowledgments   ix

Introduction   1

   I   The Early Nineteenth-Century Medical World   5

   II   Education for a Profession   40

   III   Careers in General Practice   90

   IV   The Formation of a Professional Elite   136

   V   The Struggle for Status and Income   194

   VI   Medical Entrepreneurship and Professional

        Order   244

Conclusion   283

Appendices   289

Notes   299

Bibliography   361

   1. Official Documents   361

   2. Other Manuscript and Printed Primary Sources   364

   3. Secondary Literature: Medical Profession,

       Medicine, and Science   372

   4. Other Secondary Literature (selected)   379

Index   385

Tables and Appendices

Tables

1   Education of Fellows of the Royal College of Physicians, 1800–1889   50
2   Education of Fellows of the Royal College of Surgeons, 1800–1889   51
3   Percent of Public School Men among College Officers, London and Provincial Practitioners, in the Royal College of Physicians, 1800–1889 (by date of Fellowship)   54
4   The Growth of the Medical Curriculum in the Nineteenth Century   62
5   Sources of Medical Degrees among Fellows, RCP, 1800–1889   67
6   Apprenticeship Premiums, Society of Apothecaries, in Selected Years   70
7   Estimates of the Cost of Medical Education   74
8   Educational Background of London Hospital Appointments to Full Surgeoncies, 1800–1855   142
9   Social Origins of Physicians (FRCP), Surgeons (FRCS), and Registered Apothecaries' Apprentices in the Nineteenth Century   198
10   Physicians' Connections with Aristocrats, Baronets, and Knights, 1800–1890, by Date of Fellowship, RCP   202
11   Estate Values of Heads of Medical Corporations Who Died between 1856 and 1928   208

12 Tariffs of Medical Fees for General Practitioners
    (Sydenham Medical District, 1867, and Shropshire,
    1870), Based on House Rental (i.e., "Class of
    Patient")   211
13 A Fee Schedule Based on Practitioners'
    Qualifications   212
14 Income of Medical Men in Five Selected Provincial
    Towns, 1910 and 1911   217
15 The Foundation of Specialist Charity Hospitals,
    Dispensaries, and Infirmaries in London and Great
    Britain to 1890   262
16 The Foundation of Medical Societies in London,
    1800–1900   268
17 The Foundation of Specialist Medical Periodicals in
    the United Kingdom in the Nineteenth Century   270

                            Appendices

A. Medical Licensing Bodies and Licenses and Degrees
    in the United Kingdom in the Nineteenth Century   289
B. Social Origins of Physicians (FRCP), Surgeons
    (FRCS), and Registered Apothecaries' Apprentices
    in the Nineteenth Century   291
C. Basic Organizational Structure of a Hospital and
    Medical School   295
D. The Growth of Staffs in the London Teaching Hos-
    pitals, 1855–1889   296
E. The Foundation of General and Specialist Peri-
    odicals in the United Kingdom in the Nineteenth
    Century   298

Acknowledgments

I AM indebted to many people for their assistance in the completion of this book. At the head of the list are the archivists and librarians, whose help is vital in the life of every scholar. My grateful thanks go to Mr. L. M. Payne, Librarian of the Royal College of Physicians of London, for his assistance in my research, and to David A. Pyke, M.D., FRCP, Registrar of the College, for his cooperation. The records of the Royal College of Physicians are cited here by permission of the College. Mr. Eustace Cornelius, Librarian of the Royal College of Surgeons, gave me gracious assistance at many stages of my research in the Surgeons' archives. Their records are cited here by the kind permission of the President and Council of the Royal College of Surgeons of England. Thanks are also due to Mr. Ernest Busby, Clerk and Registrar of the Society of Apothecaries, for his cooperation in the use of the archives of the Society.

Dr. N. J. M. Kerling, Archivist of St. Bartholomew's Hospital, gave me valuable assistance in my use of the hospital's manuscript collections. Miss E. D. Mercer, former Head Archivist, and the staff of the Greater London Record Office helped me in my work with the records of St. Thomas's Hospital deposited there. The records of St. Thomas's Hospital are cited here by the kind permission of St. Thomas's Hospital.

The staff of the Wellcome Institute of the History of Medicine deserves thanks for their kindly interest and highly competent assistance. All scholars in British history, myself included, must be thankful for the aid of the staffs of the

British Library, the Public Record Office, the National Register of Archives, Somerset House, the Guildhall (London), and the Bodleian Library.

Friends and colleagues gave me useful suggestions, bibliographical references, cogent criticism, and a wealth of moral support along the way. Among the many who gave helping hands were Dr. Alexander M. Cooke, Dr. Richard D. French, Professor Gerald Geison, Ms. Barbara P. Kaplan, Professor Herbert H. Kaplan, Professor Paul W. Kuznets, Professor Martin Ridge, Dr. Jeffrey L. Berlant, Professor Walter Arnstein, and the editors of the University of California Press. I owe a special debt of gratitude to Professor Hans Rosenberg who, in his seminar, opened the door of social history for me.

The clerical assistance of Miss Debra Chase was excellent, and she deserves warm thanks for her good service.

Financial support for research on this project in England came from the Sigmund Martin Heller Travelling Fellowship in History of the University of California, Berkeley, the American Association of University Women, and the Office of Research and Advanced Studies of Indiana University, Bloomington. I am deeply grateful for their support.

Assistance, guidance, and encouragement came from my teachers, Professor L. Perry Curtis, Jr., Professor Sheldon Rothblatt, and Professor Neil Smelser. They gave me suggestions and criticisms in the early stages of this work which were of great value in shaping it. Professor Curtis deserves particular and special thanks. From first to last, his substantive suggestions and his encouragement, his generosity and kindness, were illustrative of the best help that the intellectual and scholarly world has to offer.

Many helped, and this book is better because of their willingness to share information and ideas, to debate, and to criticize. Its shortcomings, however, are my own.

Introduction

WHEN Dorothy Sayers's famous fictional detective, Lord Peter Wimsey, suspected the truth, that the eminent surgeon Sir Julian Freke, Kt., GCVO, KCVO, KCB, MD, FRCP, FRCS, had murdered his old rival Sir Reuben Levy, he could scarcely believe the evidence of his own investigation. He refused to reveal the name of his suspect to his friend Mr. Parker, for fear he might be wrong: "I say I *may* be wrong—and I'd feel as if I'd libelled the Archbishop of Canterbury."[1] Such reverence for medical science and medical men, a commonplace of the twentieth century, had no part in the thinking of aristocrats or ordinary folk a century earlier.

The advancement of the medical profession is part of the larger story of the "rise of the middle classes" which took place in the wake of the industrial revolution. Unlike the working classes, whose fate was so intimately tied to industrialization and urbanization, the middling ranks of nineteenth-century English society have received relatively little attention from historians. Part of that neglect results from the enormous diversity encompassed by the term "middle classes." In addition, the nearly limitless volume of source material available poses monumental problems for the would-be historian of this segment of Victorian society. Occupation, a central feature of social identification in industrial society, offers an instrument for dividing the "middle classes" into coherent sub-groups for closer historical examination.

The medical profession in the nineteenth century can be studied from a variety of perspectives. Its legislative history, its professional institutions, and its relations with government, armed services, and the new agencies of poor law and public health—all these provide legitimate foci for examining the history of the profession. Indeed, important work has been going on in these areas for the past decade. Advances in medicine and related sciences during the Victorian years offer another important avenue to knowledge of the profession. Intellectual historians and historians of science are finding the nineteenth century a field well worth tilling.

˙ Finally, the categories and concepts of the social sciences can provide an analytic framework for a study of Victorian medical life, and this approach provides the structure of the present work. The Victorian era was a time of expanding economic opportunity and, concomitantly, an age of social aspiration and social mobility. A sociological approach to the history of the Victorian medical profession leads to the exploration of such issues as social origins, education, career patterns, income, life style, intra-occupational friendship and enmity, and the internal dynamics of professional life in the careers of medical men individually and collectively. These men—for few women managed to enter the profession during the Victorian era—found closed doors and open options, smooth paths and difficulties, the fear of failure and the pleasure of success. At one level, the social history of the medical profession is the story of men's efforts to make a living and a mark on the world. At the same time, the history of the medical profession is a group's history. Shared occupational status meant shared problems and joint efforts through group formation, concerted action, and legislation, to find solutions to their shared problems and gratification of their shared desires. Out of individual ambition and collective effort, medical men transformed their profession.

The central temporal focus of this study is the period between two major items of medical legislation, 1858 to 1886. It was a period of relative calm in the profession, preceded by the decades-long battle for medical reform which had culminated in the Medical Act of 1858. With that legislation, medical qualification was defined and the institutional structure of the profession was given at least a form of unity. But it was

2

precisely when the major battle for legal reform of the profession was over that medical men had to face other fundamental issues in the conduct of their individual and collective careers. The year 1886 marks the passage of the Medical Act Amendment Act and as such denotes the legal and symbolic integration of medicine and surgery, and the integration of general practitioners in the institutional structure of the profession. These legislative dates encompass a period when the profession's internal relations and its relationships with lay society were redefined in significant ways.

The geographical focus of this study is London. Although Edinburgh, Glasgow, and Dublin had been distinguished centers of medical science and practice before the nineteenth century, London became the locus of power, international prestige, and wealth for the profession by the early Victorian era. London was the center of medical education and practice. The most important hospitals, the most prestigious medical corporations, and the most lucrative, influential, and honorific medical careers were found there. It was the arena in which the ambitions of medical men were often whetted, frequently frustrated, and occasionally brilliantly realized. Opportunities for local influence and prominence were available in the large provincial towns, and the establishment of medical schools in Liverpool, Manchester, Bristol, and elsewhere opened up the opportunities for distinction and eminence that made London so attractive. But these provincial developments followed the London pattern, and medical men turned to London for models of success in the profession.

One of the central themes explored in this study is the changing character of medical prestige and the evolution of medical men's authority—over their work, their patients, and the organization of their professional lives.* Some might argue that authority and prestige in medicine grew with such

*For much of the theoretical underpinning for this work I am indebted to Eliot Freidson, *Profession of Medicine. A Study of the Sociology of Applied Knowledge* (New York, 1970). See especially pp. 23, 47, and 71 ff.

3

scientific innovations as vaccination, anesthetics, and antisepsis. Such an assertion implies that occupational prestige and authority grow out of the efficacy of the work performed. However true this may be in the twentieth century, efficacy was not the standard by which Victorian medical men and laymen judged the status of an occupation.

The demonstrable efficacy of medical practice was not the source of the profession's prestige and authority, any more than the status of the Anglican clergy derived from the demonstrable effectiveness of prayer and ritual.[2] Prestige and authority derive, rather, from the social evaluation placed on the work itself, regardless of the effectiveness of specific treatment. Increasing secularization, including a greater concern with physical health, human life, and productivity, provided a social environment in which knowledge of the human body, even in the absence of effective treatment, began to have significance, and in which medical men could make claims for the supreme importance of their work. Only in such an environment could medical men move from a position of dependency on lay patronage and lay values to a position of independence and authority over their own work. How they achieved that end is the subject of this book.

Since this book went to press two articles have appeared that lend support to certain aspects of this work. They are: Ivan Waddington, "General Practitioners and Consultants in Early Nineteenth-Century England: The Sociology of Intra-Professional Conflict," in: *Health Care and Popular Medicine in Nineteenth Century England, Essays in the Social History of Medicine*, ed. John Woodward and David Richards (New York, 1977), pp. 164–188; and Ian Inkster, "Marginal Men: Aspects of the Social Role of the Medical Community in Sheffield 1790–1850," in ibid., pp. 128–163.

I

❦

The Early Nineteenth-Century
Medical World

BEFORE the passage of the Medical Act of 1858, the organizational structure of the medical profession was in a state of near-chaos.[1] There were nineteen different licensing bodies in the United Kingdom by the early nineteenth century, and the rules governing their recognition were a tangle of conflicting rights and powers.* Medical men practiced with university degrees, various forms of medical licenses, sometimes a combination of these, and sometimes with none at all. Medical training varied from classical university education and the study of Greek and Latin medical texts, on the one hand, to broom-and-apron apprenticeship in an apothecary's shop, on the other—and sometimes involved no recognizable education at all. Quacks, "empirics," and drug peddlers practiced freely with no legal sanctions against them, while a physician in London could be disciplined by his College for preparing and selling a prescription to his patient.

The key to understanding the structure of the early nineteenth-century medical profession is to be found in a commonplace of medical history: the separation of medical men into three orders—physicians, surgeons, and apothecaries.[2] These three orders took corporate form in the Royal College of Physicians, the Royal College of Surgeons, and the Society

---

*See Appendix A for a list of medical corporations and universities and their licenses and degrees.

of Apothecaries, and they defined the social structure of the profession and, in theory at least, the division of medical labor.

The three orders of medical practice reflect the social division of medical practitioners into three status groups or estates. Social theorists such as Max Weber and T. H. Marshall have described the stratification of society according to estates as one of the characteristics of pre-industrial society.[3] The primary characteristics of estates are their legal rights and duties, their claims to traditional and historical legitimacy of privileges, a tendency toward membership by birth, exclusiveness of membership and functions, and material monopolies. Estates, like castes, are sometimes associated with specific occupations, occasionally having a monopoly over some trade, craft, or service, and their members are usually prohibited from taking up occupations other than those defined by their estate membership. Early Victorian medical practice was organized according to status groups of just this sort, with differing duties, legal privileges, and social ranks. Thus, while it is convenient to speak of medical practitioners collectively as "the medical profession," the unity implied by such a term is scarcely evident in the structure of early nineteenth-century medical life.[4]

I

The oldest medical corporation in England was the Royal College of Physicians of London, whose charter dated from 1518.[5] The College had a monopoly over the practice of "physic," that is, internal medicine, in London and its environs and was charged with the general oversight of physicians in all of England.*

The College granted two types of license for practice in London before 1858, the Fellowship (FRCP) and the License (LRCP). Men in line for the Fellowship held the interim title of Candidate. Only Fellows enjoyed the full rights granted to

---

*Similar corporations existed in Scotland and Ireland. See Appendix A for a complete list.

physicians by the College charter—exemption from municipal assizes, juries, inquests, "watch and ward," and military service and taxation, as well as powers within the College such as the right to vote in College elections and to hold College office. Fellows also lived under certain prohibitions: they could not belong to any other medical corporation, nor could they engage in trade. Thus, a physician could not practice surgery (the province of the surgeons' corporation), and he could not "practice as an apothecary" by compounding or selling medicines, even to his own patients.[6] A Fellow had to practice only as a "pure physician," examining patients, diagnosing disease, and prescribing medications which an apothecary or druggist then dispensed. If a physician decided to include surgery and drug dispensing in his medical practice, he had to resign his Fellowship or face the possibility of a fine or expulsion.[7] Hence, at the highest levels of collegiate life, the charter maintained the distinction between physicians and other orders of practitioners.*

While London physicians were required to be licensed by the College, provincial physicians had the option of affiliating with the London College or not. They could take the Extra-License of the College but were not prosecuted for practicing without it. Licentiates and their provincial counterparts were free to "practice generally," unrestricted by the rules that governed the Fellows.

By act of Parliament the practice of physic was reserved only to "those persons that be profound, sad and discreet, groundedly learned, and deeply studied,"[8] and, from Tudor times to the nineteenth century, this meant men with university degrees. This university education set the physicians apart from the other orders of medical practitioners. The College made distinctions, too, between graduates of English universities and those from other parts of the kingdom. Physicians with Scottish or Irish medical degrees might hold the License or Extra-License, but only graduates of Oxford

---

*W. H. Stone was the first medical man to hold both the FRCS (1856) and the FRCP (1863). See *Plarr's Lives*, s.v.

and Cambridge were eligible for the Fellowship.* The exclusion of Scottish and Irish university graduates from the Fellowship had nothing to do with the quality of medical education in those institutions. Indeed, the Scottish universities
provided medical education distinctly superior to that of Oxford or Cambridge. However, the experience of collegiate life
in Oxford or Cambridge gave medical students, it was argued, an education in morals and manners that made them fit
candidates for the Fellowship. The criteria for election, then,
were as much character and breeding as they were a man's
achievements in medicine.[9] Shared educational background,
the common experience of Oxbridge life, and membership in
the College and in a single occupation made the London
physicians a distinct social group.

The number of physicians was small. In 1800 there were
a total of 179 Fellows, Licentiates, and Extra-Licentiates in
England. By 1847 this number had grown to 683, of whom 76
percent resided in London.† Their considerable growth aside,
the College of Physicians represented less than 5 percent of
all medical practitioners in England at mid-century. Size,
however, was no measure of their strength. Their ancient collegiate foundation, their tradition of classical learning, the absence of trade or craft functions in the physician's work—all

---

*Degrees from Trinity College, Dublin, could be "incorpo-
rated" at Oxbridge, but this was only infrequently done. Table 1,
on page 50, shows the university affiliation of the Fellows of the
Royal College of Physicians in the nineteenth century. See also: Sir
George Clark, *A History of the Royal College of Physicians of London*
(Oxford, 1966), II, 663.

† Figures are drawn from Clark, *A History*, II, 738–739, and
from the Census and Medical Directories cited in A. H. T. Robb-
Smith, "Medical Education at Oxford and Cambridge Prior to 1850,"
in *The Evolution of Medical Education in Britain*, ed. F. N. L. Poynter
(London, 1966), pp. 50–51. Of the 14,700 medical men practicing in
England in 1850, there were 1,700 who claimed status as physicians.
Although the College did little to enforce its monopoly in London,
80 percent of all London physicians practiced with some College
license. However, only 23 percent of provincial physicians bothered
to affiliate themselves with the College.

these contributed to the position of the Royal College of Physicians as the most prestigious of the medical corporations.

Although surgery was, in practice, as ancient a medical art as "physic," its institutions and the nature of surgical work gave it a rather different character in the early nineteenth century from that of the learned physicians. The distinguishing feature of the surgeon's work was that it involved cutting, manipulation, and the treatment of disorders on the outside of the body. A surgeon performed operations, set broken bones, and treated accident cases, skin disorders, and some forms of gynecological ailments. Much of a surgeon's work, even after the advent of anesthetics, demanded speed, dexterity, and physical strength, as well as expertise. It was skilled manual labor, and the eighteenth-century phrase, "the craft of surgery," suggests something of the antecedents of this branch of the profession.[10]

Since the middle ages, surgeons in London had been organized in a guild. In 1540 they joined with the barbers to form the Barber-Surgeons' Company of the City of London. This union lasted until 1745, when the surgeons established a separate City company. In 1800 the surgeons received their charter as the Royal College of Surgeons of London. A new charter in 1843 made them the Royal College of Surgeons of England and established, in addition to the Membership (MRCS), the higher surgical rank of Fellowship (FRCS). The College did not have a monopoly over surgical practice, but in other respects it resembled the College of Physicians in being a legally defined group whose membership was controlled and whose occupational functions were defined. The change of name from Company to College, the severance of ties with the City of London, the new designation of officers as President and Vice-President (instead of Master and Wardens), and the institution of the Fellowship all indicated the movement of the surgeons away from craft guild traditions to the more elevated status enjoyed by the prestigious College of Physicians.

Perhaps the most important difference between the physicians and the surgeons had to do with their forms of education. Unlike the physicians, surgeons were not university-educated men. As was traditional among craftsmen, surgeons learned their skills by apprenticeship. Their training was necessarily practical and not at all classical or theoretical as the physicians' reputedly was. Only in the early nineteenth century, in the wake of John Hunter's remarkable achievements in comparative anatomy and pathology, did surgeons begin to enjoy the prospects of a reputation as men of science, and, by implication, perhaps, as men of learning. The claim of surgery to scientific status was new-born in the early nineteenth century, and most surgeons were practical men rather than researchers and theorists in this branch of medicine.* Without the reputation for classical learning which the physicians enjoyed, the surgeons' new charter and new titles represented improved status but scarcely parity with the College of Physicians.

The Royal College of Surgeons was much larger than the College of Physicians. At mid-century, over 8,000 practitioners held a surgical license. Of these, only some 200 were Fellows of the College.[11] The FRCS was not exclusively a London license, and those who held it practiced in all parts of England. A surgeon could become a Fellow by election or by examination, but the Fellowship did not lead automatically to membership in the inner circle of College power. The Council, the governing body of the College of Surgeons, was made up of London surgeons who practiced only the pure art of surgery.[12] Only the elite few could afford the luxury of a practice limited to surgery alone. In order to make a living, most members of the surgeons' corporation had to prescribe and dispense drugs as well. Increasingly in the nineteenth century, these surgeon-apothecaries qualified themselves for medical practice by taking a second qualification from the

*Sir Zachary Cope, The Royal College of Surgeons of England. A History (London, 1959), pp. 30–32. The surgeons were slow to pursue these scientific interests. Hunter's collection of anatomical specimens, bequeathed to the College, was stored for many months before finally being put on display; access was limited to two afternoons a week for only a few months of each year, and relatively few persons attended.

Apothecaries' Society. This corporation constituted the third of the medical estate groups.

The historic traditions of the Apothecaries' Society linked them with trade.[13] Before 1617 apothecaries had been a part of the Grocers' Company of the City of London. In that year they obtained a royal charter as the Society of Apothecaries. Their privileges and functions were, like those of other City companies, defined by their charter: they were responsible for the supply, compounding, and sale of drugs in London. At that time in their history they were not medical practitioners but druggists. The practice of prescribing "over the counter" by the apothecaries and the failure of the physicians to provide necessary medical care to the great masses of the population brought the apothecaries of the seventeenth century more and more into the practice of medicine as well as the drug trade. In the early eighteenth century they gained legal sanction, over the protests of the physicians, to prescribe medicines, but they were not allowed to charge for their advice; they could be paid only for the medicines they sold. The Apothecaries Act of 1815 legitimized the practice of medicine by apothecaries and authorized the Society of Apothecaries to grant a license (the LSA) for medical practice in England. Apothecaries, like surgeons, were trained by apprenticeship.

The LSA was a popular qualification among early nineteenth-century medical men. Between 1815 and 1834 the Society granted the license to over 6,000 medical men. Over half of these practitioners also held the MRCS.[14] Multiple affiliation and mixed practice was, however, prohibited to the elites of the Apothecaries' Society, the Freemen. Like the pure physicians and pure surgeons, the small group of Freemen maintained the exclusiveness of their practice and constituted a separate, privileged group. Only Freemen could practice in the City of London or within a seven-mile radius. Freemen could invest in the Society's drug trade, earn a dividend on their investments, and purchase chemicals from the Society's laboratory at a discount.[15] Sons of Freemen gained the freedom of the society "by patrimony." The Apothecaries' Society, like the Colleges of Physicians and Surgeons, had its own coat of arms, ceremonies, dress, and rituals.

The medical profession in early nineteenth-century England consisted, in brief, of three distinctly organized, legally defined status groups practicing "the profession of physic," "the craft of surgery," and the "apothecary's trade." These three orders, ranked hierarchically according to the value society placed on their modes of practice, constituted an occupational division of labor, but they also defined a pre-industrial form of social structure and stratification. When medical reforms were proposed, the corporations of London resisted change, a policy which could be seen as the product of jealousy and small-mindedness. The corporations have been accused of short-sighted defense of their own corporate privileges.[16] While it is certainly true that the officials of the three corporations were concerned with maintaining their legal privileges and monopolies, the recognition that the medical corporations were also status groups suggests a further reason for their rigidity than simple greed and jealousy. The position of the physicians and surgeons as members of Colleges with royal charters set them apart from the practice of medicine as carried on by the apothecaries. The Apothecaries' identity as a "trading company," their historic origins in the Grocers' Company, and their "tradesmanlike" practice of medicine from a shop, all marked them as men of a status inferior to that enjoyed by the physicians and desired by the surgeons.[17] The separation of the orders was not only an arrangement of occupational monopolies; it defined the social order and men's social status as well.

II

Beside the medical corporations, another group of institutions came to play a central role in medical life in the nineteenth century—the hospitals. The oldest hospitals in London, St. Bartholomew's (founded in 1123) and St. Thomas's (founded in 1207), had originally been established as charities for the needy, infirm, and aged, as well as for the sick. The eighteenth century saw the foundation of five additional general hospitals specifically for the care of the sick poor: Westminster Hospital (1719), Guy's (1721), St. George's (1733), the London Hospital (1740), and the Middlesex Hospital (1745). Between 1800 and 1850 Charing Cross Hospital, University College Hospital, King's College Hospital, and St. Mary's Hospital came into existence. Other institutions for the care of the sick poor, such as eye hospitals, maternity charities, and government-sponsored "fever hospitals" and insane asylums, also appeared in the late eighteenth and early nineteenth centuries; but these eleven general hospitals are of particular significance because they were the institutions which, during the first half of the nineteenth century, became the centers of medical teaching in London.[18]

Funds for these charity hospitals came from two sources. The older foundations were supported in large part by endowments and income from land. The later foundations relied to a much greater degree on income from annual charitable subscriptions received from the public. Laymen, from the ranks of trade to the aristocracy, found gratification and material rewards from their connections with the hospitals. As contributors they became governors of the hospital and thus participated in the policy-making and administration of the charity. Businessmen who contributed to the hospital might expect a share of the hospital's trade to come to them, and contributors in all ranks had the right to nominate patients for admission to the hospital wards, frequently their servants or employees.* Neither hygienic nor pleasant, the early nineteenth-century hospital was the resort of those who could not afford to pay for private medical care. Those with means were cared for at home.

The medical staff of each hospital was elected by its board of governors and was composed of up to four physicians, four surgeons, and one apothecary, together with assistants in each rank. Hospital posts did not usually carry a stipend, but there were benefits for the medical men who held them. As a charitable endeavor, service on the hospital staff

---

*Some hospitals refused admission to their wards to all except accident cases and those with letters of reference from subscribers. For a discussion of hospital charity, see: John Woodward, *To Do the Sick No Harm. A Study of the British Voluntary Hospital System to 1875* (London and Boston, 1974), Chapters 3 and 5; and David Owen, *English Philanthropy, 1660–1960* (Cambridge, Mass., 1964).

was an expression of a medical man's civic and humanitarian concern. Hospital posts also brought medical men connections with the prestigious lay patrons (and potential patients) on the board of governors, and they provided extensive clinical experience. An appointment to the staff of a hospital was considered an honor and provided the basis for a growing private consulting practice.

In an informal way, the hospital was a place of medical education at the beginning of the nineteenth century. Medical students came to the hospitals from Oxbridge and from apprenticeships in the provinces or London. They walked the wards and observed the practice of the hospitals' physicians and surgeons in the hospitals. The hospital only supplemented the formal institutions of medical education. At the universities, students of physic devoted themselves to the classical medical texts, theories of disease, symptoms, *materia medica*, and treatments. Apprentice surgeons and apothecaries learned the practice of their respective arts of diagnosis, operative techniques, and the prescribing and preparation of drugs at their master's side.

Fundamental changes in the conceptions of diagnosis and disease, together with developments in the sciences of anatomy and physiology, had far-reaching effects on medical science and practice. The scientific development of these changes falls outside the purview of this study, but they include the growth of knowledge about the relationship between symptoms, physical signs, and the findings of morbid anatomy, and the resultant shift away from mere "history taking" in diagnosis to the "invention of diagnosis by [the] physical examination" of the patient.[19] Less reliance was placed on the patient's description of his own symptoms and more importance placed on the medical man's evaluation of the physical signs of disease which he observed in the patient. In a subtle way, authority about the patient's physical condition shifted from patient to doctor as the doctor became less dependent upon the patient for knowledge of the patient's condition.[20] As a result, training in anatomy and physiology and experience at the bedside became increasingly important aspects of a medical student's life. Medical education changed to meet these advances in the science of medicine. Medical students who had formerly received only haphazard exposure to anatomy and physiology turned to the private anatomy schools like the Windmill Street School and the London School of Anatomy for systematic lectures and demonstrations in these auxiliary sciences. Members of the hospital staffs, too, began offering instruction in these subjects in the hospitals. The early lecture courses were the private enterprises of individual medical men; the hospital was simply a convenient place to teach. In the decades before 1850, one London hospital after another incorporated the lectures into the structure of the hospitals and brought them under the administrative control of their boards of governors. Similarly, clinical experience was formalized and made a part of the curriculum. The hospital had become a medical school.[21]

The rise of the hospitals as centers of medical education brought about changes in the structure of the profession itself. First, while apprenticeship continued to be a common mode of medical training until the 1840's, and was practiced by some until the 1880's,[22] the isolated, one-to-one relationship of apprentice and master became only one part of the total experience of medical education, and progressively a less important one. Oxbridge medical students, too, came to London to participate in hospital life, and thus began to emerge from their classical and theoretical milieu. In short, medical students began to share the same basic educational experiences and to develop a sense of group membership that mitigated the effects of corporate separatism. Second, hospital teaching brought physicians and surgeons together in a single institution. As members of the hospital and medical school staffs, consulting physicians and surgeons were participating together in an increasingly important function outside the spheres of their separate corporations. Their joint activities tended, in the long run, to undermine the isolation of the corporate elites and brought them into closer association with each other.

The importance of this new institutional role for physicians and surgeons is reflected in the growth of the term "consultant" to refer to those who held hospital appointments. Such usage reflected the development of a new distinction within the medical hierarchy—the distinction between those who held hospital and medical school posts and those who did not. By mid-century this division among medical practitioners was becoming more important than the corporate distinctions that divided physician, surgeon, and apothecary.[23] The consultants of the teaching hospitals—whether physicians or surgeons—became recognized as a separate group from the rank and file of medical men. A gradual development, rooted in early nineteenth-century changes in medical education, it took fifty years or more to be reflected in the institutional relationships of physicians and surgeons.[24] Nevertheless, the emergence of the consultant marks an important phase in the development of the medical profession's modern stratification: the "lower" grade of ordinary practitioners and the "higher" grade of consultants.[25]

Hospital physicians and surgeons were drawn largely from the leadership of the London Colleges. Thus they came to enjoy not only the prestige accruing to them as leaders of the medical corporations, but also the high status of those who were the leaders of medical education in the nation. Hospital teaching, consulting work, and corporate power were the marks of an increasingly visible and important medical elite. At the same time, since hospital teaching was displacing private apprenticeship as the core of medical education, practitioners without hospital posts lost their place and role in the training of medical men.

III

Parallel to the evolution of the hospital and consulting elite was a growing homogeneity among the rank and file of medical practitioners, those outside the elite circle. Their links to their respective corporations were, in the first place, not strong. Although licensed by the College of Surgeons or the Apothecaries' Hall, they had no power within the corporations, and they were relegated to distinctly inferior status. At the College of Surgeons, for example, an ordinary

16

Member could not be invited to dine with the Fellows, and he was required to enter the College by the back door.[26]

In spite of corporate and theoretical separation of functions among the three orders of practitioners, medical care was, for the rank and file, less compartmentalized in everyday practice. Apothecaries dispensed and prescribed, but they also performed minor surgical operations such as dental extractions and bleeding. Surgeons operated, but they also prescribed medicines for internal disorders. Physicians, except for College Fellows, also engaged in what came to be known as "general practice." These multiple functions carried out by medical men were reflected in the changing patterns of licensing. After the Apothecaries' Act of 1815, medical men who engaged in prescribing and dispensing were required to take the License of the Society of Apothecaries, whatever other license they held. While the Membership of the Royal College of Surgeons was not a legal requirement for surgical practice, it had apparently become "the general rule" by the 1830's for practitioners who held the LSA to take the MRCS qualification as well.[27] Holders of these two licenses "practiced generally"—that is, they practiced both medicine and surgery.

Changes in nomenclature also reflect developments in the structure of medical society. At the beginning of the century it was common custom to refer to medical men according to their corporate affiliation—physician, surgeon, apothecary, and later apothecary-surgeon. The term "general practitioner" emerged in the first thirty years of the century to refer to men who practiced medicine and surgery, whether dually licensed or not. This term, and other designations unrelated to corporate membership, largely replaced the traditional terminology.* This shift in language suggests that the

---

*The common usage may be seen in various Victorian novels. For example, the senior Pendennis was an "apothecary," in W. M. Thackeray's *Pendennis*; Mr. Candy, in Wilkie Collins's *The Moonstone*, was a "surgeon." Anthony Trollope uses "medical man" and "London physician" in his novels, *Dr. Thorne* and *Barchester Towers*. The generic use of the term "doctor" was not universal until late in the century. In this study the terms "medical man" and "medical practitioner" are used as general terms for persons engaged in medical

medical man's functions were becoming more important than his corporate affiliation. The new designation also points up the distinction between the general practitioner's status and function and those of the pure physicians and pure surgeons, and it indicates the weakening and breakdown of ties between the rank and file members of the corporations and their respective elites. Medical men were being identified with others who practiced as they did, without regard to the technicalities of licensure.

More concrete evidence of the breakdown of the corporate order can be seen in the unprecedented growth in the early nineteenth century of medical organizations and societies outside the established structures of the profession. Such societies were not a new phenomenon in the nineteenth century. Medical book clubs, social clubs, and a few societies devoted to medical science had existed in the eighteenth century, devoted to the pursuit of intellectual exchange and social intercourse.* Some drew their memberships exclusively from a single medical order,[28] while others claimed members from all segments of the profession. The proliferation of medical associations in the first half of the nineteenth century may reflect, in part, the growth of a medical population in any given locale large enough to sustain activities designed to further professional intercourse and mutual assistance. Hence there appeared such associations as the Society for the Relief of Widows and Orphans of Medical Men, the Lyceum

---

practice, whether as consultants or general practitioners. This is done to conform with the most common Victorian usage and to avoid any implications regarding the practitioner's status *vis-à-vis* the M.D. degree.

*For example, the Medico-Chirurgical Society, the Hunterian Society, and the Medical Society of London. See: Clark, *A History*, II, 554, 556, and 643–644. These organizations deserve further study than can be given here, but they seem to have been the preserve of the London elite, serving as a place for introductions and professional connections among consultants. See, for example, the membership lists in Norman Moore and Stephen Paget, *The Royal Medical and Chirurgical Society of London. Centenary, 1805–1905* (Aberdeen, 1905), pp. 3 and 18.

Medicum Londinense, the Medical Society of London, and a variety of student medical societies. In the provinces, the Lincolnshire Benevolent Medical Society, the Worcester County and City Medical Society, and a host of other local groups were established.[29]

Many of the societies which appeared from the turn of the century onward were formed in order to achieve professional goals which the corporations ignored or opposed. The London corporations often seemed indifferent to the needs of the great mass of medical practitioners, and extra-corporate societies worked to bring about changes in practitioners' relationships with the corporations or to remove specific sources of grievance. One example of such an association was the General Pharmaceutical Association of Great Britain, founded in London in 1793. This organization has been called "the first expression of group-consciousness of the new general practitioner in England,"[30] but it was an association of London apothecaries, members of one medical order. The Association collected information about the state of medical practice in England and made proposals for medical reform. Their efforts were effectively thwarted by the leadership of the Society of Apothecaries. The Licentiates and Extra-Licentiates of the Royal College of Physicians organized the Society of Collegiate Physicians in order to press the College leadership for improved status within the corporation, and the Surgeons' Association was a similar organization within their College.[31]

The appearance of reformist medical associations which cut across corporate lines marked a new departure in medical organization. They indicate important changes in the structure of the medical profession, both in the country and in London. That provincial practitioners tended to neglect corporate distinctions in their local organizations was not surprising. Since the London leadership was often both geographically and functionally remote from them and their local professional concerns, the corporate separatism of London had far less force in provincial regions. Provincial hospital physicians and surgeons, together with general practitioners, formed their own societies which provided a forum for professional discussion, social intercourse, and medico-political activity.

However, these mixed associations also began to appear in London, in the very shadow of the Royal Colleges. One of these early London organizations was a group known as the Associated Faculty. Formed in 1805, its membership came from both the Royal College of Physicians and the College of Surgeons. Its members were concerned with regulating medical practice in England, improving the educational standards of the profession, and elevating the social character of the profession by excluding "mean and low persons" from entry.[32] No democrats, they supported the notion of hierarchy within the profession. At the same time, however, they advocated opening up practice in all branches of medicine to all qualified practitioners, rather than limiting "the sphere of medical duty by coercive statutes."[33] Their proposals for ending the separation of physic and surgery met with immediate opposition from the medical corporations. The College of Physicians saw their proposed bill as a "design . . . directed to . . . the subversion of the existing authorities in Physic, and the depression of the rights, rank, and importance of the Physician."[34] The members of the Associated Faculty fought until 1811 for reform before resigning themselves to failure. Their organization, however, marks a first step in the direction of breaking down the separation of the medical estates.

The following year saw efforts for reform renewed. In 1812, London apothecaries met to protest taxes on glass, a burden to dispensers of bottled medicines, but they moved quickly from this specific problem to the more general matter of medical reform. Out of the meeting grew the Association of Apothecaries and Surgeon-Apothecaries.* While the name

* Their grievances, like those of the General Pharmaceutical Association before them, stemmed from the encroachment of druggists and chemists on their medical practice, and they saw the need for proper controls over unlicensed practice and for an agency to control the practice of apothecaries, surgeon-apothecaries, and midwives. Such grievances and the creation of the Association reveal the conviction that the corporations, left to themselves, were not interested in these problems of the rank-and-file practitioners—problems

of the association reflects the continued affiliation of general practitioners with their own corporations, it also reveals the willingness of medical practitioners to combine without regard for corporate alignments, for purposes of united action. In 1813 this new organization went further and proposed legislation for the regulation of general practice in England and Wales through a new licensing body, composed of men from the Royal Colleges of Physicians and Surgeons and the Society of Apothecaries, together with a number of general practitioners. Such an act would clearly have broken down the lines of division between physicians, surgeons, and apothecaries at the top levels of organization; it would also have blurred the distinction between the elites of the corporations and their rank and file. Not surprisingly, the corporations refused to cooperate and the bill was withdrawn. The Association then proposed a revised bill which placed responsibility for licensing apothecaries directly and solely in the hands of the Apothecaries' Society and left the privileges and separation of the corporations entirely unchanged. The new bill, adopted in 1815, was entitled "An Act for Enlarging the Charter of the Society of Apothecaries in the City of London, granted by His Majesty King James the First, and for better regulating the Practice of Apothecaries throughout England and Wales" (55 Geo. III, c. 194).[35] The title of the act is significant: the Apothecaries' Act was intended as a continuation and extension of the organization of medicine as it was laid down in the seventeenth century.

The passing of the Apothecaries' Act of 1815 has been hailed as the beginning of medical reform, the first step in the progress toward modern medical education and organization, and the triumph of reformers who, from 1793, had attempted to bring a new order into the medical profession in England.[36] Although the act extended the licensing power of

---

with which the elites of the profession did not have to contend. See: S. W. F. Holloway, "The Apothecaries' Act of 1815: A Reinterpretation," *Medical History*, 10:2 (1966), 119; and W. H. McMenemey, *The Life and Times of Sir Charles Hastings, Founder of the British Medical Association* (Edinburgh and London, 1959), p. 67.

the Apothecaries' Society to all of England and Wales, it was in other respects a disappointment, when not a source of dismay, to the men who had worked for reform. The efforts of the apothecaries and surgeon-apothecaries to unite the corporations in the responsibility of training and licensing its general practitioners were thwarted, and the results of the great medical reform were the continued legal separation of the medical estates and the perpetuation of the inferior status of the apothecary. He was still to be "the phisicians' cooke."[37] Although these efforts at united action fell short of their goals, they mark the beginnings of a century of action on the part of men for whom the old order was inadequate to their needs and incongruent with their professional lives.

Despite the essentially "reactionary" character of the act, one of its (albeit unintended) consequences was the merging of the identity and roles of surgeon and apothecary. The act required that all medical men who prescribed and dispensed drugs in England and Wales have the License of the Society of Apothecaries. Hence surgeons who had previously practiced with only a license from their College were now required to hold the LSA in order to engage in general practice. Thus this legislation accelerated the process of breaking down the distinctions between the ordinary surgeons and apothecaries. What had been occasional, informal practice before 1815 became institutionalized after the Apothecaries' Act among the rank and file of medical practitioners, and the evolution of the general practitioner, dually licensed, whose place in the profession was defined in terms of function rather than corporate affiliation, was well on its way.

The Royal College of Physicians had, for the most part, succeeded in keeping itself separate from the taint of licensing general practitioners, and the Royal College of Surgeons, while licensing them, denied them influence within the College. What remained, and grew, after 1815, was a body of men who continued to be dissatisfied with the organization of medical practice. Licensed by two corporations, their position was anomalous; they were "a hybrid class."[38] They held two licenses but had no sense of identification and no corporation dedicated to safeguarding and advancing their interests and status. They were relegated to inferior positions within the corporations and neglected by their leadership. After 1815 many associations specifically for general practitioners were formed. These groups, many of them based in London, were often expressly hostile to the corporations, and they sometimes specifically excluded consultants from membership. Among these organizations were such groups as the Metropolitan Society of General Practitioners in Medicine and Surgery and the old London-based British Medical Association (which was founded in 1836 and subsequently died).[39] Some general practitioners organized associations based upon particular forms of medical employment and the specific problems these entailed. Thus, the need for a united voice and the control of competition in their own ranks led Poor Law Medical Officers to form a professional society. The failure of the Colleges to promote the interests of Army and Navy medical men led them to organize their own associations as well. Another group of this sort was the Association of Medical Officers of Asylums and Hospitals for the Insane.[40] Unable to rely on the corporate elites to advance their cause, medical men organized in order to act more effectively in their own behalf.

Of the London associations that aspired to national significance and leadership among general practitioners, several openly opposed the exclusive privileges of the London corporations. The old British Medical Association and the National Association of General Practitioners, for example, worked for the creation of yet another corporation—a College of General Practitioners—hoping thereby to advance the status of the lower orders of medical men. They attempted to resolve the anomalous position of the general practitioner by creating another corporation to accommodate this new breed.

The period from 1815 to 1858 saw the continued attempts of the provincial general practitioner to find a voice for himself. Local provincial medical societies which flowered in this period drew their membership from specific geographical regions and provided associations with which medical men could identify and through which they might voice their opinions on matters of medical politics on the national level.

These organizations made no distinction between the general ranks of practitioners and the few hospital consultants and College Fellows in their ranks. Their existence testifies to the failure of the London corporations to provide national leadership for the profession and to the rift between the London medical world and the provincial practitioner. Because provincial practice was almost always general practice, the provincial societies are another reflection of the growing tensions between general practitioners and the London consultants who reigned supreme both in the corporations and in the great London hospitals.[41]

The most important of the provincial societies was the Provincial Medical and Surgical Association, founded in 1832 in Worcester by Charles Hastings and his colleagues at the Worcester Infirmary. Although it began as a strictly local organization, it became the core of a nationwide association of local societies and acted as spokesman for provincial practitioners in the long and complicated activities of the profession in the search for medical reform.[42] Its purposes were originally "friendly and scientific," but it soon found itself in the middle of national medical politics. It took a conciliatory position toward the London corporations, partly at least out of the recognition that no reform legislation had any hope of success without the cooperation of the London medical establishment. Thomas Wakley, the editor of the *Lancet*, strongly criticized the Provincial Medical and Surgical Association for its overt friendliness toward the London corporations. At the same time, other practitioners avoided joining the PMSA for fear that such an act would be considered an expression of opposition to one of the Colleges. Dr. Andrew Carrick, the Association's president in 1833, insisted that the Association was not an oppositional body. But he had to acknowledge that strife was indeed a part of medical life: it was his hope, he said, that "jealousy and hatred, that unseemly speck and blemish, shall [be] washed from the fair face of our humane and charitable profession."[43]

While the PMSA was not antagonistic to the London corporations, some of its members recognized the alienation that existed between their interests and those of the leadership in London. Dr. Carrick encouraged the members of the Association to exercise their influence judiciously for the improvement of medical education and practice:

> By acting with unanimity and kindly feeling towards one another, and with uprightness, humanity and manly independence, to the world at large, we shall best succeed in producing for ourselves that protection and encouragement for our useful services which the legislature is either too fully occupied otherwise, or too indifferent about the matter to attend to; and which the corporate bodies are, perhaps, too much interested in withholding.[44]

He expressed the view that the ancient corporations, once important in the elevation of the profession's prestige, had not kept pace with the changes in, and needs of, the profession. And at the very least, many medical men felt that the problems of provincial medical men were different from those of London. What is clear, however, whether the term used is "London," "the corporations," or "the consultants," is that there was, both in London and outside, a division between the prestigious and influential men at the top of the profession and the ordinary practitioners.

Outside the PMSA, others were less gentle in their statements about the rift between the elite and ordinary medical men. A Portsmouth surgeon expressed his sense of this division in a letter to the *Lancet* in 1837. He described his own local medical society as "an association for extending and enforcing the homage due from humble . . . medical practitioners to their lords and masters of the provincial hospital."[45] This practitioner's statement indicates that the rift between hospital consultant and private practitioner was not a phenomenon of London alone; in the provinces, too, the inequality of rank was noticed and resented.

A symbol of the conflict within the profession may be found in that constant overseer, critic, and scourge of the medical establishment, the founder and editor of the *Lancet*, Thomas Wakley. Born in 1795, the son of a west country farmer, Wakley was a medical practitioner in the East End of London. He founded the *Lancet* in 1823 and used the journal to attack the medical leadership (particularly in the College of Surgeons, whose license he held) and to agitate for reform. His politics, both medical and general, were radical, and his language was often flamboyant, frequently bitter, and sometimes extraordinarily vicious. To some he is a hero of medical reform; others see him as a distasteful troublemaker.[46] He never missed an occasion to attack the officials of the Colleges, often in highly inflammatory language. In the *Lancet*, for example, the leaders of the Royal Colleges were labelled as "crafty, intriguing, corrupt, avaricious, cowardly, plundering, rapacious, soul-betraying, dirty-minded BATS."[47] Wakley saw nepotism, monopoly, and conspiracy everywhere. When, for example, the PMSA took a conciliatory position toward the London corporations on matters of reform, Wakley saw it as the result of the fact that Charles Hastings, the leader of the PMSA, had a brother (a solicitor) who was married to the sister of an influential Fellow of the Royal College of Physicians who had, no doubt, bought Hastings off with the offer of a Fellowship in the Royal College if he would kill any efforts at reform.[48]

Wakley's views and his rhetoric were sometimes extreme, and he can scarcely be viewed as a typical representative of the medical men practicing in England in the early Victorian period. His views deserve a brief examination, however, for they provide further evidence of the divisions within the profession, and there can be little doubt that he was an often-heard and frequently influential spokesman for those who had no other voice in the medical world. While he spoke in terms of conspiracy and monopoly and fought for radical democratization, he nevertheless touched the problems that others might have expressed more moderately: the need for a greater voice for the ordinary practitioner within the profession; the need for protection of qualified medical men against the competition of the quack; and the discrepancy between the status and privileges of ordinary medical men and those who enjoyed place and power in the London corporations.

He charged the corporations with exercising their power and using the licensing fees of the small practitioner for the benefit of their own cliques. Many would probably have agreed with him as to the existence of such practices. Wakley differed from his contemporaries in his proposed solutions. He sometimes advocated the creation of a separate corporation for general practitioners; at other times he envisaged an entirely new corporation that would include medical men of all ranks within its councils. What he always fought for was the participation of the masses of medical men in the selection of their leaders. He attacked the Council of the Royal College of Surgeons for being a self-perpetuating body. The Council chose its own new members, without any reference to the interests of its rank and file. Wakley fought for political power for ordinary practitioners, while others worked to improve the education and social status of medical men. Some did not object to the distinction and power achieved by the few and felt that prestige accrued to all members of the profession from the honors given to its leadership. They supported a hierarchical order within the profession and believed that its leadership was best qualified to select its own successors. Even when Wakley's opinions differed from theirs, he gave voice to the dissatisfaction felt by the rank and file; he revealed the sense of estrangement, alienation, resentment, and sometimes open hostility that existed between ordinary members of the profession and the men of power. Wakley by his words, the new medical associations by their existence, bore witness to the failure of the corporate elites to meet the needs of rank-and-file medical men.

Many of the local societies that appeared in the early Victorian years joined forces with the Provincial Medical and Surgical Association. This organization, renamed the British Medical Association in 1856, became the voice of provincial medicine. In London, societies came and went, few of the general practitioners' organizations surviving beyond 1858. Fierce conflicts over their relationship to the corporations divided these groups, brought Wakley's curse upon them, and led to their extinction. Individual practitioners, torn between their need for affiliation and their unwillingness to oppose the corporations, turned to the BMA or were left without support.

In terms of both medical practice and corporate affiliation, the old estate order was disintegrating and the new division between consultant and general practitioner was becoming the central fact of the medical hierarchy. However incomplete these changes were by 1858, they were, nevertheless, indicators of the new structure of medical society, a structure based less upon corporate separation than upon the differential rank of those who held positions in the teaching hospitals and the colleges and who practiced "pure" medicine or surgery, and, below them, those who held no honorary offices and whose practice was a mixture of medicine, surgery, and the dispensing of drugs. For both groups, corporate identity still existed, but the day had drawn nearer when the words "medical profession" would have more significance than any corporate designation. Still divided within, physicians, surgeons, and apothecaries had taken the first steps toward becoming a single profession.

It is much simpler to recognize the symptoms of this change in the structure of medical practice than it is to explain its causes. The Apothecaries' Act alone cannot account for the merging of medicine and surgery in general practice and the new sense of solidarity among general practitioners. The auxiliary sciences of anatomy, physiology, and pathology brought medicine and surgery closer together, and medical education became more integrated partly, at least, in order to provide training in these increasingly important branches of medical knowledge.[49]

Increased demand for medical care may have brought pressure on medical practitioners to qualify for practice in all branches of the healing art. Meteoric population growth in Britain in the late eighteenth and early nineteenth centuries may have contributed to demand. One might also speculate that changing attitudes toward sickness and death might have increased reliance on medical attendants. It is also possible that the services of a medical man may have been one of the status symbols of the growing industrial and commercial middle classes in this period, and the status value of superior qualifications would not have been lost on the practitioner eager to improve his income. Certainly medical men with multiple qualifications could offer the whole range of medical care to those patients who, while concerned for the status or training of their practitioner, could not afford the higher fees of the pure physician or surgeon.

Competition from unqualified medical practitioners may have provided another impetus to surgeons or apothecaries to expand their range of practice. It is impossible to say with certainty whether there was any significant increase in the number of unlicensed practitioners in England from the late eighteenth century on,[50] but licensed practitioners were certainly worried about the threat from this quarter.* Fear of losing out to the unqualified practitioner might have driven the apothecary to obtain a surgeon's license or the surgeon to qualify as an apothecary as a way of competing more effectively for patients.

Licensed medical men also, of course, competed with one another, and the race for practice may have influenced medical men's ideas about the virtues of "purity" of corporate affiliation and practice. If the profession was growing faster than the population, or if medical men's fees were not keeping pace with the cost of living, then increased practice was necessary to maintain the medical man's standard of living. Under these circumstances, double qualification as an apothecary-surgeon allowed a practitioner to meet all the needs of his patients, thus obviating the necessity of calling in another practitioner when such action meant, at best, sharing, and at worst, losing his patient to his competitor.

Whether changes in the structure of medical society were the result of changes in medical science, social attitudes, or the nature of the medical marketplace, there is no doubt that the medical profession was suffering the upheavals of social change. Whatever the causes, the results were clear: while the

*The new medical associations discussed above reflect their worry.

old tripartite division of health care continued, it did so in attenuated form. The more important developments were the emergence of general practice, a sign of growing cohesiveness among rank-and-file members of the various corporations. At the same time, the alienation of general practitioners from the consulting physicians and surgeons of the hospital and College elite provided the foundations for continued tension and conflict within the profession for decades to come.

IV

Side by side with medical men's efforts at organization, and partly a product of the same discontents, there were a number of attempts to reform the medical profession through parliamentary legislation. The agitation for reform began not long after the passage of the Apothecaries' Act in 1815 and continued until the final passage of the Medical Act of 1858. Between 1840 and 1858 seventeen different bills were introduced into Parliament, most often as private members' bills, in attempts to reorganize medical education and licensing in the kingdom. The failure of all but one of these medical reform bills reveals the conflicting interests and needs of the elites of the corporations, on the one hand, and those of the rank and file, on the other. Parliamentary handling of the matter of medical reform also reveals some of the attitudes of Victorian society toward the profession and toward the place of medical science in the life of the English public.

Although reform had been in the wind for decades, the first proposal appeared in 1840 when Thomas Wakley, Henry Warburton, and Benjamin Hawes introduced their bill into Parliament.[51] Their "Bill for the Registration of Medical Practitioners, and for establishing a College of Medicine and for enabling the Fellows of that College to practise Medicine in all and any of its branches and hold any medical appointment in any part of the United Kingdom" defined qualified practice, created a system of medical registration, prohibited unregistered persons from practicing medicine, and created a medical council and a College of Medicine. Even as amended, the bill was unsatisfactory in several respects, but it lost the support of the medical corporations because it virtually destroyed the three orders of medical practice and placed the governance of the profession (through postal ballot) in the hands of the profession at large. The proposed College of Medicine was a thinly veiled effort to replace the existing corporations with a new all-encompassing medical body. Nationwide election of representatives to the medical council would have taken the power to select the profession's leadership out of the hands of the London elites and given it to the general practitioners. The destruction of the old corporations was an issue on which general practitioners themselves did not agree, the more extreme among them supporting such a move, the more moderate willing to see their continued existence. The democratization of the profession through the election at large of its representatives was more widely favored among general practitioners. It obviously extended their powers at the expense of the monopolies of the corporate elites. The issue of whether general practitioners should have a voice in the election of their professional leadership, not new in 1840, was to arise again and again in the next forty years. Whenever it was discussed, it revealed anew the deep division which existed between the rank and file and the corporations to which they belonged.*

Likewise the restriction of unqualified practice was of major concern to general practitioners, and it was in their interest to see strong restrictive legislation. The leaders of the corporations, on the other hand, had little interest in the control of unqualified practice, inasmuch as it had little effect on their positions, prestige, or practice. Sir James Graham's bill,

*Representation of the general practitioner continued to be an issue, both in the corporations and in the profession as a whole, until the 1880's, when the first general practitioner sat on the Council of the Royal College of Surgeons and when the Medical Act Amendment Act of 1886 provided for the election at large of a representative of the profession at large to sit with those of the corporations and universities on the GMC.

introduced in 1844, brought these differences to light. His bill would have reorganized the profession through the creation of a "Council of Health and Medical Education" which would have regulated examinations, supervised medical education, and registered all licensed practitioners. The Royal Colleges were, in general, enthusiastic, for the bill did not touch the privileges of the corporations. Its only provision regarding unqualified practitioners was to bar them from public employment. From the viewpoint of the public, prohibition of unlicensed practice constituted excessive government interference in the liberty of individuals to choose whatever form of medical attendance they wished, and it was entirely antithetical to the principles of laissez faire and the free operation of the market. General practitioners objected to Graham's bill for its failure to deal effectively with "quackery" and because it left general practitioners without power in medical education and licensing.*

A revised bill, introduced by Graham in 1845, "For the regulation of the Profession of Physic and Surgery," went far toward satisfying general practitioners' demands for medical reform, and in so doing lost all the support of the corporations. The new bill not only made it an offense to assume a medical title fraudulently, but in the amendments to the act, Graham included provision for the creation of a new College of General Practitioners in Medicine, Surgery and Midwifery. It further provided that general practitioners should participate in the examination of students for qualification. While the general practitioners approved the bill because it increased their power and status in the profession, the corpo-

---

*Graham's bill was the occasion for the Apothecaries' Society to present itself as the spokesman for the general practitioner. See: Society of Apothecaries, *An Address by the Society of Apothecaries to the General Practitioners of England and Wales on the Provisions of the Bill "For the Better Regulation of Medical Practice Throughout the United Kingdom"*... (London, 1844), pp. 3 ff., 24, and 30. See also: *A Manifesto by the Medical and Surgical Association of the Borough of Marylebone*, 2nd ed. (London, 1844), pp. 5 and 13–14. Both these pamphlets insist on the importance of limiting unqualified practice, and both reflect the view that Graham's bill was hostile to general practitioners.

rate elites objected to it on precisely those grounds.* By bringing general practitioners into the examining boards, the bill would give power to those who were inferior representatives of the profession—"imperfectly educated, all engaged in the trading, money-making parts of the profession, and not one in a hundred of them distinguished by anything like science or liberality of mind."[52]

In most of the bills for medical reform the question of the registration of medical practitioners was a central issue. A single medical register implied the equality before the law of all "Registered Medical Practitioners." The notion of all medical men as equally qualified was a "revolutionary" idea,[53] in direct contradiction to the idea of qualification as embodied in the three corporations and the three medical estates. The corporations did not usually object to the establishment of a medical register unless the bill at the same time provided for complete uniformity and standardization of medical qualifications (such as that proposed in Wakley's bill of 1847). By the same token, the general practitioners objected to a register which published the distinctions which existed among the various ranks of medical men. They considered it a way of perpetuating the inferior status of the majority. Representatives of the Colleges might voice their objection in terms of the idea that a general register would undermine the quality of the profession by discouraging advanced medical qualification, but implicit in their objection was disapproval of the levelling which would make Fellows of the Colleges equal (in terms of official recognition) with the rank and file of general practitioners.[54] At issue in the standardization of medical education and the famed "single portal" idea of medical qualification was the notion that the distinctions among the corporations would disappear, that the corporations' power over medical education and licensing would be lost, and that the government's powers over the profession would be "dangerously" increased.[55] However much de facto merging there

---

* As in the 1840 bill, there was pressure from the G.P.'s to include members of their ranks in the "Council of Health" and in examining bodies.

was among medical men, the corporations were not prepared to see the legal end of their privileged status.*

One reform bill after another was presented in Parliament, only to meet the objections of the corporations or the attacks of Thomas Wakley, and petitions came from various medical groups favoring or opposing each bill. Such war over reform suggested to some Members of Parliament the possibility that the profession was incapable of uniting except to dispose of any measure for reform. Some, wearied of the fruitless efforts at reform, concluded that medical legislation was impossible and proposed that all efforts be dropped and that the profession be left free to "fight it out." It became clear, as one bill followed another, that the issue of medical reform was a complex, often muddled one in which the deep divisions within the medical profession were exposed to public view. In the end, these disagreements divided the nonmedical parliamentary reformers as well.[56]

The medical reform act which finally passed in 1858 was the "Bill to regulate the qualifications of Practitioners in Medicine and Surgery." It was prepared by W. F. Cowper, President of the Board of Health, and John Simon, Medical Officer of the General Board of Health.† With minor amendments, the bill received final approval in the House of Commons on the 29th of July and the royal assent on August 2, · 1858. The Medical Act of 1858 (21 and 22 Vict. c. 90) was scarcely the radical reform measure hoped for by Wakley

---

* In Headlam's 1855 bill, two separate registers were proposed, one for physicians and one for surgeons and apothecaries.

† This bill was the sixteenth to be introduced. A seventeenth bill was introduced by radical M.P.'s Duncombe (Wakley's successor) and Butler. They called it a bill "To Define the Rights of the Medical Profession and to Protect the Public from the Abuses of the Corporations." See Charles Newman, *The Evolution of Medical Education in the Nineteenth Century* (London, 1957), pp. 187–188. Royston Lambert, *Sir John Simon, 1816–1904, and English Social Administration* (London, 1963), pp. 463 ff., describes Simon's role in the act. Alexander M. Cooke, *A History of the Royal College of Physicians of London*, III, 804 ff., has a concise summary.

and his followers. Many more moderate advocates of reform were less than satisfied, too. The act defined a "qualified medical practitioner" and created a General Council of Medical Education and Registration (commonly known as the General Medical Council or GMC) where, for the first time, representatives of the medical corporations were united in a single official body and given joint responsibility for overseeing medical education and licensing in the United Kingdom. Branch councils for England and Wales, Scotland, and Ireland were created to oversee affairs within each country. The General Medical Council was accountable to the Crown through the agency of the Medical Officer of the Privy Council. The act put an end to anomalies such as the power of the Archbishop of Canterbury to grant medical licenses and the lack of uniformity in the recognition of Scottish and Irish qualifications in England.

The act further provided for the registration of all qualified practitioners and the annual publication of a medical register by the GMC. The register was to list all medical men together, without regard for their differential qualifications. In spite of these new institutions and the abolition of some outstanding grievances, the Medical Act of 1858 left a great deal unchanged. The privileges and powers of the corporations were left intact, as was the hierarchical order of the profession. The GMC itself had largely supervisory powers, and its membership was made up of representatives of the Royal Colleges, the Apothecaries' Society, the universities granting medical degrees, and a number of Crown nominees. There were no seats specifically designated for the representation of general practitioners.

The power to grant licenses remained in the hands of the corporations, as did the setting of educational requirements for candidates and the bestowing of honorary distinctions such as the Fellowships of the Royal Colleges. The GMC's role in education was advisory, and since the corporations' own representatives sat on the Council, their ideas and influence were to be prominent. Efforts of reformers to establish a single basic qualification in medicine, surgery, and midwifery

35

bore fruit in the act only in the form of an enabling clause. Power to take such a step was left in the hands of the corporations and universities.

Qualified medical men gained only partial protection from competition with unlicensed practitioners. The latter were not prohibited from practice but only from government employment. All practitioners, qualified and unqualified alike, were prohibited from using the titles of physician, surgeon, apothecary, or doctor, without the appropriate license. Parliament's failure to grant licensed medical men a monopoly over the practice of medicine and the care of the sick suggests that, beneath the issues of patients' liberties and laissez faire, legislators put little faith in scientific expertise and in the medical license as proof of that expertise. Medical men themselves seemed to see the issue more in terms of protection from competition than in terms of the superior claims of medical science.

Despite the fact that all registered medical practitioners had equal status in the new *Medical Register*, the act did not, as some have suggested, "end . . . the rigid hierarchical division of the profession."[57] It is true that the Medical Act brought the three orders together under the umbrella of the GMC and the *Medical Register* and thereby took one more step in the dismantling of the old order of medical society. But the disintegration of the estate structure had begun long before, and it was being replaced by a new medical hierarchy of consultants and general practitioners which was to survive all of the formal and informal efforts at reform.*

The medical profession was legally defined and technically united by the Act of 1858, but the privileges, powers, and internal structure of the old corporations were untouched by the legislation. A new legal framework for medical practice in England was created by the act, but within this

*Charles Newman says the survival of medical hierarchy saved Britain "from the professional defects of countries on the other side of the Atlantic where . . . general practitioners on the staff of hospitals are still holding up professional developments" (*Medical Education*, pp. 190–191). Cf. Thomas McKeown, "A Sociological Approach to the History of Medicine," *Medical History*, 14:4 (1970), 346–348.

framework the distinctions of rank remained, and hierarchy was preserved.* Perhaps most important, power over professional education and licensing was left squarely in the hands of the London elites. Added to their powers in the corporations and the hospitals was their new status as members of a government agency charged with the supervision of medicine in the whole kingdom. Without the endorsement of law on their superior knowledge and without absolute protection of the state against competition from the "quacks," medical men of the rank and file were left in a somewhat anomalous position. The elites of the profession had extensive powers over the possibilities for advancement within their ranks, but success in practice depended on the decision of patients as to the value of the medical license.

Whether one defines a profession as an occupation with "a prolonged specialized training in a body of abstract knowledge, and a collectivity or service orientation," or whether one defines it as a "special type of occupation" which is "autonomous and self-regulating," it should be clear that medicine in 1858 was not truly a profession.† One could, in theory, argue that *physicians* were professional men by either of these definitions, but it would be an absurdity to define Victorian health

*The Medical Act itself provided for the extension of that hierarchy within the Royal College of Physicians through a new license for the qualification of general practitioners. With the establishment of the new LRCP in 1861, there was created in the Royal College of Physicians a body of practitioners whose status was analogous to that of the Members of the Royal College of Surgeons. They had no corporate privileges, no powers within the College, and were even refused access to the College library. The new LRCP brought the College into direct competition with the Society of Apothecaries for the licensing of G.P.'s.

† The first definition is that of William J. Goode, "Encroachment, Charlatanism, and the Emerging Profession: Psychology, Medicine, and Sociology," *Am. Soc. Rev.*, 25 (1960), 902–914, quoted in: Freidson, *Profession of Medicine*, p. 77. The second definition is Freidson's, ibid., p. xx and passim. For a comment on the changing nineteenth-century usage of the word "profession," see: Sheldon Rothblatt, *The Revolution of the Dons. Cambridge and Society in Victorian England* (New York, 1968), pp. 90–91.

care service as a whole on the basis of the characteristics of a minute portion of its practitioners. While medical men disagreed among themselves as to the degree of their membership in a single occupational group, the public had begun to identify them with one another, and, with the legal unity of 1858, they must be judged in terms of both legislative and popular acknowledgment of their affiliation.

The "medical profession" in 1858 was a hybrid agglomeration of learned, university-educated physicians, surgeons in transition from an old craft to a new "science," and apothecaries who claimed the practical skills of physic and surgery while drug sales wedded them to trade. While the Medical Act of 1858 granted the "medical profession" control over entrance to the *Medical Register*, the GMC did not have "the exclusive right to determine who [could] legitimately do its work and how the work should be done."[58] The untrained and unlicensed "quack" continued to be an accepted source of health care. Victorian society in 1858 had limited confidence in the power of medical "science" and serious reservations about medical men's social authority and prestige.[59] The fruits of their lack of commitment to establishment medicine were the limited advantages granted to the "medical profession" by the 1858 act.

Moreover, in the matter of self-regulation, the "profession" of medicine was only beginning the process of extended control, not simply over licensing but over the behavior of men in practice.[60] True, the corporations had for long laid down rules for the behavior of their elites, but the rank and file of the corporations were left to themselves, expected only to keep to their place. In the mid-Victorian years, the GMC and the Colleges began to regulate the behavior of all registered practitioners and to sanction those who did not conform.

Perhaps more important, the standards of occupational expertise were not the sole, nor even the primary, criteria for the judgment of "professional" qualification and performance. Qualification and advancement on the basis of classical studies and social status betrayed claims that skill was the foundation of medical life and practice. Among laymen and medical men alike, the practitioner was judged more by who he was than by what he did.[61] Such criteria as classical learning, liberality of mind, the graces and style of the gentleman, and lay society's favor were the standards by which Victorian medical men evaluated each other.

The mid-Victorian period saw the first steps toward autonomy and self-regulation in medicine. The process was a slow one, and one in which the values of scientific knowledge held a back seat. Medical practice, most vulnerable to the dictates of a doubting lay public, continued to be defined and carried on in the ambiguous context of "quack" competition and too frequently oriented to the values, taste, or whims of patients. In the institutions of elite medical life, the foundations existed for the extension of professional control over practitioners. In the realm of medical education, by circumstance and by design, the elites of the profession began to build a system of autonomy and central control that would eventually build a profession.

II

Education for a Profession

STEEPLECHASES in the dissecting room, cheating on the Latin examination, flirting with the barmaid, gin-and-water until three o'clock in the morning, these were the stereotypical activities of the medical student of the 1840's.[1] By the 1880's the press presented a new image of the medical student: surrounded by books, a model of a human skull at his elbow, he labored over his studies with gravity and decorum late into the night.[2] The transformation of the medical student's popular image suggests that, in the course of the Victorian years, medical students buckled down to work. A careful look at changes in medical education during the course of the century suggests that medical students had indeed earned their image. The new image was the product of discipline—not only the self-discipline of study but also the command of the profession over those it was training for admission to its ranks.

Throughout the mid-Victorian era, those who entered medical training were a motley group. Mixed motives dictated the choice of a profession; diverse attainments marked their pre-medical education; and uncertainties clouded their professional goals. By experiment, imitation, and necessity, the faculties of the London medical schools began to shape this heterogeneous group of medical students into a body of professional men.

I

Victorian medical memoirs offer little evidence that a dedicated altruism provided a common motive for the study of medicine. Nor was love of science a very common basis for electing to study medicine. Given the history, character, and image of medical practice, little wonder that, from the prospective student's point of view, a scientific orientation was neither a necessary nor even secondary consideration in the choice of a career. The medical students' decisions reflected extrinsic considerations of economics, family ties, and personal taste. Practicality and particularism were the rule.

Victorian families seem to have varied greatly in the freedom given to sons to choose an occupation. Parental temperament may have been a factor in this variation, but the family's economic, occupational, and social circumstances proved more important considerations. Predictably, the most common background for the Victorian medical student was that of a medical family. Systematic information is available for three groups of Victorian medical men: Fellows of the two Royal Colleges and apprentices of the London Apothecaries' Society. Of these, 22.4 percent of physicians, 11.7 percent of surgeons, and 35.2 percent of apothecaries were sons of medical men.* Many others claimed uncles, grandfathers, or older brothers in some branch of the profession. Victorians themselves sometimes described such succession in terms of "inheritance."[3] Such a judgment, however, does little to explain how family relationships served as a fundamental part of medical careers.

The occupational training of young men by their fathers and uncles was quite common. For example, Henry Cline, Jr., was apprenticed to his father, a Surgeon at St. Thomas's Hospital. The senior Cline taught his son the principles of his craft and took him into the hospital where he gained practical experience at his father's side.[4] Perhaps Sir Astley Cooper, Surgeon to St. Bartholomew's Hospital and a leader of early nineteenth-century surgical education and practice, offers the most famous case of family medical training. His apprentices—Frederick Tyrell, Aston Key, and Bransby Cooper—were all his nephews.[5] But obscure medical men as well as

---

*See Appendix B for details. These figures, based on data regarding elites, are atypical, probably showing less father-son succession than was taking place in the profession as a whole.

41

famous ones carried on the tradition of family education. The apprenticeship records of the Apothecaries' Society reveal that, of the total of 1,241 indentures registered during the period 1817–1889, at least 26 percent were apprenticeships between relatives—fathers and sons, uncles and nephews, or older and younger brothers.* The records of the Royal College of Surgeons, while less complete, show a similar trend.†

The pattern of inheritance in the early nineteenth-century medical profession rested on a sound economic basis: the younger generation could be educated in family medical apprenticeship with a minimum of cost, while the choice of an occupation without family connections could lead to hundreds of pounds in educational expenses. For families of limited means, such economies must have been compelling.[6] Even in the mid-Victorian years, as the medical schools became paramount, students sometimes took a year or two of pupillage with a family member as a means of saving up to £75 or £100 in tuition and living costs.‡

*Information drawn from monthly entries in: Society of Apothecaries, Court Minute Books, Vols. 10–17, 1816–1893. In computing this statistic, the master apothecary was assumed to be a maternal uncle when the apprentice's middle name corresponded to the surname of the master (e.g., Albert Godwin Brown, apprenticed to Robert Godwin). Only occasionally are relationships indicated in the entry. This figure constitutes a minimum, since relationships between apprentice and master are not always detectable.

†See *Plarr's Lives* for biographical data. A few physicians are known to have been apprenticed to relatives.

‡In the 1870's and after, medical men urged the advisability of a year or two of private medical study with a private practitioner, both for its "moral" benefits and for its value in learning the rudiments of private practice. See: William Dale, *The State of the Medical Profession in Great Britain* [Carmichael Prize Essay] (Dublin, 1875), p. 44; and Charles Bell Keetley, *The Student's and Junior Practitioner's Guide to the Medical Profession*, 2nd ed. (London, 1885), pp. 12–14 and 27. Cf. Charles Newman, *The Evolution of Medical Education in the Nineteenth Century* (London, 1957), pp. 224–226. Some medical schools gave sons of their own hospital medical officers free tuition. See: St. Thomas's Hospital, Minute Books of the Grand Committee (H.1/ST/A6/12), 6 August 1850, p. 136.

Economic motives also influenced students who did not come from medical families. Sons from families of limited means may have chosen to study medicine instead of another profession because it was less expensive. Jukes De Styrap observed that medicine was thought to be a "cheap profession."* V. S. (later Sir Victor) Horsley chose on this basis. Victor wanted to be a cavalry officer, but his father, a musician, could not afford to send him into the Army and suggested medicine as a less costly alternative.[7]

Perhaps medical education seemed particularly accessible to men of modest means because, unlike university men or those destined for Army or legal careers, medical students could take measures that cut educational costs to a minimum. If a medical student lived at home, studied with a local practitioner, and did his clinical work at a nearby hospital, he could reduce the financial burden on his family. In fact, a medical student could even support himself. After a year or two of training, he could find work as an assistant to a qualified medical man, serve as a coach to first-year medical students, or enjoy some other tasks related to his future career. John Bland-Sutton earned enough to cover his fees and completed his education with virtually no financial help from his father.[8] Thomas Heckstall Smith supported himself while in medical school by writing for the *London Medical Gazette*.[9] Charles Bell Keetley, FRCS, suggested to prospective medical students that they seek employment as assistants to medical men as a way to earn enough to cover educational expenses, indicating that Sutton and Smith were not isolated cases.[10] Thus, for frugal and industrious young men, as well as sons in medical families, medicine held the appeal and the opportunity of inexpensive training.

Even if educational costs played a negligible part in career choice, being a medical man's kin was thought to be

*Jukes De Styrap [MKQCP Ire.], *The Young Practitioner: With Practical Hints and Instructive Suggestions . . . for His Guidance on Entering into Private Practice . . .* (London, 1890), p. viii. Others were equally sure that this idea was a delusion and that medicine was in fact both costly and difficult to enter. See: *Confessions of an English Doctor* (London, 1904), p. 27.

both an advantage and an influence in a young man's career choice. William Rose, Jr., the son of a Buckinghamshire surgeon, was not trained by his father, but his biographer records:

> He was nursed in an atmosphere of the healing art. Long before he entered as a medical student at King's College he had learnt from his father, the leading surgeon in High Wycombe, something more than the rudiments of the profession, with the result that having the end in view, he was able to appreciate more thoroughly than the younger and less experienced students the meaning and bearing of the teaching facilities which a great medical school affords.[11]

Obviously sons entered their professional training with knowledge and skills learned informally in the process of living in a medical household. Moreover, their familiarity with the workings of professional life gave them a sense of ease about entering the profession that might not exist for others to whom medicine was entirely new. The sons of medical men were expected to do well in their studies because of their family background or, as some thought, "inheritance" of knowledge.[12] One of Arthur Conan Doyle's fictional characters —the son of a medical man—put it succinctly: "I was born inside the machine and I have seen all the wires."[13] There was more to medical practice than anatomy, *materia medica*, surgery, and therapeutics, and sons of medical families had been partially socialized before they entered the profession. The son in a medical household selected a career in which he had a sense of assurance and advantage.

There were, of course, other reasons why Victorian practitioners gravitated toward a career in medicine: chance, illness, curiosity, and a somewhat casual interest in science, health, or disease. H. E. Counsell claimed that his choice of medicine came about "quite by chance." But his uncle was a doctor, and his mother suggested that he might like to follow in his footsteps. When Counsell evinced some interest, a neighborhood general practitioner who had been a Guy's student, agreed to write to the Dean of the Medical School on his behalf.[14] S. H. Snell attributed his choice of medicine to the fact that his father enjoyed leisure-time scientific pursuits.* John Bland-Sutton was the son of a taxidermist and naturalist. His father stimulated his interest in natural history and gave him early instruction in comparative anatomy and physiology. Later, when being treated for an infected wound by the family doctor, young John quizzed him about the nature of the injury, and the practitioner responded by giving him a dried dissection of a forearm. Sutton studied it and decided to become a surgeon, "feeling convinced," he comments, "that my knowledge of comparative anatomy would be useful."[15] Sutton's utilitarian decision to put knowledge to some use was perhaps more common among medical students than the devotion to science displayed by William Henry Stone. His father, Rector of Christ-church, Spitalfields, wanted Stone to follow a clerical career, but the young William pursued scientific studies independently from an early age and, after studying at Balliol, entered medical training.[16]

Frequent childhood illness sometimes led, directly or indirectly, to a medical career. As a youth, John Beddoe suffered from dyspepsia and began reading physiological chemistry as a result. His interest in diet led him to correspond with a medical man about the subject, and the Beddoes' family doctor, noting his interests, urged him to take up medicine as a profession.[17] In an age when pure science was not an avenue to occupation and income, some medical men chose their occupation as a way of bringing their interests and their need to earn a living into some sort of alignment.

A consuming passion for science was not, however, a prerequisite for electing medicine as a profession. Sir John Simon, FRCS, who eventually became Medical Officer to the Privy Council, Surgeon to St. Thomas's Hospital, and President of the Royal College of Surgeons, provides an excellent case. His father chose surgery as a career for him, and he entered medical studies in 1833. After qualifying, Simon became Demonstrator of Anatomy at King's College. He spent

*Sidney H. Snell, *A Doctor at Work and Play* (London, 1937), pp. 1, 2, and 7. As a schoolboy he won a prize in chemistry, indicating his serious interest and ability in science. Until the 1870's, when science was introduced into the schools, interest in science was much more dependent upon the home environment.

his spare time, however, reading books on metaphysics and oriental languages and looking at prints at the British Museum. Under the stimulus of a fellow-student's example, Simon began to think that independent work in medicine and science was a necessary part of his professional advancement. Only then did Simon begin scientific work in earnest. In his *Recollections* he records, "I think I may claim that, by 1847, I was learning to feel an interest in science." By that date he had written four essays on medical and scientific subjects, won the Astley-Cooper Prize for his article on the thymus gland, and been elected a Fellow of the Royal Society for his research on the thyroid gland.[18]

Sir Benjamin Brodie, Bart., FRCS, a President of the Royal College of Surgeons, was outspoken in his view that neither passion nor talent for science was a necessary or even desirable prerequisite for medical careers:

> Others have often said to me that they supposed that I must have had, from the first, a particular taste or liking for my profession. But it was no such thing; nor does my experience lead me to have any faith in those special callings to certain ways of life which some young men are supposed to have. For the most part, these are mere fancies. . . . The persons who succeed best in professions are those who, having (perhaps from some accidental circumstances) been led to embark in them, persevere in their course as a matter of duty, or because they have nothing better to do. They often feel their new pursuit to be unattractive enough in the beginning; but as they go on, and acquire knowledge, and find that they obtain some degree of credit, the case is altered; and from that time they become every day more interested in what they are about. There is no profession to which these observations are more applicable than they are to the medical.[19]

Brodie, long a teacher of surgery, observed that many medical students found their studies "distasteful" or "repulsive," but he thought that interest in the profession grew with practical experience. Another medical man absolutely denied any youthful interest in medicine. He rejected the myth of the "born doctor," labelling that notion an "illusive but popular legend."[20]

Other Victorian observers, taking a somewhat different line, insisted that scientific interests, and even intelligence,[21] counted for less in a medical career than a man's personal characteristics. H. B. Thomson advised fathers that "It is . . . an error to send a young man to this profession simply because he displays an early taste for chemistry bottles, or fitting together dead men's bones; he ought to show more practical qualities than a simple love of science."[22] Thomson cites such traits as tact, discretion, and the ability to act with decision and to inspire confidence as primary considerations for those contemplating a medical career. Conversely, a bad temper, an "anxious disposition," intemperance, "want of cleanliness," and "defects of manners" could seriously hinder successful relations with a patient and his family, and thus success in the profession.[23] A medical man's knowledge or technical skills took second place to his facility in personal relationships.

These observations by Brodie, Thomson, and others find their reflection in the lives of those who achieved success in their careers with neither devotion to science nor commitment to a suffering public. Dr. Thomas Watson, the President of the Royal College of Physicians, spoke of one such man in his Presidential Address to the College in 1866. Dr. Reginald Southey (the younger brother of the poet) had died that year, and Watson's eulogy described his career:

> It would be incorrect to speak of him as a great physician. I doubt whether he ever had that true love of his profession which is essential to the making of a great physician; but he possessed a large share of that useful faculty which we call . . . common sense . . . which, in the business of life, often stands a man in better stead than deep or abstract science.[24]

Southey, a handsome, active man, of great kindness and good judgment, became a favorite among aristocratic families in the north and a successful London practitioner as well. Sir William Jenner, on a similar occasion in 1885, said of another Fellow: "At the bedside his diagnosis was neither [ms. illegible] nor always accurate but he was notwithstanding a good practitioner for he never forgot that it was the patient and not the nominal disease he had to treat."* Jenner went on to praise the good physician for his "sterling probity" and his kind-heartedness.[25]

If some thought love of science unnecessary to medical careers, others knew that more mundane motives were frequently at work in the choice of the profession of medicine. The eminent Sir Benjamin Brodie recalled that he was disposed to take up a career in medicine because of the "great reputation" which his cousins and an uncle had achieved in the profession.[26] John Beddoe, looking for a livelihood, asked Charles Hastings' advice about a medical career. Hastings, the founder of the BMA, responded with an old proverb: "a physician does not get bread until he has no teeth wherewith to eat it."[27] In 1890 Jukes De Styrap warned prospective medical students against entering the profession for the prospects of wealth, a living, or social distinction. He labelled these motives ill-founded and ignoble. Wealth, he said, could be found more easily elsewhere; a mere living was a prostitution of the healer's ideal; and, as for social distinction, the medical man has no time to cultivate the "graces and opportunities without which social distinction cannot be won."[28] The fact that De Styrap needed to warn young men of the invalidity of these motives suggests that they continued to be a factor in the choice of medical careers.

Clearly, cost, convenience, family influence, and the hope for income and prestige outweighed talent and ability in the decision to study medicine.

II

Medicine may have been termed a "liberal profession" in the nineteenth century, but such a designation should not

---

*Sir William Jenner, Presidential Addresses (RCP Mss.), Vol. 1, 1885, pp. 3–4. These are Jenner's remarks regarding Dr. Alexander Tweedie. He also praised Tweedie for his power of prognosis, which was, he said, "rarely erroneous. I have heard him say early in a case that a patient will die and yet be unable when time had verified his prognosis to say why he had come to that conclusion."

obscure the fact that, for most medical men, their occupation was still tied to the traditions of trade and skilled craftsmanship. Nowhere is this more obvious than in the general education of Victorian medical practitioners.

Victorian secondary education could be obtained in a variety of public and private ways, and the education of nineteenth-century physicians, surgeons, and general practitioners reflected this diversity. Private tutoring, proprietary schools, grammar schools, the new Victorian public schools, and the great foundations—all of these provided secondary education in the nineteenth century. The cost of such education ranged from free to very costly, and family means, ability, and, in the case of the grammar schools, the interests and concerns of the local community determined a young man's options.[29]

Records of the educational backgrounds of Victorian medical men are far from complete; the only systematic records are those of the two Royal Colleges regarding the education of their Fellows, recorded in *Munk's Roll* for physicians and *Plarr's Lives* for surgeons. Those elected to the Fellowship of the Royal College of Physicians, the most select group within the profession, constituted less than one percent of the profession in the nineteenth century. Between 1800 and 1889, of the 756 physicians elected to the Fellowship, 101 (13.3 percent) attended one of the nine Clarendon Schools or one of the new foundations (see Table 1). Among the somewhat less select body of men who made up the Fellows of the Royal College of Surgeons, the record of public school attendance is still more meager—51 out of 2,452, or 2.1 percent were educated at a public school (see Table 2). The largest proportion of public school men in these two groups were those who were educated at the day schools, St. Paul's and Merchant Taylor's. While their numbers were, in absolute terms, rather small, there was a marked increase in public school education among surgeons in the latter half of the century.* If public school education was uncommon among the

* Public school education among physicians shows a relative decline in the latter half of the century, perhaps reflecting the College's

TABLE 1 Education of Fellows of the Royal College of
Physicians, 1800–1889

	1800–49 Percent	1850–89 Percent	Average 1800–89 Percent
SECONDARY EDUCATION			
Public school	18.7	10.3	13.3
Grammar and major proprietary schools[a]	10.4	23.9	19.2
ARTS DEGREES:			
Oxbridge	27.0	17.4	20.7
London University	—	2.6	1.7
Other English universities	—	—	—
Scottish universities	—	1.9	1.2
Irish universities	3.0	1.9	2.3
Foreign	—	0.5	0.3
All arts degrees	30.0	24.2[b]	26.2
MEDICAL DEGREES:			
Oxbridge	61.7	20.4	34.9
London	0.9	28.9	19.1
Other English universities	—	0.7	0.5
Scottish universities	27.0	38.3	34.3
Irish universities	3.0	1.9	2.3
Foreign	6.5	7.8	7.3
M.D. Lambeth	—	0.2	0.2
All medical degrees	99.1[b]	98.1[b]	98.8[b] (756)

SOURCE: compiled from *Munk's Roll*, III and IV, by date of
FRCP.

[a] Major proprietary schools: See T. W. Bamford, *Rise of the
Public Schools* (London, 1967).

[b] Off because of rounding.

TABLE 2 Education of Fellows of the Royal College of
Surgeons, 1800–1889

	1800–49 Percent	1850–89 Percent	Average 1800–89 Percent
SECONDARY EDUCATION			
Public school	1.1	4.8	2.1
Grammar and major proprietary schools [a]	4.6	13.2	6.9
ARTS DEGREES:			
Oxbridge	0.3	9.3	2.8
London University	0.2	1.2	0.4
Other English universities	—	0.1	[b]
Scottish universities	0.7	0.9	0.7
Irish universities	0.2	0.8	0.4
Foreign	0.4	0.6	0.4
Unknown	[b]	—	[b]
All arts degrees	1.8	12.9	4.8
	(33)	(86)	(119)
MEDICAL DEGREES:			
Oxbridge	0.4	7.2	2.3
London	2.0	22.1	7.4
Other English universities	0.3	4.8	1.5
Scottish universities	14.4	10.4	13.3
Irish universities	0.3	1.9	0.7
Foreign universities	2.6	3.2	2.8
Unknown	0.5	—	0.4
All medical degrees	20.5	49.6	28.4
	(367)	(330)	(697)
(Total Fellows)	(1787)	(665) [c]	(2452)

SOURCE: *Plarr's Lives*, by date of MRCS.

[a] Major proprietary schools: See T. W. Bamford, *Rise of the Public Schools* (London, 1967).

[b] Percentages below 0.1 not shown.

[c] Includes only those FRCS's who died before 1930.

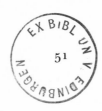

51

highest ranks of medical men, it was probably extremely rare among the rank and file of medical men in nineteenth-century England.

Attendance at a major proprietary school or grammar school was far more common among nineteenth-century medical men. The records show that 19.2 percent of physicians and 6.9 percent of surgeons who were later to become Fellows were educated in these establishments. For the remainder of the Fellows in the two Colleges, early training was a patchwork of education at home by fathers, older brothers, tutors, or occasional governesses, at schools run by clergymen, or at other proprietary establishments.

A few examples will illustrate the variety and combinations of educational experience of Victorian medical practitioners. C. J. B. Williams's clergyman father educated him entirely at home.* Peter Eade, the son of a surgeon in Acle, Norfolk, received his early education with a governess, after which he went to the Proprietary Grammar School in Great Yarmouth, some eight miles from home.[30] George Makins was a day pupil at the school of a Miss Earl near his home in suburban London. He then studied with a Mr. Bradley at Winkfield Rectory and completed his studies at a cathedral school.[31] Less typical cases indicate the ingenuity of Victorians in educating their children. In the Budd family, the father died young and left his wife with eight sons to rear and educate. She "skinned flints" to educate the first, and he in turn educated his brothers.[32] John Postgate, FRCS, was born in 1820, the son of a Scarborough builder. Apparently without prospects, he took employment as a grocer's boy when he was eleven years old. Later, while employed as a "surgeon's boy" earning 2s.6d. a week, he taught himself Latin, chemistry,

---

policy of electing to Fellowships a proportionately greater number of medical men from universities other than Oxbridge. These may have been less likely to have attended public schools.

*C. J. B. Williams, *Memoirs of Life and Work* (London, 1884), p. 40. Sons of professional men commonly got part, if not most, of their preliminary education at home.

and botany, and proceeded to study medicine at Leeds and later in London.[33]

Conventional historical wisdom has it that professional men and their children in the Victorian period were educated mainly in the public schools.[34] However true this may have been for some professions, it was not the case in medicine. Of the 101 Fellows of the Royal College of Physicians (elected between 1800 and 1889) who were educated in the public schools, 58 were sons of professional men. But almost 200 professional men's sons who became FRCP's were not educated in public schools.* A similar pattern appears among Fellows of the Royal College of Surgeons. Thus, while professional men were more likely than others to send their sons to public schools before beginning medical training, the converse is not true. Professional men's sons who took up medicine were, in the vast majority of cases, not educated at public schools. Some fathers specifically eliminated public school education for those of their sons who were destined for medicine. Charles J. B. Williams was the son of a clergyman whose brothers were educated at public schools before entering careers in the Church and the law. It had been decided early on that Charles, a younger son, would enter the medical profession, and he was educated entirely at home until he entered the University of Edinburgh for his medical training.[35]

While public school education was by no means a prerequisite for entry into the profession, it seems to have been an advantage to those who had had it. Two-thirds of the public school boys who eventually became FRCP's succeeded in establishing themselves in London, the most competitive place for medical practice and career-making† (see Table 3). Moreover, public school men had a better chance to reach positions of leadership in the profession. While 46 percent of

---

*Drawn from *Munk's Roll*. Cf. Tables 1 and 2, above.

† It is possible that some public school men who entered medical practice never became Fellows and thus fall outside the source of these statistics. It is difficult, therefore, to establish absolutely the relationship between public school education and medical careers.

TABLE 3 Percent of Public School Men among
College Officers, London and Provincial Practitioners,
in the Royal College of Physicians, 1800–1889[a]
(by date of Fellowship)

Categories of Medical Men	1800–29 Percent	1830–59 Percent	1860–89 Percent	Total Percent
Royal College officers	10.5	25.0	26.4	20.6
London physicians without college office	[1.0]	14.7	12.4	13.3
Provincial physicians	25.9	16.2	4.6	10.2
Other[b]	[1.0]	—	—	[1.0]
Total public school men elected FRCP	16.1	15.2	11.0	13.3 (756)

SOURCE: *Munk's Roll.*

[a]Figures in square brackets designate absolute numbers, not percentages.

[b]In practice abroad or in the military.

London Fellows without public school education became officials of the College of Physicians, 57 percent of former public school men became College officers.* Similar tendencies appear among surgical Fellows in the latter half of the century.

It is possible only to speculate about the reasons for the success of public school men in the profession. They may have been particularly ambitious men, the sons of ambitious families, and the same drive to "improve" that sent the son to public school also drove him to strive for success in his profession. Possibly the status that gave the young man access to public school education prompted others in his profession to see him as a desirable leader and representative of the profession. Perhaps the "old school tie" operated to bring young men from the public schools into positions of professional power. Whatever the virtues of the public school for the fu-

*This was more likely the case in the latter half of the century. From 1800 to 1850, public school men seem to have gravitated more often toward provincial (or "county") practice.

ture medical man, they seem not to have been related to the medical and scientific aspects of his profession. One Victorian doctor expressed the view that public school education gave a man mental discipline, "correction" and polish of character, "intellectual rivalry," and "a gentlemanly standard of conduct."[36] Such qualities might have little bearing on a man's practice of medical science, but they made the future medical man a "medical gentleman" and a sought-after representative and leader of the profession.

The question of public school education raises the larger issue of the importance of a "liberal education" in the lives of the Victorian middle classes. A liberal education met both intellectual and social needs. A good secondary education was considered an aid to future study: "those whose minds have been formed by a good preliminary education will, on the whole, be found to be more diligent, and to gain knowledge more readily than others."[37] However important its intellectual value, the social value of liberal education was even more central. H. B. Thomson, in advising young men on the choice of a profession, urged that those who chose to practice medicine "should be possessed of such a degree of literary acquirement as may secure the respect of those with whom they are to associate in the exercise of their profession."[38] For Thomson, liberal education brought status to, and respect for, the medical man, whether from his colleagues or from his patients.

Thomson's opinions had wide currency within the profession. Sir Benjamin Brodie, Bart., FRCS, in an address to medical students in 1843, emphasized the importance of "general cultivation" as the basis for a medical man's acceptance in "society."[39] Three decades later, William Dale, in his prize-winning essay on the state of the profession, stressed in a similar way the importance of a liberal education for medical men: it is, he insisted, the "education of a gentleman," and its purpose is "to enable him, in after life, to mingle amongst all classes of the community with equal ease." The question of general education bore directly on a man's "general status and position" within society.[40] The matter was stated in personal terms by a Victorian doctor, James Vaughan-Hughes, in his reminiscences of his youth. The son of an Anglican cleric, he received a good classical education at home: "hence we were well founded in what was then deemed the *sine quâ non* of a gentleman's education, and . . . [when] we reached the age of thirteen, . . . we were sent off to public school to continue our plodding."[41] A liberal and classical education was the mark of the mid-Victorian gentleman. For medical men, it was the basis for a claim to genteel status and the key to social acceptance.

Leaders of the profession were concerned about the educational backgrounds of its members. In the British Medical Association, arguments were frequently put forward for increasing the requirements in general education for men entering the profession. At the BMA Annual Meeting in 1868, the out-going president, Dr. William Stokes, called for increased standards of "moral and religious cultivation and general intellectual advancement." Higher standards of general education would, he admitted, exclude "a certain order of candidates" from medical practice, but it would work "greatly to the advantage of . . . [the] social position" of the profession.[42]

During the course of the nineteenth century the licensing bodies and the General Medical Council made efforts in the direction of improving the standards of "general culture" within the profession.* Licensing bodies instituted preliminary or "arts" examinations for medical students registering with them. These examinations varied greatly, both in the

---

*Phrases like "general culture" and "liberal culture" are common in discussions of the need for improving the non-technical education of medical men. See, e.g., T. C. Allbutt, *On Professional Education. With Special Reference to Medicine. An Address Delivered at King's College, London, on October 3, 1905* (London, 1906), p. 10 et seq., for an excellent discussion of the issues and implications of the place of "culture" in professional education. See also: T. C. Allbutt, "Medicine in the 19th Century," *Bull. of the Johns Hopkins Hospital*, 9 (December, 1898), 277–285 [reprinted with explanatory notes by A. M. Chesney in *J. Medical Education*, 31:7 (1956), 460–468]; and T. C. Allbutt, *The Need for a Liberal Education in Medicine* (London, 1889). Cf. Keetley, *Guide*, pp. 18, 48 ff., and 52 ff.

subjects tested and in the standards required for passing.* For advanced qualifications, the arts examinations set higher standards, requiring competence in English language and literature, mathematics, Latin, and elementary physics, along with Greek, logic, or a modern foreign language. But even in the 1880's, English and elementary natural philosophy (i.e., basic anatomy) were enough to begin medical training.[43]

The effectiveness of many of these examinations in keeping "uncultured" men from careers in medicine is doubtful indeed. Sir George Turner, who studied at St. George's Hospital in London in the 1870's, found among his fellow-students both public school men and some who were so poorly educated that they barely managed to enter medical school.[44] In 1898 Timothy Holmes, a surgeon with many years' service as an examiner for the Royal College of Surgeons, made similar observations about the state of general education within the profession. He thought that the arts examination of the College had failed in its purpose: candidates for the Fellowship often took the advanced arts examination after "a few months' 'coaching' in little bits of French, Latin, and algebra." Even after the College had introduced improvements in educational requirements, "there is still much to be desired in the general education of our students; . . . the proportion of those who spell badly, and still more of those who could not put four or five Latin words together decently, would be, if not so high as in those days [i.e., the mid-nineteenth century], still far higher than it ought to be."[45] By "cramming," many medical students managed to pass the examinations without having had the sort of liberal education that the profession sought in its students and future colleagues.

Liberal education beyond secondary schools was, of course, the province of the universities. Except for Oxford, which required the B.A. of all candidates for the M.D. degree, an arts degree was nowhere a prerequisite for medical

*Newman's account in *Medical Education*, pp. 50–55 and 108, is impressionistic, and very little else has been done to study the general education of medical men.

studies.[46] Most future medical men entered medical training immediately after completing their secondary schooling; only a very few took arts degrees, and those were among the elite. Among Fellows of the Royal College of Physicians, over 26 percent held the B.A. or M.A. degree. In the Royal College of Surgeons, Fellows who held arts degrees numbered 4.8 percent. (See Tables 1 and 2.)

The reasons for taking an arts degree before entering on medical studies paralleled those advanced for a good secondary education. Dr. Hugh Rayner, pressing the advantages of the Oxford B.A., said, "There is no doubt that the Arts degree gives a medical man a higher social standing."[47] Some objected that university education was a waste of time and money, that an early start in professional life, especially in surgery, was a distinct advantage in the pursuit of a successful career. In the *British Medical Journal* in 1884, the editor argued that such was not the case: "experience after all shows that a longer and more costly training is worthwhile, for it raises a man's status in the eyes of the lay world," and the medical man enjoyed "not only more social privileges but also a higher fee."[48] Not all medical men viewed university education in quite such utilitarian terms. Sir Henry Acland, FRCP, valued a liberal education less for its professional advantage than for its personal and moral value. In an address to the BMA in 1869, he argued that it served to "discipline the faculties" and gave the professional man the benefits of "the light of general culture."[49]

Some university students tried to combine their arts studies with preliminary medical training, but they were urged not to divide their time this way. T. G. Davy's advice to those in pre-professional studies was to concentrate on the honors degree: "A first will help him far more afterwards than a fragmentary knowledge of elementary medicine and surgery. A fellowship gives a man a start in life which is unequalled by any other advantage. This should be a word enough for the wise man."* When the senior Acland con-

---

* In Keetley, *Guide*, p. 55. A good degree leading to a fellowship was, of course, a source of income for the fellow, too. See also: Keet-

sulted Sir Benjamin Brodie about the education of his son Henry, Brodie told him to "Send the boy to Oxford, and let him pay there no attention to his future profession, but do as he would if he were going into Parliament like you. When he has taken his degree, send him to me and I will tell him what next."[50] In Brodie's view, the university offered general preparation for public and professional life.

A combination of circumstances militated against the arts degree for most medical men. Not required by any licensing body for medical qualification, it resulted in delays before a man could begin practice. In a family of small means, the delay meant economic disadvantage. The cost of university study was an additional deterrent. Few had the support of exhibitions or scholarships, and families of modest income could scarcely afford the costs of education and life in Oxford or Cambridge for their sons. Few families were either able or willing to take the advice of men like Brodie, but for those who did the careers of their sons were often eminent. In the Royal College of Surgeons, for example, a Fellow with a B.A. was almost three times as likely to be elected to College office as the man without that degree.*

While some of the most prominent members of the profession may have enjoyed the luster of a liberal education, the great bulk of the profession had a general education of markedly less distinction. Classical education, the mark of the Victorian gentleman, was not the standard among ordinary general practitioners. The image of the Victorian professional man as a gentleman of liberal learning, subsequently trained in professional skills, applies to only a few in medicine. For the rest, their patchy preliminary education gave little support to the claim that medical men belonged to a "learned profession."

The concern of medical leaders for the character of gen-

---

ley, *Guide*, p. 49. Very few medical men who bothered to take the B.A. took only a pass degree.

*Among Fellows with the B.A., 14.3 percent were elected to College office between 1800 and 1889; without the B.A., 5 percent. Computed from *Plarr's Lives*.

eral education in the profession is significant for the way it reveals their orientation toward the approval of non-medical society. Adherence to the standards of gentlemanly society reflected their search for status and respect in terms of liberal learning instead of scientific skill. In the 1880's the profession instituted the preliminary scientific examination, to test future medical students' knowledge of matters directly related to their professional studies. Only then were medical students expected to begin their studies with a knowledge of physics, chemistry, and biology.[51]

III

After completing his general education, a young man began his formal medical training—what one Victorian called his "bread-winning and technical studies."[52] The minimum curriculum for qualification changed radically during the nineteenth century. These changes can be described generally as an increase in the amount of formal course work, lectures, laboratory work, and supervised practice, and a decline in the amount of time spent in simple observation and in private surgical and medical practice. Each licensing body set its own minimum requirements, but in general it is fair to say that at the beginning of the century one year of academic training and four years of practical (apprenticeship) experience was characteristic of the kind of education most medical men had. After 1815 the Society of Apothecaries required five years of apprenticeship for the LSA. Courses in anatomy, physiology, chemistry, *materia medica*, and the theory and practice of medicine, together with six months of hospital practice were obligatory. Lecture courses and hospital practice could be done simultaneously, and it was possible to complete the formal requirements in a single year. Similarly, the Royal College of Surgeons in the early nineteenth century required two courses of anatomy (lectures and demonstrations) and one year of hospital practice, all of which could be completed in one year of academic instruction. The remainder of an apprentice's time was spent in his master's private practice. Even within the universities the requirements for a medical degree were minimal and not rigorously structured, medical

60

studies being left to the discretion of the student and his knowledge of the demands of the examiners for his future license.[53]

By 1835, course work had been extended to such a degree that two and one-half years of academic studies were typical of most formal curricula. This minimum time in lectures and laboratory work remained constant for much of the century, but the number of optional courses for medical students grew, and recommendations for extended studies were issued from time to time by the General Medical Council.*

The curriculum of medical education expanded in two ways. First, subjects originally included in one course were separated and offered in separate courses. For example, most medical schools offered anatomy and physiology (with dissections) in one course of lectures in 1815. By 1855, anatomy and physiology were offered separately, the latter course including general physiology and morbid anatomy. By 1884, physiology, practical physiology, and morbid anatomy were three separate courses. Similarly, a single course in chemistry in 1815 became two courses by 1884, one in chemistry and one in practical chemistry.[54] (See Table 4 for further details of course expansion.)

In addition to the courses resulting from the subdivision of older courses and the additional time required for the

---

*Keetley, *Guide*, p. 12; and Newman, *Medical Education*, pp. 107–108 and 218–219. With the decline of apprenticeship, most medical courses took four years. After 1885 the standard medical course was five years (Newman, *Medical Education*, p. 207). Despite developments in the curriculum, the quality of much mid-nineteenth-century medical education was not very high. A series entitled "The Physiology of the London Medical Student," *Punch*, 1 (1841), 177, lampooned English medical studies: "[T]he knowledge of the natural class and order of a buttercup must be of the greatest service to a practitioner in after-life in treating a case of typhus fever or ruptured blood-vessel. At some of the Continental Hospitals, the pupil's time is wasted at the bedside of the patient, from which he can only get practical information." Information in the *Select Committee on Medical Education* (1834) makes the *Punch* lampoon look all too realistic.

TABLE 4 The Growth of the Medical Curriculum in the Nineteenth Century

1815: LSA, MRCS	1855: LSA, MRCS	1884: LSA, MRCS, LRCP
Anatomy (lectures, demonstrations) (MRCS)	Anatomy (with dissections)	Anatomy (with dissections)
Anatomy and physiology (LSA)	Physiology (including general physiology and morbid anatomy)	Physiology Practical physiology Morbid anatomy
Chemistry (LSA)	Chemistry Practical chemistry	Chemistry Practical chemistry
Materia medica (LSA)	Materia medica Botany Forensic medicine	Materia medica Practical pharmacy Botany (LRCP, LSA only) Forensic medicine
Theory and practice of medicine (LSA)	Theory and practice of medicine	Theory and practice of medicine Clinical medicine
	Theory and practice of surgery	Principles and practice of surgery Clinical surgery Practical surgery
	Midwifery	Midwifery and the diseases of women
Hospital practice (MRCS, LSA)	Hospital practice	Hospital practice Service as clinical clerk, dresser

NOTE: This chart includes only the minimum medical and surgical curriculum required for general practice. Optional subjects such as ophthalmology, children's diseases, laryngology, dermatology, and the like were included in the general medical courses, but could also be studied in special courses in special hospitals and later in the general hospital medical schools as well.

SOURCES: Charles Newman, *The Evolution of Medical Education*, p. 74; *London and Provincial Medical Directory*, 1855; and *BMJ*, 1884, ii, 504–505. Cf. H. Hale Bellot, *University College London, 1826–1926*, Chart 6.

study of an expanding body of knowledge in these areas, the medical curriculum was also expanded by the introduction of new courses. By 1835 courses in morbid anatomy, forensic medicine, midwifery, and the diseases of women had become a part of the medical curriculum required by the Society of Apothecaries.[55] Some of this material had been taught informally in apprenticeship, and thus some of the new courses institutionalized and formalized the haphazard "curriculum" of apprenticeship.

Medical education also expanded because of the breakdown of the traditional medical orders. The growth of general practice required that a medical man be trained in both medicine and surgery. The Apothecaries' Society required a course in the principles and practice of medicine in 1815 for what was essentially a license in "physic." By 1885 they also required courses in surgery for the LSA, in recognition of the fact that the LSA was a general practitioner's license. Similarly, the Royal College of Surgeons began to require the theory and practice of medicine as part of the training for the MRCS.*

The initiatives for innovations in the medical curriculum sometimes came from the medical corporations.[56] More often, however, they came from the staffs of the medical schools themselves. From the beginning, medical men had dominated medical and surgical teaching. They had brought their teaching into the hospitals, where it was institutionalized in the 1820's and 1830's. While ultimate control over hospital policy was in the hands of the laymen on the boards of governors, doctors controlled much of medical school policy, planning, and growth.[57] Just as individual apothecaries and surgeons had exercised control over their apprentices, so the staffs of the medical schools developed and extended their power over the students they taught. Through the medical corporations they set the requirements for licensing, and through the hos-

---

*Newman, *Medical Education*, pp. 17–20 and 153. In 1800 the MRCS required only surgical training and no formal training in medicine ("physic") at all, although holders of that license often engaged in general practice.

pital medical schools they defined the expanding curriculum of required and elective professional studies.

From the standpoint of medical students, the establishment of medical schools and the growth of the curriculum at first expanded their options but, in the long run, brought them under the firm control of their seniors in the medical world. At the beginning of the nineteenth century the question of education was relatively simple: for the few who intended to become physicians, education at Oxbridge or one of the Scottish or Irish universities was the rule.* For the mass of medical students, apprenticeship to a surgeon or apothecary for five years or more led to qualification.[58] This education in private practice might have been supplemented by a course at one of the private anatomy schools and some informal work in the hospital, observing the consulting physicians and surgeons at their work; but the core of medical education in this period was the one-to-one relationship of master and apprentice in the surgery or the apothecary's shop.

For a time, in the first half of the nineteenth century, the new hospital medical schools co-existed with the private anatomy schools, and an apprentice could compound his education by mixing the three types of educational experiences. The increasing importance of clinical experience and bedside teaching in the curriculum brought the hospital to the center of a student's educational life. Apprentice surgeons, apprentice apothecaries, and university students from Oxbridge all gravitated to the London hospitals for the wealth of clinical experience with patients and their diseases that could be found there. By the 1850's, private education in the anatomy

---

*Some reported that foreign degrees could be purchased in the Tottenham Court Road. See Robert H. Belcher, *Degrees and "Degrees." Or, Traffic in Theological, Medical and Other "Diplomas" Exposed* (London, 1872), pp. 5 and 16 ff.; and Newman, *Medical Education*, p. 135. A few went abroad for medical degrees in France, Belgium, and Germany; others studied abroad for brief periods. See: Alexander M. Cooke, "The College and Europe" [The Langdon Brown Lecture, delivered at the Royal College of Physicians, October 1968], *Jour. Roy. Coll. Phys. Lond.*, 4:2 (1970), 97–113.

schools was co-opted or destroyed by the hospital medical schools.[59]

Growing requirements for course work and hospital experience in the first half of the century undermined the importance of apprenticeship as an institution of medical education. Even while a student might be formally indentured for a five-year apprenticeship, he spent more and more of those years in the lecture halls, dissecting rooms, and hospital wards, and less and less time in his master's private practice. With the decay of apprenticeship, private practitioners without ties to the hospitals lost the status and income that came from a role in medical education. Some fought a rear-guard action in the 1870's and 1880's, urging that a year of pupillage to a private practitioner offered special benefits to medical students: it provided a period of personal transition and socialization to medical life, and it was a practical way to learn the basic terminology of anatomy, physiology, and therapeutics before beginning course work in earnest.[60] While a few medical students continued to elect a year of private pupillage, the battle for private medical education was lost, and the hospital medical schools dominated medical education and medical students' lives.

By 1860 an almost dizzying array of medical schools could be found in London: St. Bartholomew's Hospital Medical School, St. Thomas's Hospital Medical School, St. Mary's, the Westminster, Charing Cross, Guy's, St. George's, the London, the Middlesex, University College, and King's College—all these institutions offered full programs of medical education. In addition, provincial medical education was growing apace, offering alternatives to metropolitan schools.[61]

Even within the framework of the medical school, students did not simply enroll, complete courses, and qualify. Some, of course, pursued their studies from start to finish in a single school. But others, and perhaps many, picked and chose among the lecturers and courses offered in various institutions, taking anatomy at one medical school and forensic medicine at another. George Makins, for example, was a student at St. Thomas's Hospital in London, but he took his botany and *materia medica* at the Middlesex Hospital because the St. Thomas's lectures in those subjects were given at 8 A.M. He specifically chose Middlesex because two of the surgeons there were old friends of his father.[62]

Medical schools cooperated in this supermarket approach to medical education by offering itemized fees for individual courses as well as a single total matriculation fee. This practice put the medical schools and individual teachers in the position of competing with each other for students. It was an advantage to the cash-poor student, who could begin his education at an inexpensive provincial school near his home and finish his course work and hospital practice in a London hospital.

The opportunities for provincial medical education also expanded in this period, and a student might elect to study medicine at Manchester, Durham, Liverpool, or Bristol. Oxford and Cambridge continued to lure students who wanted to pursue a medical degree in an environment of "splendid opportunities both for social and general literary and scientific culture."[63] With the mid-Victorian reforms of Oxbridge medical education, those universities gained a reputation for fine theoretical work in medical science. By the 1880's the Oxbridge medical man was trained in the inductive method, experimental techniques, and skills in generalization to prepare him to deal with "the difficult and complicated questions raised in the medical art and science."[64] The practical and clinical side of university medical study could best be found in London.

From its inception, the University of London was known for the strength of its medical curriculum and its clinical resources. By the 1880's it enjoyed "the highest reputation for difficult and searching examinations."[65] The establishment of a university in London, cheek by jowl with the London hospitals, allowed students to pursue both a university degree and clinical experience. The meteoric rise of the University of London may partly be attributed to the way it met the needs and desires of medical students.

The dominance of the University of London may be as-

TABLE 5 Sources of Medical Degrees among Fellows,
RCP, 1800–1889

Dates	Oxbridge Percent	London Percent	Scottish Percent	Other[a] Percent
1800–09	85.2			14.8
1810–19	83.3			16.7
1820–29	75.0		19.4	5.6
1830–39	62.3		33.3	4.4
1840–49	35.3	2.9	42.6	19.2
1850–59	15.0	23.0	46.0	16.0
1860–69	19.0	30.4	46.8	4.2
1870–79	18.7	30.0	39.3	12.0
1880–89	29.9	32.0	21.6	16.5

SOURCE: *Munk's Roll.*
[a]Provincial English Universities, Ireland, foreign degrees,
M.D. Lambeth, and no degree.

sessed most effectively in the patterns of university education
of Fellows of the Royal College of Physicians. Throughout the
century, of course, a substantial number of the College's Fellows came from the ancient universities. During the first three
decades of the nineteenth century, 75 percent to 85 percent
of all Fellows elected had been educated at Oxbridge. From
the 1820's onward, the College embarked on a policy of electing a larger number of Fellows and bringing a larger number
of provincial physicians into the Fellowship. The result was an
increase in the number of men with Scottish degrees among
Fellowship holders (see Table 5). Within a decade of the
foundation of London University, its graduates began to be
elected to the Fellowship of the Royal College of Physicians.
By the decade 1880–1889, the largest single group of new
Fellows were those educated at the University of London.
Among Fellows of the Royal College of Surgeons the importance of London University was even more marked. The
FRCS did not require any university medical degree, and in
the first half of the nineteenth century only 20 percent of
those elected to the Fellowship had earned the M.B. or M.D.
degree (see Table 2). Between 1850 and 1889, almost 50 percent of those achieving the Fellowship held a medical degree,

and nearly half of those were London graduates. From the medical student's point of view, the University of London offered the best of both worlds. Students did not have to choose between a medical degree and extensive clinical experience (or the compromise of Oxbridge study and London practice). For those who had no hope of Oxbridge medical education, London made available a university medical degree and metropolitan medical education at the same time.

The University of London offered the teaching staff distinct professional advantages as well. In Oxbridge, medical teaching played a small and relatively insignificant part in the curriculum of those institutions. In London, especially at King's and University Colleges, medical teaching was a far more central and important part of academic life. At Oxbridge, the weight of tradition diluted the significance of medical teaching; in London, the lack of tradition gave greater influence to the teachers of medicine, surgery, and allied science. The establishment of university medical education in London marked the beginning of the end of the division between the elite education of the physicians and the practical education of the surgeons, the end of the gap between university and hospital. Only two hospital medical schools were affiliated with the University of London in the nineteenth century, King's College Hospital and University College Hospital. But they made a beginning, and in the twentieth century all eleven great teaching hospitals became affiliated with London University. Thus, the elites of the London medical and surgical establishment, who controlled the Colleges, the General Medical Council, and the curriculum of the hospital medical schools, gained a foothold in what was to become the major academic institution for the training of medical men.

IV

The cost of medical education deserves special scrutiny, for the Victorians seem to have held contradictory views regarding the relative costliness or cheapness of professional training in medicine. As we have seen, some elected a medical career because they thought it economical, and indeed for medical men's sons it was. On the other hand, some contemporary observers—frequently cited in the historical literature—mentioned figures of £500 to £600 for apprenticeship or medical school, including educational and living expenses. Indeed, a few Victorian writers suggested that £1,000 or more might be needed to pay for tuition, living expenses, and the costs of getting established in practice.[66] Such a figure implies that medical men must have been recruited from among the prosperous classes of society, for the ordinary artisan or shabby-genteel professional man could scarcely afford such educational expenses for his son. If these figures are accurate estimates of what most medical men paid for their education, then they make nonsense of the profession's worries that medicine might attract a socially inferior breed of man.

The figure of £600 for four to five years of medical study is an accurate one, but only for the best available medical education. Apprenticeships with leading surgeons at the beginning of the century carried a fee of five hundred guineas. For education in a hospital medical school, that figure is also accurate, even as late as 1884. In the London hospitals, fees were over £100 for all lectures and hospital practice; London living costs were estimated to be about £100 a year for a single medical student living relatively comfortably; and miscellaneous expenses for books, equipment, and examination fees brought the total to £600.* A careful look at the records indicates that these figures apply to a minority of medical students. With care, medical education either in apprenticeship or medical school could be had for much less.

The Apothecaries' Hall registered all apprenticeships between London apothecaries affiliated with their society and their students. The vast majority of apprenticeships cost less than £500, and some carried only nominal charges. The results of a survey of apprenticeship fees paid by apprentices

---

*Keetley, *Guide*, pp. 12–15. A. F. Street says that medical education, strictly speaking, was cheaper in Oxbridge than in London, but the social benefits of Oxbridge could not be had "on the cheap" (in Keetley, *Guide*, p. 51). The expenses of Oxbridge social life put educational costs there above that of an ordinary London medical training.

TABLE 6 Apprenticeship Premiums, Society of Apothecaries, in Selected Years

	Premium	1820–21	1846–48	1869–72	Total
[1.]	No fee (relatives)	12	16	13	41
[2.]	0–5s.	14	10	20	44
[3.]	5s.–£100	3	8	7	18
[4.]	£101–200	9	1	1	11
[5.]	£201–300	11	3	—	14
[6.]	£301–400	6	1	—	7
[7.]	£401–500	1	—	—	1
	TOTAL	56	39	41	136

SOURCE: Society of Apothecaries, Court minute books, 1820–21, 1846–48, 1869–72, monthly entries.

and their families in sample years are given in Table 6. Group 1 in this table represents apprenticeships between relatives, for which no fees were charged. Some of the no-fee apprenticeships in Group 2 may also have been contracts between relatives; the records do not always identify family apprenticeships. Over 60 percent of all apprenticeships registered in these sample years involved only nominal fees or no fees at all.

Family apprenticeships were, of course, predictably without premium. Why unrelated individuals should arrange an indenture with minimal fees involved is not, from the master's point of view, so easily explained. Perhaps a medical man took a student in order to have his assistance in a practice. The medical apprentice could sweep the surgery or shop (which some did) and, with some training, could prepare drugs and pull teeth. Perhaps the fee-less indentures represent private arrangements among friends in which an exchange of favors, not mentioned in the contract, was the basis of the service: a medical man might take a clergyman's son as his apprentice in exchange for the general education the cleric gave to the apothecary's children.

Whatever the motives and arrangements, the fact remains that most apprenticeships in this sample cost less than the stereotypical five hundred guineas. Of all those in the sample, only one-fourth involved fees of more than £100, and those apprenticeships represent a declining proportion of all indentures during the century. Such a reduction reflects the declining value of private medical education, the decreased time students spent in private study, and the loss of the private practitioner's role in medical education.

When lecture courses first appeared, they were, as apprenticeship had been, the private arrangements of individual medical men. Students paid the lecturer involved, and each teacher made his own arrangements regarding the character, duration, and location of the lecture series. The foundation of London hospital medical schools transformed the relationships of teachers and students. Courses were no longer the ventures of individual medical men but became part of a coherent curriculum offered by the medical school. Students paid their fees not to the teacher but to the school officials, and the medical teachers were, in turn, paid out of the medical school coffers.[67] It seems very likely that these patterns of institutional, rather than personal, payment resulted in freeing the medical teacher from the obligations and dependency that must have been involved in the direct payment relationship. He had been, in some sense, an "employee" of his pupil. The advent of the medical school gave him relative freedom from his students and tied him more closely to his peers and the institution.

Students, too, lived under a new social order in the medical school. The lecture system ended the individual tie between the medical student and his teacher. No longer did a student bind himself to his master with the promise that "the said Apprentice his said Master faithfully shall serve, his Secrets keep, his lawful Commands every where gladly do."[68] In the medical school he was only one of many students. He had continuing relationships with his student peers and with the institution as a whole rather than with any single teacher. He gained a new sense of membership in a corporate group, that of medical students and future professional men—a sentiment not greatly fostered in private apprenticeship. Such social experience laid the foundations for his sense of membership in the larger profession. Where the traditional apothecary or surgeon, trained in isolation, might easily have felt himself to be an independent and isolated craftsman or tradesman, the new education of Victorian medical men fostered a sense of membership in a common profession. The medical school was the parent of group-consciousness, of profession-consciousness.

The existence of private anatomy schools gave medical students in the first half of the century some flexibility in educational budgeting. Hospital medical schools announced fees for all course work and for clinical practice, but allowed students to enroll in their schools for only part of the course work or hospital practice. Westminster Hospital Medical School was typical. In 1855, fees for individual courses ranged from two to seven guineas. The total cost of course work there was 42 guineas, and hospital practice carried an additional fee of £27.6s. However, a student could save one-sixth of his course fees by going to a private school. The Grosvenor Street School of Anatomy and Medicine, for example, charged 35 guineas for all required lectures, a saving of seven guineas.[69] With the disappearance of all the private anatomy schools by the 1860's, the hospital medical schools had a monopoly over the teaching of medicine in London.

In view of the expansion of the medical curriculum, it is not surprising that educational costs rose in the mid-Victorian years. The minimum fee a student could pay in a London hospital medical school in 1860 was £73.10s. By 1884 the minimum was £105. The respective maximum fees at those two dates were £105 and £120.[70] While the fees rose, the cost differential between the least and most expensive London schools narrowed in this period. Provincial medical schools, growing in numbers in the Victorian years, were less expensive than those in the metropolis. Their rates tended to be one-third to one-half those of London, ranging from £65 to £90 for all hospital and lecture fees.*

The cost of maintenance was a more complex factor in

---

*Keetley, *Guide*, pp. 14–15. Newman, *Medical Education*, p. 122, cites a figure of £52.10s. for fees at Queen's College Birmingham in 1858.

the total cost of medical education. If a young man lived at home, parents still bore the costs involved in supporting him, but they were notably less than those involved in providing separate housing and boarding accommodations. Families of students living near a medical school could take advantage of their proximity and support their sons at home. When a student had to live away from home, the cost of maintenance was a significant part of the cost of education.

One author, writing in 1885, estimated the cost of maintenance at £400 for four nine-month terms away from home, covering room, board, and pocket money (see Budget A, Table 7). His figures are computed on what he considers "usual" costs for board and room: shared housing (for two) at 25–30s. a week, a total of £50–60 per year, with the remaining £40–50 allocated for food and pocket money. Alternatively, a student might pay a combined fee of 37s. a week for food and lodging, a total of £75 a year, with the £25 remaining for pocket money.[71] The same author suggests that minimum room and food costs might amount to 15–18s. a week for lodging (£30–36 for nine months) or combined room and board for a minimum rate of 25s. a week, or £50 for the year. With pocket money on the minimum budget reduced to £15 or £20 a year, the total annual maintenance cost would be £50 to £70 a year, or £200 to £280 for four years. Under the more austere budget, a student could reduce his total expenditure for medical education from £600 to from £330 to £410 (see Budget B, Table 7).

Given these fairly detailed data regarding educational costs in 1885, it is possible to estimate what educational costs might have been in 1860. If a family of six could live very modestly on £100 a year,[72] an unmarried student might live similarly on one-third to one-half that amount. This would mean that a student's living expenses would be £35 to £45 for a school year, a total of £140 to £180 for four years of maintenance, and a total educational cost of £230 to £270 for a London medical education in 1860 (see Budget C, Table 7).

All writers on the subject indicate that medical education, and living expenses generally, were less costly in provincial towns.[73] Thus, a student seeking the cheapest possible medi-

TABLE 7 Estimates of the Cost of Medical Education

A: Moderate Budget, London, 1884		B: Minimum Budget, London, 1884	
Hospital fees	£105–126	Hospital fees	£105
Books and instruments	15	Books and instruments	15
Exam fees (double qualification)	28– 35	Exam fee (LSA only)	6
GMC registration fee	5	GMC registration fee	5
Subtotal	£133–181	Subtotal	£131
[Tutors, optional £7–10 per term]			
Board and lodging, 4 years @£100 p.a. (room @ 25– 30s./wk. or room & board @ 37s./ wk., plus pocket money)	£400	Board and lodging, 4 years @£50–70 p.a. (room @ 15– 18s./wk. or bd/rm @ 25s./ wk., plus pocket money)	£200–280
Total	£533–581	Total	£331–411

C: Minimum Budget, London, 1860		D: Minimum Budget, Provincial, 1860	
Hospital fees	£65	Hospital fees	£50
Books and instruments	12	Books and instruments	12
Exam fee	6	Exam fee	6
GMC registration fee	5	GMC registration fee	5
Subtotal	£88	Subtotal	£73
Board and Lodging	£140–180	Board and Lodging	£110–150
Total	£228–268	Total	£183–223

SOURCES: *London and Provincial Medical Directory*, 1860; C. B. Keetley, *The Student's and Junior Practitioner's Guide to the Medical Profession* (London, 1885), pp. 14–15; J. A. Banks, *Prosperity and Parenthood* (London, 1954), pp. 59, 75; E. H. Hunt, *Regional Wage Variations in Britain, 1850–1914* (Oxford, 1973), pp. 91–92.

cal training would look to a provincial medical school for his education. Taking into account all the ways for reducing expenses, it seems probable that a man might be able to obtain training outside London, and on a sparse budget, for something like £185 to £300 for four years, instead of the oft-quoted £600 (see Budget D, Table 7). Such a figure seems a more reasonable amount for a family of modest means to spend for a son's medical education. Moreover, it is a feasible amount for a student to earn supporting himself through medical school, as some were able to do. Typically, parents paid for the education of their sons, but financial assistance sometimes came from other relatives, too.[74] A few entered medical training with scholarships, prizes, or exhibitions from grammar or public schools.

One of the by-products of the creation of the medical school was the introduction of institutional support for medical students. Medical schools established cash prizes for outstanding performance on the entrance examinations, and later they began to extend a system of scholarships and awards for performance in particular courses or as grants for needy students, at the discretion of the staff. In 1860 for example, Charing Cross Hospital Medical School offered "Free Scholarships" to "sons of professional men, or of gentlemen in a corresponding station of society, of reduced circumstances, and all are to have had a good preliminary classical education fitting them for the medical profession."[75] St. Thomas's Hospital gave similar prizes to entering pupils "to encourage and reward a good general education."[76] In 1875 the Middlesex Hospital Medical School offered two entrance scholarships, one at £20 and one at £25 per annum, each for two years' tenure. Students completing their third year were eligible to compete for the Brodrip Scholarships, worth £20 and £30, and several other awards were offered for various categories of students in the medical school as well.[77] A combination of these prizes sometimes provided full support to a medical student. In the early 1860's William Warwick Wagstaffe, Sr., received two entrance scholarships, one in classics and mathematics and one in natural science and modern languages, and was able to carry on his studies at St. Thomas's without any expense to his parents.[78]

Within the context of collective medical education, the staffs of the hospital medical schools found the means for improving the character and quality of medical students.[79] They used the system of entrance prizes to recruit the sons of gentlemen into the profession. Such quality control had not been possible in private apprenticeship, but their corporate roles as medical school teachers gave them new power over the next generation of medical men. Certainly, they used that power to foster the values of non-medical, socially genteel Victorian society. But the important point is that power now came into the hands of medical men, and they exercised that power collectively for the improvement of the profession.

V

Financial considerations may have placed limits on the choices young men and their families made about medical education. Within these limits, decisions about medical education were taken, during much of the nineteenth century, on the basis of such criteria as family, friendship, and connection. Such bases were predictable ones in the days of apprenticeship, when an apothecary or surgeon had only a few students and their relationship was an intimate one, working together from morning until night. Such arrangements also grew out of the traditional assumption that families and friends had obligations to each other that extended beyond the private sphere. A master surgeon or apothecary took on a relative or the son of a friend as his student in preference to a stranger because their relationship implied obligation and loyalty on both sides. Even where financial considerations need not have been an issue, indentures between relatives were made because of the advantages of personal ties between the apprentice and master. Edward Cock (1805–1892), the son of a Lloyd's underwriter and grandson of a wealthy London merchant, was apprenticed to his uncle, the famous Sir Astley Cooper.[80] Family ties gave the would-be medical student access to these prestigious teachers. The teachers, in turn, saw the education of their nephews as an advantage, since family ties gave them greater control over their students. Friendship between the master and the apprentice's family functioned in a similar way.[81]

A young man's medical career depended heavily on the assistance his master could provide: connections, influence, advice, and professional employment. The most costly and influential apprenticeships were those with hospital surgeons or apothecaries, since the apprentices of men with hospital appointments had first claim to openings on the hospital staff. Apprenticeships based on family and friendship kept these benefits among intimates. This pattern of succession through apprenticeship continued until the 1830's and 1840's; by the 1850's the system was dead. The last surgeons to be appointed under the apprenticeship tradition were Samuel Solly and John Birkett. Solly, indentured in 1822, became Assistant Surgeon at St. Thomas's in 1841 and full Surgeon in 1853. Birkett became Assistant Surgeon at Guy's in 1849 and Surgeon in 1853.[82] The expansion of the medical school and the growth of the curriculum undermined the independent authority of individual medical teachers. Instead, the staff became jointly responsible for the medical education of all their students.

Despite the new institutionalization of medical education, personal relationships and extrinsic considerations continued to play an important role in a student's choice of medical education. After serving an apprenticeship in Stepney, Walter Rivington (1835–1897) chose to study at the London Hospital, where his cousin, T. B. Curling, was Surgeon.[83] Richard Quain's studies at the Aldersgate School of Medicine were, at least in part, motivated by the fact that his brother, Jones Quain, was a teacher there.[84] And James E. Lane (1857–1926) was a student at St. Mary's Hospital; his great-uncle, Samuel Lane, had founded the hospital, and his father was a Surgeon there.[85] Some students chose a medical school because a relative—father, older brother, or uncle—had been a student there earlier. This was the case with Dennis Hovell (1818–1888) at the London Hospital, John Hammond Morgan (1847–1924) at St. George's, and the Adams brothers at the London Hospital.[86]

In the absence of family ties to a school, students chose on the basis of friendships within the school and came to their medical studies with introductions to the staff from their connections. George Makins enjoyed both sorts of ties in his student years. He chose St. Thomas's Hospital Medical School partly, he said, because it was convenient to his train connection. But he also had an uncle on the Board of Governors. He attended some lectures at the Middlesex Hospital, and his reasons are typical: "I went to Middlesex because my father in his young days had been a lecturer on chemistry there and still had friends in the persons of Campbell de Morgan and T. W. Nunn, two of the surgeons there."[87] When the prospective student had no "connexion," his choices were likely to become arbitrary, and he suffered anxiety at the lack of any relationship between himself and the medical school he was to enter. John Bland-Sutton felt keenly the lack of advisers and connections, and he eventually chose Middlesex after having read in the newspapers of the "clever" action of one of the Middlesex house surgeons in saving a man from drowning in the Thames.[88]

That relational ties were significant in students' decisions about medical school may be inferred from these examples. It is explicit in Charles Bell Keetley's discussion of how young men chose a medical school. Writing in 1885, Keetley enumerated the bases on which students selected a medical school:

> A youth usually goes to some particular place for one or more of these reasons:
>
> 1. His father, or the surgeon with whom he has been a pupil, went there before him.
> 2. He knows, or can get an introduction to, some member or members of the staff.
> 3. As a moth flies to the candle, though luckily without the same serious consequences, he is attracted by the glitter of names on the list of medical officers. . . .
> 4. He prefers a large hospital; or
> 5. He prefers a small one.[89]

Keetley elaborated on this list to suggest that students also chose medical schools because they liked hard work—or wanted to avoid it, or because a school had a reputation for its gentlemanly students.[90] Keetley's itemization of students' motivations is a fascinating one, both for what he includes and for what he leaves out. The most important considerations are the connections between the student and the medical school through family, friends, or introductions. Missing from Keetley's list is any reference to the quality of medical education offered by the medical school. Item 3 might be considered an oblique reference to quality, if the "glitter" of reputation is an index of superior medicine and science.

Keetley attempted to educate his readers by pointing out some of the technical and medical considerations which should be involved in the selection of a medical school. He advised "diffident men of moderate ability" to go to the smaller medical school, where "offices, prizes, and clinical work are more easily obtained."[91] In a small school, such a man would enjoy close social ties with his fellow students, individual attention from his teachers, and a "happy home" for the course of his medical training. On the other hand, "persons of exceptional ability have more scope to show their talents" at the great centers of medical study, where they can attract the attention of the influential teachers.[92] What is remarkable about Keetley's discussion of the choice of a medical school is that he found it necessary, as late as 1885, to urge students to consider their own talents and abilities when choosing a school. His assessment indicates the continuing existence of familial and private criteria for career decisions in a profession where careers were presumably open to talent.

The continuing concern of prospective medical students with having "connexions" with a medical school came from the fact that those associations shaped not only the years of medical study but a man's whole career. As an apprentice and his family might have felt more comfortable when the son was indentured to a family friend, so a medical student probably entered medical school with greater assurance if he had some friend within it. Family ties must have given the young student some sense of acquaintance in what otherwise could be a strange and alien environment. Parents could rest easier, knowing that their connections provided a surrogate family to keep an eye on the lad in the notoriously unruly milieu of medical school in London, a frequently dangerous city.

Beyond medical school, "a young man about to start in life often derives help from the support of the staff of his school," Keetley observed.[93] A brilliant medical student might gain the assistance of the staff on his own. For most students, however, that was a risky way to plan one's future life, and connections of family and friendship offered traditional, known, and more certain foundations for a future claim to a teacher's assistance. It is not surprising that talent was slow to replace connection as the basis for choosing a medical school. If a medical student had to depend on his teachers, it was better to rely on family and friends than to depend on the objective evaluation of one's talent by strangers.

Keetley advised medical students that the greatest influence for their future careers came from the great medical schools: "The influence of the staff of a great school is usually, when compared with that of the staff of a small one, even more than proportionally great."[94] For "great schools" one can read London, and the young men who chose the London medical schools, whether because of connection or ambition and a conviction of talent, found themselves in the glittering center of English medical life.

VI

Once a young man and his family had chosen a suitable plan for his medical training, all that remained was to pass the "arts" examination and register as a student with a medical corporation or university. After 1858 he also registered with the General Medical Council. He then began attendance at his chosen medical school. He went to lectures and spent the requisite number of months in the dissecting room observing the hospital's demonstrator of anatomy performing dissections. After the supply of cadavers was increased by changes in the law,[95] a student not only studied prepared dissections in the museum and observed the anatomists operating on the dead body, but he also did his own anatomical studies. After completing his introductory courses, he began his studies of medicine and surgery and spent time in the wards of the hospital, on his own or with staff members who lectured at the bedsides of patients. When an operation was performed, he and his classmates made their way to the surgical theater to observe. A particularly difficult operation or a specially skilled surgeon often filled the theater to capacity with eager students.[96]

Victorian medical schools introduced an interim examination in which the basic medical sciences—anatomy, physiology, botany, and *materia medica*—were tested. Advanced studies in these subjects, together with examinations in the principles and practice of medicine and surgery, were covered in the final examinations.

In social terms, the coming of the medical school brought changes in the lives of London medical students. In apprenticeship, a student lived at home or with his master. In the early days of the hospital medical schools, students had found lodgings, either alone or with friends, in the neighborhood of the hospital. In the early Victorian period, medical faculties, concerned about the students' unruliness and lack of discipline, began to introduce "collegiate" residences affiliated with the hospital medical schools. The faculty at St. Bartholomew's Hospital Medical School, for example, did a thorough study of the costs and conditions of medical student living arrangements, and then they proceeded to establish a residential college where students could live, dine, and study.[97] Here students lived in an environment not unlike the Oxbridge colleges. They were supervised more carefully than they could have been in "digs." Their hours were defined and their behavior was regulated by rules set down by the medical school administration.[98] In yet another area of medical life, students were thus brought under the corporate discipline of the profession. In addition, the isolation of independent, solitary apprenticeship was replaced by the community life of the college residence. With this came new organizations and associations that further integrated the students into a student body.

By mid-century most of the medical schools had student clubs or societies which combined debating, lectures, scientific papers, and purely social activities. All the clubs provided an opportunity for students to get acquainted with each other. Medical students were encouraged to participate in their hospital society in order to gain experience in leadership. Debating, lecturing, or presenting a paper helped the student to "acquire the art of thinking and speaking when standing up before an audience."[99] Holding an office in a medical school club was thought to "teach . . . a little knowledge of business and of human nature, and train . . . for more important positions of a similar kind."[100] There was, a student was to discover, more to a medical career than the techniques of diagnosis and treatment. The poor student, whose time was consumed in studies and employment, may have had little opportunity to participate in this aspect of professional training. But for those who could afford it, the medical school's auxiliary activities provided an early training ground in leadership and corporate professional life.

Sporting clubs—cricket, football, rowing—also became a part of life in the London hospital medical schools, perhaps in unconscious imitation of Oxbridge. More than one medical student's activities and prowess in the athletic realm brought him recognition as a sportsman and introductions that benefited him in his professional career.[101] Masonic lodges also appeared in a number of the London medical schools.[102] Clubs and societies brought students into closer association with one another and fostered their further integration into the community.

A student's social life outside the structure of sports and clubs depended on his private interests and connections in London. S. T. Taylor, in his diary of mid-Victorian medical studies, records having spent his leisure time visiting relatives, enjoying the popular entertainments London offered, and engaging in the inevitable sessions of student gossip.[103] Some students, with introductions to the staff, were entertained in their teachers' homes.[104]

Along with cooperation and growing collegiality in the medical school, there was competition as well. Students spent time preparing for the examinations which could lead to honorary medals and cash prizes. By the end of the century these competitions had become a major part of student life. As one observer put it, "All the year round, and in every class of academic, institutional and professional training, men are winning prizes, losing prizes, competing for prizes or scratching for those competitions. . . ."[105] Cash awards offered the short-range benefit of support for the cost of medical training. But prizes, whether cash or a gold or silver medal, brought long-term career benefits as well. S. Squire Sprigge, a medical man and later editor of the *Lancet*, judged that "success in after-life is found in large proportion among those whose performances as students have commended them highly to examiners and have earned them prizes."[106] The biographical records of the Royal Colleges support his judgment; many leaders of the profession had won prizes during their student days. Those who judged success in terms of income evaluated prizes in the same way. C. B. Keetley urged students to compete, saying that prizes and honors "have a value far exceeding their intrinsic worth. A gold medal worth £5 has, before now, led to an income of a thousand a year."[107]

While there was certainly some relationship between prizes and future success, the nature of that connection is not entirely clear. On the one hand, prizes might simply have distinguished those men who had mastered most thoroughly the subjects of the medical curriculum and, in later life, put that learning to most effective use as good, and therefore successful, doctors. But success was often more dependent on a man's manners and social style than on his skill or learning, and thus no simple rational equation between prizes and success can be made. Victorian observers of the prize system saw other elements involved. Sprigge noted that the prize system encouraged students to greater efforts by appealing to "an honourable as well as to an inevitable spirit of rivalry."[108] The prizeman was likely to be a competitive and ambitious man. The same spirit that enabled him to compete successfully for prizes might also have given him an edge in the race for practice and professional success.

While prizes may have reflected the abilities or drive of

the successful competitor, they also created a relationship between the winner and the medical school staff. The prize examinations gave the staff the chance to identify the talented, industrious, and ambitious students from the herd of aspirants seeking notice in the large medical classes—a problem not faced in the one-to-one relationship of apprenticeship.[109] There, the fact of indenture bound teacher and student in a relationship of patronage. In the medical school, it was the prize system that engaged the whole staff in bestowing honor and future favor on the winning student. As Sprigge observed, "our educational schemes are largely founded on the promotion of the prizeman and the nurture of the successful examinee."[110]

A prize brought the medical student the attention of the medical press as well as that of the medical school staff. News of prizes appeared in the *Lancet*, the *British Medical Journal*, and other professional periodicals. When a young medical man began practice and applied for medical posts in his community, his prizes may have served as a form of advertising that would serve him in good stead, contribute to his income, and perhaps even lead to a "thousand a year." Like the recommendation of one's master, the medical school prize served as an institution's endorsement of the new medical man.

Whatever import prizes may have had for the public, their impact on the competing medical students was, at the first level, in their relationships with their teachers. Medical apprentices of an earlier day might have labored to please their masters. New generations of medical students learned that the judges of the examination papers and the leaders of the hospital had power over them.

In his last year of medical studies a student was required to serve at least three months as a clinical clerk to a hospital physician or a dresser to a surgeon. These posts involved the basic care of medical and surgical patients in the wards under the supervision of the house physicians and surgeons, who were in turn responsible to the senior staff. (See Appendix C for a chart of the organizational structure of a hospital and medical school.) Such undergraduate posts provided essential care to in-patients and important experience for the student. Clerkships and dresserships brought the closest relationships a student had with the medical teachers. Students who came to the medical school with connections on the staff often served under those "friends" during this period of practical work.

Beyond the immediate educational value of these posts, they often had far-reaching career effects. Clerks or dressers serving under the same houseman became known as a "firm." They often kept close ties, both personal and professional, long after medical school. Such friends could be a source of patients or consulting work. As valuable as peer relationships may have been, connections with the senior staff could be even more important. When George Makins was in his fourth year of medical study he became a dresser to Sir William MacCormac, Surgeon at St. Thomas's Hospital. "This appointment," Makins records, "was the commencement of a friendship which lasted the whole of MacCormac's life and materially influenced my entire career."[111] Makins enjoyed patronage and assistance from the senior man. His testimony reflects the experience of a number of medical students whose associations in medical school paved the way to a prosperous future. On a less elevated scale, William B. Page enjoyed similar assistance. Page served as one of Sir Astley Cooper's dressers, and Cooper, when asked to recommend someone for a junior post in a new hospital in Cumberland, nominated the young Page.[112] Senior men recommended their dressers and clerks to military posts, private medical service with aristocratic families, and a variety of other appointments that helped them start their careers.

Upon the completion of his medical studies, typically at age twenty-one or twenty-two, the student took his examinations for qualification. A single license was the minimum needed for admission to the *Medical Register*, but a double qualification, one in medicine and one in surgery, became increasingly common. General practitioners usually took the MRCS and LSA, or, after 1861, the MRCS and the new

LRCP. In a survey carried out in 1885, the GMC found that, of those students who entered medical training in 1871 (a total of 1,253), 30 percent had not qualified for practice by the time of the survey. Of the 877 who completed their professional studies, only 12.5 percent had a single qualification, while 87.5 percent had at least two.* The Council found that those who took only one license completed their medical training, on the average, after almost six years of study, while those who took two or more licenses received their first license in less than five years.[113] Such data suggest that students who had to be self-supporting or who had other problems in completing their education tended to settle for a single qualification and to move immediately into practice. Conversely, those students who were more advantaged or able tended to finish sooner and to gain, in the long run, superior qualifications. The fact that most students took longer than four years to complete what was considered a four-year program suggests that perhaps many students were self-supporting while studying medicine and thus could not work full-time at their studies.

For many of those destined for general practice, formal medical education ended with their qualifying examinations. Some continued their studies on their own, preparing themselves for additional licenses while carrying on a private practice.† A number of students did not enter private practice immediately but continued their education for a year or two either abroad or at home. Some went to the continent to study some special medical subject. Paris was a favorite place for such studies in the 1850's, but by the 1880's Vienna and the

---

*General Medical Council, *Minutes of the General Medical Council, of its Executive and Dental Committees, and of its Branch Councils, for the Year 1885*, Vol. XXII (London, 1886), pp. 135–137. [Hereafter GMC, *Minutes.*] Of those who had only one qualification, about 60 percent were English licensees, 25 percent Irish, and 15 percent Scottish.

†See A. J. Cronin's description of his studies for a second qualification while working as a colliery surgeon in Wales, in his autobiography, *Adventures in Two Worlds* (Boston and Toronto, 1935), Chapter 18.

German cities were the focus of English travels abroad, where they learned about pathology, dermatology, and gynecology in the hospitals and medical schools of continental Europe.[114]

Postgraduate service as a houseman was another way of continuing one's medical education. In the early nineteenth century such posts were usually held only by those who planned consulting careers. With the increased numbers of hospitals in the nineteenth century, house posts became a common form of postgraduate education for general practitioners as well.[115] Service in a maternity hospital, for example, gave a general practitioner good experience in obstetric cases, an important part of a general practitioner's work and a good, though not prestigious, source of income. A post as resident in a provincial hospital paid a small stipend so that, in addition to its educational value, a newly qualified man had the beginnings of an income.

Personal connections played a part in these post-qualification studies, as they did in other elements of medical education. George Makins was elected House Surgeon at the Greenwich Hospital "mainly," he said, "as the result of the support of an old friend of my father's" who was a member of the hospital's Board of Governors.[116] Fortunate young men whose fathers held senior posts in hospitals frequently gained junior positions there. This was most common in provincial hospitals, where competition was not so keen as in London.[117] Even without familial connections to a provincial hospital, a young practitioner often succeeded in his bid for a residency if he was a native of the community. These appointments were so common as to suggest that a hospital's board of governors saw the sons of their own community as deserving of favor above strangers to the town.[118]

These early career decisions had a critical influence on a young man's professional life. If he had ambitions to rise to "the top of the tree,"[119] it was important to stay in London, to continue his affiliation with the world of hospitals and medical teaching, and eventually to gain appointments at the center of English medical life. If he planned to practice generally, in London or the provinces, these first appointments could lead to the establishment of a practice. In both instances, he was dependent on the ties of family and, more and more, on the ties to his medical teachers.

The medical schools of Victorian England left their mark on students in the same way that apprentices were marked by their affiliation with a particular teacher. Students developed loyalties to their medical school, to their associates there, and to the profession they entered. Discipline and competition as well as friendships bound them to these institutions. H. E. Counsell, a student at Guy's Hospital Medical School in the early 1880's and later a practitioner in Oxford, recalled his student days:

> Without any teaching from our chiefs except their example, loyalty was the essence of what we learned at Guy's then. I never heard a member of the staff speak disparagingly of his colleagues. . . . We were as proud of being Guy's men as any guardsman of his regiment. In fact, we looked with surprised scorn at any outsiders who seemed unaware that Guy's was the finest hospital in London and therefore in the world.[120]

Counsell believed that in medical training the student gained "a sense of our profession being an honourable calling, a vocation rather than a mere means of earning a living."[121] On one occasion he told the famous Jowett, "I am as proud of being a Guy's as a Balliol man."[122]

The years of medical training were years of learning the skills of a future occupation. They were also years for establishing and extending personal and professional connections —those "useful and interested friends"[123] that could contribute to a man's future career. But course work, clubs, prizes, and service also brought students into the process that socialized them to the profession of medicine. No longer was the medical student isolated, bound only to his master. The student's years in medical school, whether at Guy's or Bart's or Charing Cross, were years when the student came under the discipline and control of the elites of the medical schools. Out of the shared experiences of living and working together a new professional identity was being forged.

The centralization of medical education transformed the lives of medical teachers, too. Medical education was no longer the province of the individual practitioner in his private surgery, nor was it simply a minor subject in the curriculum of the great institutions of Oxbridge. The products of the medical schools were their joint responsibility, a reflection of their shared efforts. London, its schools, and its teachers had gained for themselves new powers over the next generation of practitioners. Whatever medical graduates did in the years after their training had been completed, however incomplete the profession's control over their behavior then might be, centralized medical education gave the elites of the medical world a time for training them not only in the skills of an occupation, but in educating students to the mores, values, and loyalties of a potentially self-regulating and autonomous profession.

III

Careers in General Practice

THE newly qualified medical man of mid-Victorian England might view with pride the license for which he had studied so hard and which represented the endorsement of a medical corporation. However, as he faced the prospect of practice, he was confronted with a lay public whose recognition of the value of qualified practice was less than whole-hearted. Many, perhaps most, people frequently relied on home remedies or patent medicines purchased at the local chemist's shop. People of all classes resorted to the unlicensed ministration of the herbalist, bonesetter, homeopathist, or midwife.[1] A general practitioner at a dinner party might blush to hear his gentlemanly host scoff at the doctor-patient relationship as a case of "the blind leading the blind" and a course of treatment as "a course of groping in the dark."[2] Medical opinion on matters of public health was sometimes ignored, sometimes not even sought. Employers of medical men treated them as employees, rather than as experts.

Lack of public confidence in the medical license was symptomatic of the more serious problem faced by the medical "profession"—it did not yet have that autonomy of the true profession which gave it "the exclusive right to determine who [could] legitimately do its work and how the work should be done."[3] For the general practitioner, this lack of public recognition of the professional meaning of his license was crucial for the way in which he approached the establishment of his career. As a prospective medical student he and his family had been warned that scientific abilities and interests were less important for his success in practice than his style of speech and the cleanliness of his person which his patients would judge. Beyond the superficialities of style, patients were known to be concerned with the morals and character of the man they might consult.[4] Whether judged by style or by character, medical men were caught in the particularism of a society uncommitted to the value of medical science and medical skills. No one felt this dependency on the social judgment of patients more acutely than the young man just starting out in practice.

I

Victorian writers advising those who planned to enter the medical profession informed aspiring young doctors that they would do well to have funds beyond those needed to cover the cost of their education. The beginning practitioner had to have capital for the rental of a house and for the supply of drugs he would stock. He also needed funds to live on in the early years of practice. The first years were likely to be lean years, for it took time to develop a practice. Even when patients came in sufficient numbers, they did not usually pay cash, and the months between the doctor's service and the payment of the annual bill could be hungry months without a supplementary source of support. The public image presented by the new practitioner in the early months and years of practice was crucial, too, for poverty and shabbiness did not inspire confidence in prospective patients.

Some young practitioners had the resources of prosperous families to tide them over the lean years. With family support, some of the difficulties of starting out in practice could also be obviated by investing in an already established practice through purchase or partnership. However, such options were closed to men with limited means. The impecunious medical graduate could take some form of temporary medical employment as a way of accumulating funds for setting up a private practice, but most of such jobs paid little and did not pave the way to fiscal comfort or security in the early years.

Perhaps by default, the poor young practitioner found it

necessary to start out on his own, to build a practice from the ground up. This was assuredly the most difficult way to begin:

> . . . taking a house, putting up a brass plate, and perhaps a red lamp, wearing good clothes, getting introductions to as many people as possible, and otherwise partly by pushing, partly by patience, making a practice, this plan can only be recommended under special circumstances.[5]

If a young man decided to enter private practice this way, he had many problems to face. He shared with his more prosperous peers the disadvantage of youthfulness and immaturity. But his lack of funds did not allow him to compensate by accumulating the paraphernalia necessary for social acceptance. The proper house, the carriage, the clothing that would all have testified to his gentility and, by extension, his respectability and trustworthiness, were out of the reach of the man without resources. A wife was "almost a necessary part of a physician's professional equipment,"[6] because women were reticent to seek advice from a bachelor medical man. But marriage without an assured income was imprudent.

In addition to these personal and social disabilities, the young medical man faced difficulties in the very decision about where he should try to establish himself. In a town where other practitioners were already well ensconced, a new man's chances for success were poor. "It cannot be done," wrote surgeon C. B. Keetley, "in a sober, slow place where the doctors already in possession are sound men well liked by their patients."[7] The experienced medical man urged the young practitioner to make a systematic survey of prospective sites. He should take into account the population of the town and, from the country directory, ascertain the number of gentry, clergy, and other medical men there. With irony and not a little pessimism, Keetley concluded that the best plan for a man starting out on his own might be "to settle in a small place where there is only one doctor on his last legs from old age, drunkenness, or consumption. The . . . plan is not likely to commend itself to anybody troubled much with nice feelings and a sense of what is due to widows and orphans."[8] Such "advice" indicates the grave difficulties which a new man faced from established competitors.

Accounts of Victorian medical men who started out poor and alone are rare. One of the few, and perhaps the most detailed, is Arthur Conan Doyle's novel *The Stark Munro Letters*.[9] The book is based on Conan Doyle's own experiences in Portsmouth, where he practiced in the early 1880's,[10] and his account gives an unparalleled record of the trials and problems of the poor beginning practitioner. The details of the novel match closely the information provided elsewhere regarding the problems of beginning practice. Neither Conan Doyle nor his Stark Munro began their careers in London, but there is no reason to suppose that the difficulties of the new practitioner were very different in the metropolis than in the large provincial town described in the novel.

Stark Munro, the son of a poor country practitioner, studied medicine at Edinburgh and then served briefly in several salaried medical posts before deciding to try his hand alone in private practice. After a survey of potential towns in which to settle, he chose "Birchespool," a "mildly manufacturing" town with a population of 130,000. He arrived there with £5.18s., a trunk, a hat box, a large brass plate to be hung outside his surgery, and his medical equipment—a stethoscope, several medical books, "and the whole science of medicine packed between my two ears."[11] He took temporary lodgings in a boarding house and began his search for a residence. He surveyed every street, marking on a map the vacant houses and the locations of other medical men, so that he could see "where there was a possible opening, and what opposition there was at each point."[12]

He found a modest house situated on the border between a well-to-do quarter of the town and a poor one. The cost was £40 a year, £50 with taxes. Short of funds, he managed to avoid paying a quarter's rent of £10 in advance by giving character references. He furnished the house, albeit sparsely, with second-hand furniture bought at auction, for a little more than £3. His bedroom had only a bed, no mattress or bedding, and he used a crate for a dressing table. His mother sent him bedding, and he made a mattress for himself.[13] Most of the furnishings went into the waiting and consulting rooms, for it was important that his patients have at least an impression of respectability. He paid an ironmonger half-a-crown to hang his brass plate, and with a one-and-ninepenny broom he cleaned his house and put his furnishings in place. A servant was out of the question. On credit he ordered £12 worth of "tinctures, infusions, pills, powders, ointments, and bottles" from the Apothecaries' Company in London.[14]

He instituted a rigid scheme of economy in his habits, cutting his living expenses to the barest minimum on which he could survive for the long lean period he knew was ahead. His daily fare and its costs are an indicator of the minimum living costs on which a man could survive in the early 1880's. His daily ration consisted of tea with sugar and milk (1d.), one loaf of bread (2¾d.), and one-third pound of bacon, or two sausages, or two pieces of fried fish, or a piece of canned beef (2d. to 2½d.). His newspaper cost him ½d. each day. His total daily expenditure for food was 5¾d. to 6¼d., or about four shillings a week. He estimated that he could live on as little as 2d. a day, but only for a short time without risk to his health. He did without butter and tobacco, and sometimes had to forego his newspaper as well.[15] Even on this narrow budget he found survival difficult: "[A]t my best I was living hard, at my worst I was very close upon starvation."[16] He wrote of his difficulties with wry wit:

> In the main, it is a dreary sordid record of shillings gained and shillings spent—of scraping for this and scraping for that, with ever some fresh slip of blue paper fluttering down upon me, left so jauntily by the tax-collector, and meaning such a dead-weight pull to me. The irony of my paying a poor-rate used to amuse me. I should have been collecting it.[17]

During his first six months in Birchespool, patients were few. His first was a kindly but addled old Army man, Captain Whitehall, whom Munro had met in the lodging-house his first day in town. His second patient was the child of an impoverished gypsy family. Instead of collecting a fee, Munro supplied the medicine free of charge and gave the family a few pence besides. "A few more such patients," he wrote, "and I am a broken man." [18] Days went by when his surgery bell did not ring, and Munro reflected on his situation:

> I was alone in a strange town, without connections, without introductions. . . . I had no one at all to look to for help. . . .
>
> On the other hand . . . there were some points in my favour. I was young, . . . energetic. I had been brought up hard, and was quite prepared to rough it. I was well up in my work, and believed I could get on with patients. My house was an excellent one for my purpose, and I had already put the essentials of furniture into it. The game was not played out yet. [19]

Munro did not give up, and patients trickled in. The old Captain sent him patients from among his cronies. Others came, mainly from the poor district, who could only afford to pay 1s.6d. a visit—"and when you consider how many one and sixpences are necessary in order to make up the fifteen pounds which I must find every quarter for rent, taxes, gas and water, you will understand that even with some success, I have still found it a hard matter to keep anything in the . . . larder." [20] At this stage his earnings were probably around £15 to £16 a quarter, and at that rate his income for the year would have been less than £70.

A few patients came to him by sheer accident. A grocer had a "fit" just as Munro was walking past his shop, and he seized the opportunity to make himself of service. He "treated the man, conciliated the wife, tickled the child, and gained over the whole household." [21] The grocer's illness was chronic, and he and Munro arranged to balance his medical fees against Munro's grocery bill. When two minor road accidents took place near Munro's house, he treated the drivers in each case, and he "ran down to the newspaper office on each occasion, and had the gratification of seeing in the evening edition that 'the driver, though much shaken, is pronounced by Dr. Stark Munro, of Oakley Villa, to have suffered no serious injury.'"[22] Munro was hopeful that these newspaper accounts would serve as a form of advertising for him:

[I]t is hard enough for the young doctor to push his name into any publicity, and he must take what little chances he has. Perhaps the fathers of the profession would shake their heads over such a proceeding in a little provincial journal; but I was never able to see that any of them were very averse from seeing their own names appended to the bulletin of some sick statesman in *The Times*.[23]

A third accident case involved one of the town's lawyers. Munro earned a guinea fee for his care, but the patient, by the rules of medical etiquette, was released immediately to the care of his own doctor. Munro had dreams of a "fair countess" slipping on an orange peel in front of his door, or of saving the chief merchant of Birchespool by some "tour-de-force," as an opening to more lucrative practice.[24] No such luck fell to him, and in the long months he had to be content to listen to "the throb of the charwoman's heart and the rustle of the greengrocer's lungs."[25]

At the end of his first six months in practice, Munro's nine-year-old brother came to live with him. He helped with household chores and answered the door. This last was an important improvement in Munro's household. He was sure that his lack of servants had lost him more than one patient: "I fancy that a doctor who opened his own door forfeited their confidence."[26] The next eight months saw his practice grow: more friends of the Captain, accident cases, newcomers to the town who came to him by chance, a few examinations for a life insurance company, and a consultation or two with a friendly nearby practitioner. Munro added to his domestic staff by subletting his basement rooms to a spinster who, in return for lodging, served him as housekeeper.[27]

The greatest source of growth in Munro's practice came as a result of the growth of his household and the consequent change in his social habits. When he had lived alone, he dared not leave the house for fear he would miss a patient, and he spent many days sitting and waiting. With his brother and the housekeeper in residence, he not only improved his image as a medical gentleman, but he also was free to leave the house and to begin to mix with the people of the town. It was in this social milieu that he found the key to building his practice:

> I learned a fact which I would whisper in the ear of every other man who starts, as I have done, a stranger among strangers. Do not think that practice will come to you. You must go to it. You may sit upon your consulting room chair until it breaks under you, but . . . you will make little or no progress. The way to do it is to go out, to mix everywhere with men, to let them know you.[28]

Munro warned his hypothetical young advisee, however, never to forget his purpose in mixing with the men of the town:

> You must inspire respect. Be friendly, genial, convivial—what you will—but preserve the tone and bearing of a gentleman. If you can make yourself respected and liked you will find every club and society that you join a fresh introduction to practice.[29]

He advocated concerts, meetings, and clubs—literary, debating, political, social, and athletic: "These are the rungs up which one climbs."[30] Munro spent time on the cricket pitch and the bowling green making connections. When a patient rang the bell, the housekeeper stalled him while his younger brother ran to him with the message that a patient was waiting.[31]

By the time Stark Munro had been in Birchespool for two years his income had risen to £270 a year. He married, and his wife's dowry brought an additional £100 a year to the family income.[32] Munro had managed to survive.

The young Munro began private practice without financial resources. His story suggests that impecunious young men, even without several hundred pounds at hand, could still make their way into practice.[33] Conan Doyle's account indicates that a practitioner might even manage with a reserve of as little as £100. He could thus afford a small house, a single servant, the time to wait for practice, and the freedom to cultivate it. With any luck, such a sum could carry a man through his first year of practice, after which he could almost live on his earnings. Munro got by, although not happily, on much less.

General practice was local practice, whether in some provincial town or in a district of London. Information about general practice in London is scarce, and, in the discussion that follows, data on general practice from all regions has been used, on the assumption that the considerations and problems of general practice in town and city were much the same. What differences there were, were a function of the greater competition of London practice and, perhaps, the greater fluidity of the population, which would tend to undermine the social base of practice. Hence, difficulties facing general practitioners in all parts of England were, if anything, more extreme in London.

Whether in London or the country, lack of funds and lack of friends constituted the most serious obstacles to building a practice. However much medical science a man had "packed between his two ears," ability was no substitute for connections that led to patients and income. Chance acquaintances might help, but in the closed social networks of Victorian England, marginal people like boardinghouse lodgers and itinerant folk scarcely served as an introduction to a community. Like the "connexions" that bound Namier's eighteenth-century politicians to each other,[34] family and friendship were the lifeblood of Victorian general practice. Funds could, to some degree, compensate for lack of connection by allowing a practitioner to buy time to get acquainted. Funds could also buy a form of introduction to the community.

II

Buying a practice was an avenue by which the financially solvent young practitioner could get a foothold in a community or neighborhood. A potential purchaser found out about practices for sale through the medical press, medical placement agencies, and personal and medical associates.[35] Prices for practices were based on the average yearly income at the time of the sale. In the 1880's, practices sold for a year or a year and one-half's purchase, i.e., one to one and one-half times a year's income. Thus, a practice with an income of £300 a year could be expected to sell for £300 to £450, while a practice worth £700 a year sold for between £700 and £1050. Some practices were thought to be "uncommonly good investments."[36] Practices offered for sale in the medical press ranged widely in price. In a single issue of the *British Medical Journal* in the year 1876, for example, asking prices ranged from as little as £100 to over £1,000.[37] While some sellers required full cash payment at the time of sale, others allowed for installment buying. This allowed a practitioner with modest savings to get a start.

Characteristics other than income per se made some practices more desirable than others and thus influenced the purchase price. The best were those which had not only a high annual income but, integral to that income, a visiting list with a high ratio of prosperous middle-class patients.[38] The higher the income of patients, the higher the fees a man could charge, and the less labor he had to expend in the pursuit of his livelihood. As Munro said, it took many small fees to pay for rent, rates, and food.

Practices differed, too, in the specific types of medical services that were expected of the practitioner. In many practices, patients looked to their medical man for their drugs as well as for diagnosis, in return for the fees they paid. When this was the case, a general practitioner had to spend part of his income on the drugs he dispensed and part of his precious time mixing prescriptions, bottling, and labelling them. In what were judged to be more "fashionable" or "good class" practices, patients took their prescriptions to the chemist's shop to be filled, and their practitioner was not involved in dispensing drugs. The non-dispensing general practice was the more costly investment.[39]

Similarly, the amount of obstetric practice made some purchases more desirable than others. While midwifery was a common part of general practice, it was disliked by most practitioners.* It was time-consuming work and, in lower-class

---

*Much midwifery was done by unqualified women and therefore had little prestige. Obstetric practice may also have been dis-

practices, the remuneration was poor. The best practices had little midwifery and that was well paid. In better practices a medical man could expect to earn a guinea or more for such service, while in poorer practices the fee was likely to be 10s.6d. or less.[40]

Like the man starting out to build a new practice, buyers of established practices were also concerned about the number of other medical men already in practice in the neighborhood of their prospective purchase. Less "opposition" meant that a practitioner could expect some growth in the practice, while an over-supply of medical men was a poor forecast for the future. One practice offered for sale in 1876 was situated in a northern city with a population of 5,000. It had an income of £800 a year, and one of its virtues was that there were "only two opponents."[41]

When the incumbent in a practice died, his heirs often sold the practice as a part of the settlement of the estate. Such practices were risky investments because the practice may have been in decline before the practitioner's death. In the time between the death of one practitioner and the arrival of his successor, patients may have turned elsewhere for medical attention. Even the most loyal of patients could not afford to wait for a replacement. These practices were, therefore, likely to be sold at bargain prices. One practice offered for sale under these conditions was said to have had an income of £132 a year at the time of the former practitioner's death. But the practice included "50 respectable patients," and the sellers estimated that the practice could "easily" be increased to £300 a year. The purchase price was £100.[42]

The purchaser of a practice bought access to a location or a neighborhood in which a practice had been carried on and,

---

tasteful to medical men because of its sexual connection and the influence of Mrs. Grundy. Exposé literature sometimes related obstetric practice with sex crimes. See, for example: W. Talley, *He, or Man-Midwifery, and the Results; or, Medical Men in the Criminal Courts* (London, 1863); and John Stevens, *Man-Midwifery Exposed* (London, 1866). The most recent study of midwifery in the nineteenth century is Jean Donnison, *Midwives and Medical Men. A History of Inter-Professional Rivalries and Women's Rights* (New York, 1977).

presumably, the benefits that came from the good reputation of the former practitioner—otherwise known as the "good will" of the patients. Purchase worked in part because of the power of human habit.[43] People knew that a given house was a doctor's residence, and they could be expected to go there when seeking medical advice, even when a new practitioner took over. Professional qualifications seem to have played little part in determining the effectiveness of purchase as an entree to a neighborhood. Sellers almost never mentioned medical licenses when they advertised practices for sale. On the rare occasion when they did, they mentioned them in connection with social qualifications required for a higher class patient clientele. As one advertisement put it, "the successor should possess high qualifications and be accustomed to good society."[44] Such standards spoke well for the quality of the practice and, of course, justified a higher purchase price.

Habit, however forceful, did not guarantee that the man who purchased a practice could expect a complete transfer of patients from his precursor's visiting list to his own. When a practice was sold, some patients might turn to already established rival practitioners in the district rather than consult a new man. Moreover, if unfortunate comparisons could be made between the personal style of the seller and buyer, the newcomer might lose practice as a result: "Suppose, for instance, an insignificant-looking, unpolished person buys the practice of a man who had made it by the force of every physical gift added to charming and cultivated manners. Is it astonishing that the patients should not troop over in a flock?"[45] S. H. Snell, practicing in a town in Essex in the last decades of the nineteenth century, assumed that patients preferred him over another practitioner because of his superior medical qualifications. When he inquired, however, he found that not to be the case. One patient came to him because she disliked the other practitioner's moustache. None seemed concerned about his superior education, and Snell records that it was "firmly brought home to me . . . that the public knew nothing, and cared less, for degrees, etc."[46]

Given the difficulties of transferring loyalties from the

old practitioner to the new one, the best purchase opportunities included a period when the incumbent and the buyer carried on the practice together. Sometimes as much as six months or a year was devoted to this period of transition. One such practice, valued at £1,100 a year, brought with it a large, convenient house at a moderate rental, high fees, and a "partnership introduction of eight months."[47] Such overlapping of old and new practitioners allowed time for patients, following their old habits of medical consultation, to meet the new man. The incumbent's introduction was a form of endorsement, which, like the recommendations of friends, was an advantage to the man entering the practice. The partnership introduction provided continuity and stability for patients and practitioner alike. There was less disruption in the minds of patients and in their habits and expectations, and therefore less chance for the buyer to lose patients in the process.

The benefits of outright purchase were, in large measure, also the benefits of buying a partnership. In exchange for a premium, the incumbent shared the medical work and the income of the practice with his new partner. Partnerships were most viable when a practice was growing too large for one man to handle, or when the holder of a good practice elected to work fewer hours and thus needed a partner to share the medical labor. The conditions of work in a prosperous partnership were better than those in practice alone. The buyer moved into an established practice, he had introductions to his patients, and he did not have to wait for income. Moreover, partnership removed the pressures on one man to remain constantly available to patients, thus easing some of the stress of private practice. Many lone practitioners feared, and rightly, that they would lose patients to their competitors if they left town for a holiday. Some medical men never went away for more than a weekend a year during much of their professional lives.[48] A partnership avoided the necessity for such undivided attention to a practice.

Partnerships were thought, too, to be a way of circumventing the whims and tastes of fickle patients: "If one sees that certain patients are getting tired of him and desire a change, he may adroitly introduce his partner, who can coyly accept them as *his* patients. Then the two partners chuckle over the little manipulation, knowing that the firm has lost nothing."* The cooperative circumstances of a partnership could overcome many of the difficulties of practice alone.

Purchase, whether of a partnership or of a whole practice, was a way of buying a place, literally and figuratively, in the community. Even though seller and buyer had never met before, the medium of cash established a tie between them that was the basis for introduction. The relation between them, vis-à-vis the patients, was one of friendship, and the old medical adviser sponsored the entry of the newcomer and fostered the transfer of good will. At the very least, a capital investment in a practice may have led patients to believe that the buyer was, ipso facto, respectable and deserving of the patients' confidence.

However well purchase worked in the best cases, there were distinct risks involved as well, and it behooved the would-be buyer to investigate as thoroughly as possible the practice he might buy. There was, of course, the question of whether or not the price was fair. The uncertainties that arose through the death of the incumbent were, perhaps, the easiest to calculate in trying to determine value for money. A seller might misrepresent the value of a practice, either by direct falsehood or by inadvertence. He could calculate the purchase price on an exceptionally good year, not representative of the typical income of a practice. He might try to hide the fact that the neighborhood or district was in the process of decline, or the economy of the town in trouble. Such facts might not be immediately apparent but would certainly affect the character of the practice and the level of income.[49] Thorough investigation could save a young purchaser from a poor investment.

*Charles Bell Keetley, *The Student's and Junior Practitioner's Guide to the Medical Profession*, 2nd ed. (London, 1885), p. 44 (emphasis his). Cf. Sidney H. Snell, *A Doctor at Work and Play* (London, 1937), p. 43. Purchase and partnership had the odor of trade about them and, perhaps for that reason, were forbidden to some elites, e.g., the holders of the MRCP and the FRCP.

Risks might also come from the personal character and history of the incumbent of a practice. Ill health might have reduced his power to sustain a practice, but more damaging yet could be the possibility of scandal or questionable medical practices. The incumbent's poor reputation could, even without his knowledge, injure the newcomer's chances of success.[50] Thus, while the personal endorsement of a respected practitioner could contribute to a purchaser's success, the reverse could also be true. Whatever his own personal and professional virtues, the buyer had to beware of a disreputable predecessor. Such problems made potential purchasers wary, and sellers tried to assure them that they had "a satisfactory reason for retirement."[51]

Many of the difficulties and dangers arising from purchase could be traced to the fact that the cash transaction had the form, but little of the substance, of a personal connection. For both patient and new practitioner, the unknown was still too large a factor in their relationship. For the patient, the new medical man was unknown, and thus untested. He might be a man of skill and probity, but the purchase did not thoroughly guarantee his qualities. Purchase might implicitly bring with it the endorsement of a man's predecessor, but only experience could assure patients that a medical man placed their welfare above his own profit. The outcome of purchase could only, finally, be known with time.

Some practitioners did not, however, have to face even the difficulties of purchase. They did not have to depend on the introduction of a stranger, nor on the habits of patients when they stepped into the vacant shoes of their predecessors. They were able to begin practice in the best situations of all. They went to the place where introductions were no longer needed, for they were already known. They went home.

III

In 1881, Nathaniel Henry Clifton, FRCS, died. In his obituary in the *Lancet*, the history of his family's medical practice in Cross Street, Islington, was recounted. Clifton's grandfather had established a practice in Cross Street in the 1770's.

From 1822 his son carried on the practice until his death in 1861, and he was followed in a third generation of medical practice by N. H. Clifton, the subject of the obituary:

> Some practices are the creation of one man. A larger number represent a principle of continuity, not to say heredity. The name of Mr. Clifton carries the people of Islington back more than a hundred years. . . . [O]ver all this time a large section of the people of Islington have enjoyed the privilege of being attended by Mr. Clifton or his immediate ancestors. . . .
>
> There is an element of permanence, a faithfulness to groove and place, in most good families, which is not to be unnoted. Cross Street, as it exists now, may not seem to passers through a romantic spot to which to fix one's existence, but to a man of Mr. Clifton's character . . . it had a claim and a charm to which the new built villa has no pretensions.[52]

These observations constitute a eulogy, not only to the deceased but to an entire family and to the loyalty, stability, and continuity that the Clifton medical family represented.

The Clifton family is not an isolated case. The records of the Royal College of Surgeons reveal a large number of families who carried on medical practices in one town, and often in one house, for three generations or more: the Crowfoot family practiced in Beccles, Suffolk, for five generations; three generations of Robert Cravens practiced in Hull from the 1790's to 1903. The Ransomes in Manchester, the Heys in Leeds, and the Bacots in London were all families with three or more generations of medical practice in one place.[53] Still more common was the two-generation family medical practice. A father established a practice in a town, and his son, after medical studies in London or at a provincial medical school, returned home to join his father as assistant, partner, and eventually successor. Robert Thorpe (Manchester), Bowyer Vaux (Birmingham), George Norman (Bath), and Thomas Griffith (Wrexham) are only four examples of Fellows of the Royal College of Surgeons who joined their fathers in practice.[54] Of all the College Fellows who entered provincial practice up to 1890, 127 (or 7.2%) entered practice with their fathers.[55] Frequently these young men followed their fathers' footsteps into provincial hospital posts as well. Three generations of Bickersteths served as Surgeons to the Liverpool Infirmary, and John Lawrence, Jr., succeeded John, Sr., as Surgeon to the Sussex County Hospital at Brighton.[56]

Even when the son did not become his father's partner in practice, the senior medical man's influence could aid the younger man's career in the same town. When John Beddoe tried to establish himself in practice in Bristol in the late 1850's, he faced just such a situation in the Fox family, father and son. Beddoe had excellent professional training as a houseman in London and Edinburgh, service as a civilian medical man in the Crimea, studies in Vienna and the Italian spa cities, and the support of Sir James Clark, a leading London practitioner. But his choice of Bristol was, he found, "imprudent." He applied for a post at the Bristol Infirmary, but it went to a man just out of medical school but "with a great local interest." Edward Long Fox, his successful rival, was the son of a Bristol medical man, and he went on to build a large practice in the town.[57]

The advantages of joining a family member in practice were striking. Keetley put it succinctly with the dictum that "he who wishes to make a practice ought to be known, and known to his credit, in the place *before* he sets up."[58] In a family practice a young man's "introduction" to the community was ready-made. Moreover, the practice was already established, and he did not have to suffer the years of hardship and meager living while waiting for his visiting list to grow.

The frequency of such patterns of family practice suggest that they were successful because patients, too, found them a satisfactory mode of medical care delivery. The medical son was not a stranger, and patients knew what they could expect from him. Patients probably enjoyed a certain psychological security in the long association of a medical family with generations of families in the town. They perhaps believed that a family connection in the community was a strong basis for honorable, reputable behavior in the young practitioner. He had both his own reputation and that of his family to uphold. For both the young practitioner and his patients, the shared membership in the community created social pressures to conduct themselves respectably—the medical man to deal honestly with his patients, and the patients to support their practitioner with loyalty and bills paid. Such "objective" measures of medical skill as the quality of his medical school, his prizes, and his degrees were secondary to historic ties between patients and a medical family.

Analogous to father-and-son medical practices were the partnerships and successions of uncles and nephews, brothers, and cousins. Robert Keate, FRCS, and William Henchman Crowfoot, FRCS, both joined their uncles in private practice and succeeded to their practices at the retirement or death of the senior men.[59] Brothers or cousins who practiced as partners shared a sense of family loyalty and family reputation, and they could establish partnerships based, frequently, on years of association and knowledge of each other's character. In 1878, officials at St. Bartholomew's Hospital estimated that 40 percent of their students had the option of joining a relative in practice.[60]

Marriage, ever a form of social and political alliance, also served young medical practitioners in the establishment and advancement of their careers. Medical students and beginning practitioners often married the daughters of their teachers, sisters of their medical school classmates, or daughters of practitioners in the places where they were attempting to establish themselves. These matches, fostered by the socializing that went on among medical men, brought clear benefits to a young man who married a woman from a medical family. She was likely to make a good "medical wife" because she knew the rigors of medical practice and the demands it made on family life. Such an alliance could also be an entree to a medical practice. For example, Thomas Warburton Benfield (1822–1890), FRCS, was employed as an assistant to John Nedham (d. 1856), FRCS, in his Leicester practice. Benfield married Nedham's daughter, became his partner, and eventually succeeded to his father-in-law's practice and to his posts at the Leicester Infirmary and at the local lunatic asylum. Honoratus L. Thomas, FRCS, H. D. Farnell, FRCS, and H. J. Rose, FRCS, made similar, professionally profitable unions.[61] Both father- and son-in-law benefited from such arrangements. The senior man had help in his practice and, by assisting his son-in-law's career, secured his daughter's future economic security. The younger man got his start in an established practice and an introduction, through his marriage, to the community and his patients.*

The pattern of family succession may have been more common in provincial practices than in London. The judgment of a medical man's character took time, and the relatively greater stability of non-industrial provincial communities allowed successive generations of practitioners to benefit from the good reputations that their medical fathers had built. In the more fluid populations of London and the new industrial towns, where both medical men and patients were more mobile, there may have been less advantage in family medical succession.

Even without the advantages of a medical family, a number of young practitioners returned to their native places to practice. The records of the careers of Fellows of the Royal College of Surgeons indicate that at least five percent of those who entered practice before 1890 went to their home towns to begin their medical careers.[62] Because information on birthplaces is far from complete, this figure constitutes a minimum. In addition, Fellows tended to be those with high career aspirations who would have tended to gravitate toward London and the larger provincial cities, where they could have a chance at a hospital career. Thus, one might guess that home-town practice might have been much more widespread among those who never achieved the rank of Fellow. Many of the benefits that came from having a relative in practice in a town came, *pari passu*, to young men whose families were known and respected outside medical circles in the place

---

*The first surgeon on record whose *wife* was also in medicine was James S. N. Boyd, FRCS. For a discussion of the role of the medical family in modern professional life, see: Oswald Hall, "The Stages of a Medical Career," *Am. J. Soc.*, 53:5 (1948), 327–336.

where they sought to establish themselves. As a son of the community, he had an "interest" there. The network of friendship and connection brought support in the form of practice to the medical man, and he was bound to his patients by life-long ties of association.

Ties of family and friendship could help a young man in other ways, too. Within a society that was largely Anglican and Anglo-Saxon, non-Anglican or non-English origins might have been a disadvantage in trying to build a practice. But ethnic or religious affiliation could also be a tie to patients, and hence a stepping-stone to practice. When Arthur Conan Doyle finished his medical education in Edinburgh, he had the option to practice in London. Relatives there who were well-to-do and well connected could have been the nucleus of a practice for him. They were Roman Catholics and "they had more than hinted that, once he had set up his own practice . . . Catholic influence would not be lacking to bring him patients."* Buxton Shillitoe (1826–1916), FRCS, came from a Quaker family in Hertfordshire and had Quaker patients as part of his London practice.[63] Caleb Williams, FRCS, and Daniel Hack Tuke, FRCP, also had practices based on their connections with the Friends.[64] The Jewish community in London was the nexus of practice for Abraham Woolf, FRCS, and G. E. Herman, FRCS. J. M. Martin's connections were Roman Catholic, and Jean Samuel Keser had French connections.[65] When the German-born Felix Semon, FRCS, first decided to practice in London, he was advised that he could build a lucrative practice among the Germans living there.[66] Nationality ties were, of course, of practical value if patients did not speak English, but, utility aside, religious, ethnic, or national ties between medical man and patient were the basis

---

*John Dickson Carr, *The Life of Sir Arthur Conan Doyle* (New York, 1949), p. 26. Carr says that Conan Doyle could not be a devout Catholic and, knowing that his patients would expect him to be, decided against London practice. Cf. Arthur Conan Doyle, *The Stark Munro Letters* (New York, 1895), p. 230, where the connection is "Wesleyan." Munro refused the aid because he felt it "low down" to use religious organizations to his advantage after having condemned them.

for a sense of kinship between them (however distant or oblique) which fostered trust. Like families, they formed a chain of introduction and friendship so that the doctor and his patients did not meet entirely as strangers.

Stark Munro's chance acquaintance, the Army Captain, helped him by sending patients his way. But chance was not the most desirable ally in starting a career. The long-standing ties of birth, family, and connection were the surest guarantees of obligation and loyalty, good will and mutual assistance. They were the foundation for successful Victorian medical practice.

IV

The Victorian era saw a prodigious growth in the number of salaried appointments available to medical men. These posts fell into two general categories—government appointments and private posts. Some appointments involved institutional care of the sick; other posts were salaried versions of private practice—as in the case of working men's provident dispensaries or sick clubs. All salaried posts had the virtue of bringing immediate income, and many provided an introduction to the community which made it "much easier . . . to make a practice there."[67] There were disadvantages to "bureaucratic practice"[68] too, especially in the way it defined a man's income or limited his freedom in practice.

Government medical employment led medical men into many arenas of practice, as Public Vaccinator, Prison or Gaol Medical Officer, Police or Militia Surgeon.[69] With the establishment of the Metropolitan Asylums Board in 1867, medical men found appointments in London's institutions for fever patients and the mentally ill.[70] The most significant growth in public medical work came in the arenas of poor law and public health, where service as a Poor Law Medical Officer or as a Medical Officer of Health was considered "a publicly guaranteed introduction to the neighborhood."[71] By the 1870's there were over 4,000 poor law officers and over 800 medical men employed under the public health system. Both types of appointment could be full-time or part-time. Salaries varied widely, but were, in any case, not munificent. A part-time poor law practitioner in the 1840's might earn as little as £5 or £10 a year, and in the 1880's as little as £30.[72] Until the 1860's, Poor Law Medical Officers had to provide the drugs used in treating their pauper patients, a further drain on an already minimal income.* Full-time service under the poor law brought higher salaries, but they were set by local boards of guardians and varied according to the guardians' generosity and public-mindedness, motives which were nearly always secondary to issues of economy.[73] Full-time Medical Officers of Health tended to fare rather better; in the 1880's some were earning as much as £500 a year.[74]

Full-time posts had the advantage of larger remuneration, but they precluded private practice. Part-time posts allowed the practitioner to begin building his practice immediately. The work was difficult, the pay never commensurate with the labor. The poor law doctor was, as a salaried employee, under the direct authority of the laymen who served on the board of guardians. His day-to-day practice was defined by the relieving officer, a layman who was charged with granting medical relief to pauper applicants. The medical man's work was defined and carried on within the considerations of public costs and laymen's judgments of need. Administrative commitment to fiscal economy often conflicted with the medical man's judgment of patients' needs, and the lay officials held the upper hand.[75]

Public appointments brought connections with the lay officials of a district or town, but they were often not so prestigious as an ambitious young practitioner might want. Joseph Rogers, the Medical Officer of the Strand Union in London, had extensive contact with the Board of Guardians there. Its members included a baker, a tax collector, a milkman, and a wholesale fruit dealer from Covent Garden. The Chairman of the Board was "the proprietor of an à-la-

*Ruth G. Hodgkinson, *The Origins of the National Health Service* (London, 1967), pp. 120, 328, 365, and 448. In 1860, new regulations provided that medicines for the workhouse infirmary were to be paid for by the parish. In 1867, under the Metropolitan Poor Act, London Boards of Guardians provided medicines for out-patients as well as in-patients.

mode beef shop," whom Rogers described as a "greasy digni-
tary," wholly uninterested in the welfare of the poor.[76] However modest, they were connections nevertheless, and they
could lead to practice among the respectable orders of lower
middle-class society.

It has frequently been said that state employment was a
source of status for medical men.[77] Certainly medical men
were often eager for such appointments and sometimes went
to desperate lengths to keep them.[78] While the employment
of medical men by the state may be a form of public recognition of expertise, it may also indicate the relatively low professional status of medicine in Victorian England. Bureaucratic
medical practice draws its status from the "authority of office"
rather than from the "authority of knowledge."[79] Given the
lack of authority of Victorian medical knowledge and medical
judgment in the public eye, state employment brought at least
a degree of authority which medical men might not otherwise
have had. The conditions of state medical employment
suggest that local and central government may have credited
medical men with technical skill but did not acknowledge
their right to independent professional judgment.

Like the social criteria which ruled private practice and
reflected the limited esteem of medical knowledge, limited
authority in public practice reveals the lack of autonomy and
independence of the mid-Victorian general practitioner. The
system of "tender," or bidding for posts, by which poor law
appointments were made until the 1840's, guaranteed that
fiscal considerations would always be considered above the
quality of a man's training or his skill. In all likelihood, the
end of the tender system only left the appointments system
open to the influence of personal connection.[80] However
forcefully the central Poor Law Board tried to regulate the
standards and quality of poor law practice, the power of local
boards of guardians in matters of appointments was paramount. In the debates over permanent versus annual appointment of poor law medical men, local boards insisted that the
threat of non-reappointment was a necessary instrument in
ensuring the poor law doctor's attendance to his duties and
his attention to economy.[81] The annual appointments system

was only one way in which the guardians expressed their distrust of doctors' professionalism and in which laymen continued to maintain control over these public servants.

In the matter of drugs for pauper patients, too, the work of the medical man was subject to constraints that left him with little independence. Policies of local boards varied with respect to drug provision, some requiring that costs be paid out of the poor law officer's salary, others providing drugs from the public purse. In the latter case, guardians were constantly concerned about the costs borne by the rates and exercised careful supervision over the medical man's prescriptions. When medical men, underpaid already, were burdened with drug costs, they were forced to choose between their professional judgment of the best drug and the inferior drug which they might more easily afford. In either case, patients expected drugs as a primary feature of medical attendance[82] —perhaps a reflection of the trading-apothecary origins of general practice. Such expectations elevated drug provisioning above medical advice and medical knowledge per se. In this respect, poor law practitioners and private practitioners alike lacked the authority of their knowledge and were subject to the standards and expectations of their patients.

In other respects, too, both poor law and public health officers worked in conditions which were defined, both formally and informally, by non-medical personnel and non-medical considerations. In their day-to-day work, Medical Officers of Health had no power to act on the basis of their findings; only their superiors, most often laymen, could act.[83] Decisions about who should receive treatment from the poor law doctor were in the hands of the relieving officer—a layman.[84] For much of the Victorian period, the official hierarchies of both poor law and public health were heavily non-medical, when they were not positively "anti-medical."[85] When inspectors, board members, guardians, and relieving officers were overwhelmingly laymen, both practice and policy were in the control of non-professionals.[86] However well such dominance may have served the public interest, the cause of professional autonomy was not advanced by medical subservience to lay control. Medical men were keenly aware

of the derogation of their status that such supervision entailed: when lawyers were appointed to supervise the administration of the public health laws in 1873, the *Lancet* branded it
an "infamous thing, that lay inspectors should have been appointed to supervise the work of medical men."[87] In the informal circumstances of day-to-day public health work, Medical Officers of Health felt constrained from the free exercise
of their professional judgment by the fact that their appointments were in the control of the very laymen who, as residents
and businessmen in their districts, might be violating public
health laws.[88]

Similar benefits and similar difficulties came to medical
men who took some salaried position in the growing number
and variety of private institutions which employed medical
men. Public and proprietary schools, asylums for orphans, inebriates, fallen women, and the insane—many sorts of charitable and entrepreneurial institutions frequently employed
medical men on a full- or part-time basis.[89] Railway companies and life assurance societies also employed medical
men, sometimes as regular members of their firms, sometimes
on an ad hoc basis.[90] Mining companies often employed a
general practitioner to provide medical care to colliery employees. Such work was burdensome, often dismal, and if the
town were entirely built around the mine, there was much
poverty and little chance for the colliery surgeon to extend his
practice to include better-paying patients from the middle
classes.[91]

Akin to the salaried appointments described above was
the contract or "club" practice which grew up in the 1830's
and after. Medical clubs, a form of self-help for the poor,
were encouraged by local boards of guardians to foster independence among the working classes of society and to forestall the possibility that the parish would have to bear the cost
of their medical care when illness kept them from work.[92]
Fraternal societies and working men's clubs sometimes established "sick clubs" for their members. Some of these medical
clubs were funded entirely from the weekly or quarterly subscriptions paid in advance by their members; others were sub-
sidized through private philanthropy. Clubs were sometimes

administered by a local poor law official, sometimes by a medical man. Some clubs had a single doctor who served all members, while others had a panel of doctors from which members selected one who provided them with medical care. The fees varied. In the 1830's some medical men were paid as little as 2s. per person per year, to as much as 7s.6d., while in the 1880's minimum fees were nearer 3s. a person. Additional fees came for "extras" such as maternity care, insurance certificates, and the care of broken bones. Some medical men served more than one sick club, and held other kinds of appointments at the same time. William Martin, MRCS, in practice in Staine, Yorkshire, in the 1880's, was Poor Law Medical Officer to the Thorne Union. He was also employed by the Manchester, Sheffield and Lincolnshire Railway and served as medical man to the Oddfellows' Club, the Union Gift Sick Club, the Foresters and Temperance Hall Clubs, and the New Vine Lodge. His poor law appointment paid £25 per annum, and the other clubs and appointments brought in varying amounts, from as little as £1.10s. a year. From these appointments he earned a total of £47 during 1888 and £50 in 1889.[93]

There seems to have been widespread willingness among medical men to engage in contract practice. Perhaps they saw it not only as a source of income but also as a way of controlling competition within their communities. Some went so far as to canvass neighborhoods in order to enroll as many individuals and families in their own club visiting lists as possible.[94] While contract practice limited the doctor's freedom by binding him to patients and to the club for a year or more, the need to make a living in the competitive environment of mid-Victorian medical practice drove many to such arrangements.[95]

Provident dispensaries were a similar form of working-class medical self-help combined with philanthropy. An out-patient clinic, where subscriptions and contributions paid for drugs and the balance of income was divided among participating medical men, the provident dispensary also limited the doctor's freedom to practice and, like club practice, drew patients away from the private practitioners in the districts they served. Both club and dispensary practice, by offering cheap medical care, tended to lower incomes for both contract and private practitioners.* In addition, charitable donors had a large hand in the election of infirmary medical officers and in medical policy. The *Lancet* described the situation in one town:

> Clergymen, benevolent old ladies, rich manufacturers, all sorts and conditions of persons, who are moved either by high motives of charity or by meaner love of ostentation and patronage, dole out guineas and become governors of the Leicester Provident Dispensary. On their vote depends the fate of the Medical Officer, and they may be called to decide purely medical and pharmaceutical questions . . . though they have no technical knowledge.[96]

In the dispensary the medical man was spared the burden of paying for drugs out of his pocket, but he had the perhaps more onerous burden of working under the rule of his philanthropic but non-professional employers. When the dispensary was entirely supported by workers' contributions, it was governed by a committee of working men—"not a pleasant matter for an educated gentleman."[97]

Whether in public employment, salaried posts, sick clubs, or dispensaries, medical men shared the fate of being subject to, ruled by, and dependent on their lay employers. Such lay dominance was possible because of the overcrowding of the profession and the consequent competition among medical men for practice wherever it could be found. The worst feature of these medical posts from a professional point of view—lay supervision of medical treatment—might have been

---

*Hodgkinson, *National Health Service*, pp. 612–618. Medical care provided under the National Insurance Act of 1911 was a form of state-regulated contract practice, the fees set at 7s.6d. per year per patient. Early plans for boycott collapsed, and thousands of medical men agreed to serve. See: Brian Abel-Smith, *The Hospitals, 1800–1948* (London, 1964), pp. 238 ff.; and Alexander M. Cooke, *A History of the Royal College of Physicians of London* (Oxford, 1972), III, Chapter 45.

corrected by including medical men on the governing boards of the agencies and institutions that hired medical men. But general practitioners were in no position to make such a demand effective. The Royal Colleges were perhaps the obvious defenders of their own rank and file in the struggle for professional independence and better pay, at least in theory. In practice the elites of London were half-hearted, when not entirely indifferent, to the needs of general practitioners serving in salaried posts.[98]

Voluntary associations like the British Medical Association and the medical press, particularly the *Lancet*, were, however, aware of and concerned about the autonomy and independence of medical practitioners and made strong efforts to improve the conditions of public employment. They were well aware of the demeaning and unprofessional character of contract practice and throughout the century raised protests against the conditions under which such practice was carried on. The medical press and the BMA objected particularly to the poor remuneration of club practitioners, despite the rise in working men's wages, and to the fact that, while the clubs were designed to benefit the poor, they were being used by those who could well afford private care. Attempts in the 1860's to organize a boycott of clubs that did not pay a minimum fee of 5s. a person had some success but were undermined by medical men who were willing to step into the posts vacated by boycotting doctors.[99]

Medical men who were aware that competition was self-defeating and unprofessional and who believed that united efforts were better than individual struggles formed organizations to promote professional solidarity and to advance their interests. The Association of Medical Officers of Health was established in London in 1856 and worked to promote sanitary science, public health legislation, and their own role in public health.[100] In 1868 the Poor Law Medical Officers' Association was established.[101] Although the officers had many and serious grievances, they had no confidence that their dissatisfaction could provide the basis for the reform of the system of medical relief "because the general public never cared for our class in any way."[102] Instead, they argued that the interests of the sick poor demanded reform in the administration and financing of poor law medical practice.[103]

These and other pressure groups worked for change; they also fostered communication among practitioners and promoted colleagueship above competition. But the efforts of medical associations towards greater professional self-determination were likely to fail as long as too many medical men in an overcrowded profession had to choose economic survival above loyalty to their peer group. In such circumstances, those who paid the salary had power over medical men. It was a vicious circle, for greater solidarity might have led to better economic and professional circumstances for all.

Medical men who began their careers alone, those who relied on the assistance of families, and those who used medical appointments as a vehicle of introduction all found themselves dependent on the non-medical world and its values for the advancement of their careers. Throughout the century some medical men, however, managed to avoid at least some of the indignities of lay dominance through service to, or favor from, their seniors within the profession. These young men were indebted, too, but they might have consoled themselves that at least part of the judgment of their worth came from men who could apply professional standards of merit.

V

Employment as a private medical assistant to an established practitioner brought professional earnings and avoided the bad odor of lay control. Young men found news of assistancy posts in the medical press and sometimes heard of them by word-of-mouth. In the 1880's, salaries for qualified assistants ranged from £60 to £120 a year, plus board and lodging. An assistant might be called upon to prepare drugs, see patients, and carry on the whole practice when his senior was away. Some employers stipulated that their assistants could not, after termination of their employment, establish a practice in the senior man's territory. These conditions prevented the young medical man from viewing such employment as a foundation for independent practice in the future. In other cases, however, assistantships led to partnerships and thus could be an excellent launching-point for a career.[104]

Unlike purchase and family practices, the partnerships between a medical senior and his junior friend illustrate patronage which allowed room for professional judgment in the selection. Medical teachers sometimes chose as a junior partner a favored student. G. A. Mantell (1790–1852), apprenticed to James Moore in Lewes, took his hospital training in London and then returned to Lewes to become Moore's partner. Similarly, C. F. DuPasquier (1811–1897), who had studied with John Nussey, afterward joined him in his London practice.[105]

Short of partnership there was a myriad of ways in which medical men helped each other on an ad hoc basis. When a patient moved from one town to another, the doctor could refer him to his friend in the new place. When a consultation was needed, friendly practitioners called on one another. When new patients came to a man whose practice was already too large, they could be referred to the struggling younger man. The association of William Coulson (1802–1877) and Buxton Shillitoe (1826–1916) illustrates well the relationship of professional assistance. The origins of the Coulson-Shillitoe connection are unknown. Both were London practitioners and, early in Shillitoe's career, Coulson seems to have found him trustworthy and called on him to care for his patients when he was out of town. Later, when a vacancy occurred on the staff of the Lock Hospital where Coulson was a consultant, he may have been influential in Shillitoe's successful candidacy for the post.* When Coulson died in 1877, he left the lease of his house and his practice in Frederick's Place, Old Jewry, to Shillitoe, as a gesture of thanks for Shillitoe's aid in his practice. Coulson's bequest led to a large increase in Shillitoe's practice and income.†

*Coulson was on the hospital board when Shillitoe was elected Assistant Surgeon. See: Lock Hospital and Asylum, and Male Hospital, Minutes of the Weekly Board, 1862–1873, Meeting of July 9, 1863, pp. 1 and 5 (RCS Lib. Ms.).

†The Coulson-Shillitoe connection, not mentioned in *Plarr's Lives*, has been pieced together from entries in Buxton Shillitoe's Vis-

Senior men could be helpful to their junior colleagues by introducing and endorsing them among a larger circle of professional men who might be of assistance. William James Erasmus Wilson (1809–1884) was apprenticed to the well-connected surgeon George Langstaff, FRCS. During his apprenticeship, he met several medical men at Langstaff's house who helped him in the early years of his career. Among them were Jones Quain, Professor of Anatomy at the University of London, Sir William Lawrence, Surgeon to St. Bartholomew's Hospital, and Thomas Wakley, editor of the *Lancet*. After finishing his medical studies, Wilson became Quain's assistant at the university, and he later served as a private tutor to Wakley's sons and as assistant editor of the *Lancet*.[106] When Joseph Hodgson, a former Bart's man practicing in Birmingham, wanted an assistant, he consulted his former teacher, Sir John Abernethy, who recommended Richard Middlemore, his dresser at the hospital. Middlemore accepted the post. Eventually he joined Hodgson on the staff of the Birmingham Infirmary and established his own private practice in Birmingham.[107]

Professional seniors could also give a young man assistance by endorsing him to patients and employers. In seeking posts or private practice, the recommendation that came by word of mouth or by letters of reference could be of great help. John Ayrton Paris (1785–1856) was fortunate enough to have the favor of Dr. Maton, a well-known London practitioner. After Paris had spent some time in London, he decided to move to Cornwall to practice. Maton arranged for him to meet all the most important families there, and Paris had a successful practice among them.[108] On a more limited scale, senior practitioners frequently nominated young practitioners for temporary service as medical attendants to travel-

iting Lists and Diaries, WHML Ms. 4507 (1856) et seq., and William Coulson's will, Principal Probate Registry, Folio 359, 17/5/1877 (Somerset House), together with Lock Hospital, Minutes, 1862–1873, Meeting of July 9, 1863, pp. 1 and 5 (RCS Lib. Ms.). Coulson also assisted his nephew, Walter John Coulson, FRCS. Walter in turn assisted George Borlase Childs, FRCS, probably a relative. See *Plarr's Lives*, s.v. See also s.v. Sir William Dalby and William Cross.

ling aristocratic families. A well-established practitioner could scarcely take the time for such service, but for a junior man the posts offered decent pay, a chance to travel, and an introduction to "good society and valuable connections."[109]

With the nationwide expansion of public and charitable institutions for the care of the sick poor in the mid-Victorian years, medical teachers had growing opportunities to give their students help in gaining these posts and thus launching their careers. The final decisions regarding hospital and infirmary appointments rested with the laymen who constituted the board of governors. Positions in hospitals, infirmaries, and other institutions were not always advertised, of course, and then some version of the "old boy" network operated. Governors might consult a medical school teacher whom they knew for a nominee, or they might offer the post to some young practitioner with connections on the board. When the governors of the new Cumberland Infirmary were seeking a medical man, they consulted John Scott, Surgeon to the London Hospital. He nominated one of his students, William Bousfield Page, and Page was given the post.[110] George Makins was appointed to the Greenwich Infirmary through his father's connection with a member of the Board of Governors.[111] When these positions were advertised, candidates were invited to submit letters testimonial with their applications. It is difficult to assess the relative importance of professional dossiers in appointment decisions, for there was always the tendency for local hospital boards to solicit applications from their medical acquaintances or to favor candidates who came from their region of the country.

In all likelihood, the growth of the medical schools transformed the character of medical patronage. Under the apprenticeship system, general practitioners in country towns had also been medical teachers, and they had had the opportunity to exercise their influence locally on behalf of their students. The rise of the medical schools concentrated powers of nomination in the hands of the regional and national elites of the medical schools and brought increased reliance on formal letters of recommendation for the burgeoning number of public appointments available to medical men.

The professional dossier was a part of medical life from at least the early nineteenth century. Letters testimonial had, of course, been used in elite circles for recommending medical men to the College Fellowships. Such professional endorsement would, on the surface, suggest that the dependency of medical men on the lay world's judgment was, at least to a degree, being redressed by the fact that laymen looked to professional men for their evaluations in these letters testimonial.

Professional dossiers would provide a useful clue to the standards by which medical applicants were being evaluated. Unfortunately, very few such dossiers have survived. One of the rare exceptions is the dossier of James Joseph Power, whose letters seem to have been assembled in 1838, when he was an applicant for the post of surgeon to the West Kent Infirmary and Dispensary. Power's qualifications included the LSA, LRCS Edin., MRCS, and some special certificates. His letters of recommendation came from some eminent members of the profession, presumably including some of his teachers. There are strong similarities in the form of the letters. They all offer general statements regarding his "professional ability," his "zeal . . . in the acquirement of Professional Knowledge & understanding," his "Practical Knowledge," and his competence "to undertake any professional appointment."[112] There is little detail regarding the candidate's skills in surgery. More important, most letters devote a major part of their space to describing Power's personal character, and some make explicit reference to their connection with Power. Francis Ramage testified to the "good conduct" of his "friend" Mr. Power. Another writer equated Power's zeal with the "exemplary rectitude of [his] moral conduct" that would make him "an honor & an acquisition to whom so ever he may be connected."[113] Power himself seems to have played on his relationship with the previous incumbent by referring, in his letter of application, to the post "vacant by the death of my lamented friend Mr. Saunders."[114]

Perhaps medical men placed more emphasis on medical skills when recommending a candidate for what might have been considered the more scientific and high-powered posts,[115] but if Power's recommendations are at all typical of the ordinary practitioner's dossier, then professional references reflected what was a fact of life for much of nineteenth-century general practice: that the non-professional standards of the lay world continued to be the standards by which medical men were judged and appointed. As long as medical appointments to the hospitals and infirmaries of England were in the hands of the lay governors and boards of guardians, it was their standards that medical men had to meet and their criteria that writers of letters of reference had to address. The professional dossier suggests a form of professional influence, and because they were required of applicants, the medical job-seeker knew that, at least to a degree, he was dependent on his professional seniors.

Medical references were perhaps most important when a young medical practitioner applied for a junior post in one of the voluntary hospitals in London or the provinces. While these posts in the teaching hospitals tended to go to young men aspiring to consulting careers, they were especially useful in provincial cities and towns as an entree to private practice. House physicians and house surgeons usually held their appointments for a year, with salaries ranging upwards from £50, plus room and board. There was little, if any, time for private practice during the year's tenure, but a man could get valuable experience and acquaintance with fellow-practitioners and the population. John Nottingham's experience is typical. Born in Yorkshire in 1810, he served an apprenticeship in Snaith (Yorkshire) before moving on to further training at Guy's in London, and in Paris. In 1837 he was appointed House Surgeon to the Liverpool Infirmary, and in 1840 he began private practice in Liverpool.[116] Nottingham, like many other young practitioners, used his house appointment as a vehicle for moving into the community. Doubtless his attachment to the Liverpool Infirmary served as a form of endorsement and helped launch his professional career.

It would be unwise to see the system of medical references as a sign of the growing authority of the medical profession. True, letters from a man's medical teachers implied some concern for medical men's judgments about a candidate. But as long as the power of appointment was in the hands of a lay board, medical men's references had to take account of their standards of evaluation. Ignorant of medical science and, all too often, more concerned with matters of personality, style, and character, laymen defined the terms of their medical employees' conduct and practice, and medical men were subject to them. Only when medical men achieved some degree of power over medical appointments was it possible for medical employees to begin to free themselves from the domination of lay society. Then medical men became the judges of other medical men. Such changes came gradually, in the last decades of the nineteenth century.

VI

For a variety of reasons, some medical practitioners found it impossible to establish themselves in private practice in England. They could find no posts likely to lead to settled practice in a town, and, rather than continue to grapple with their inability to attach themselves to a network of personal or professional patronage, they left the country—some temporarily, some permanently. The military services offered full-time paid appointments to medical men and were recommended particularly to young men "with fairly good abilities, an adaptable temperament, good health, frugal habits, and with no chance of doing great things as a town practitioner or consultant."[117] The Army, Navy, East India Company, and the Indian Army all had medical officers in their ranks.[118] A term of service offered the medical man an opportunity to practice while accumulating funds in order to begin private practice. After ten years' service he could retire on half-pay, return to England, and, if he wished, pursue a civilian medical career.[119] Sherlock Holmes's friend Dr. Watson is a fictional example of this pattern of career. Alternatively, a man might choose to spend his entire professional life in military medical service. Some experience of military medicine was common in the Victorian profession. Among Fellows of the Royal College of Surgeons, for example, one-sixth of those who entered the profession before 1890 spent some part of their professional lives in one of the services.[120] Appointment to the services came, early in the century, by an informal system of nomination, but around mid-century an examination system was introduced. Medical men served on the examination boards, but of course appointments were in the hands of the military hierarchy.

There were some advantages in military medical posts that made them attractive to the young practitioner without connections and, perhaps, without ambition. The income was fairly good. In 1885 the pay was £200 per annum plus quarters—not luxurious, but adequate, immediate, and certain. Youth was no disadvantage in military medical practice, and there was thought to be less drudgery in military practice than in some civilian posts. Except in war time, the military surgeon had time for reading and study, and there was the added benefit, in some men's eyes, of travel. In the Indian Medical Service, it was said, the military medical man had the chance to meet "good society." In short, it could be "a serviceable if not brilliant career."[121]

There were disadvantages as well. Some considered the work routine and boring, and much time was spent in administrative rather than strictly medical work. Although the pay was adequate, it did not allow a man to marry comfortably unless he had private means.[122] More serious were the issues of status and professional independence. Medical men were excluded from the officers' mess and in other respects treated as less than military "gentlemen" until the Warrant of 1884 opened the way toward their full legal status as officers. The conditions of practice were less than ideal. A military surgeon might have escaped the "dependence which exists in civil life, namely, that upon patients," but he was not, thereby, independent.[123] He was part of the military, and he lived and practiced under its discipline. Perhaps for these reasons the services had the reputation for not attracting the "ablest and best students."*

*Richard Quain, *Observations on Medical Education* (London, 1865), p. 33 and note. Quain offers as evidence the fact that the majority were Irish licentiates: between 1859 and 1864 the Army Medical Service drew 230 men from Ireland, 115 from England, and 85 from Scotland.

Short-term absence from England as a ship's surgeon could also be a way for a friendless and fortuneless young man to build up his capital. Government employment as a ship's surgeon in the Emigration Service was one such option.[124] Private steamship companies such as the P. & O. and Cunard also employed medical men on board their vessels. These posts, paying £8–10 a month, plus expenses, could be a valuable form of temporary employment. A few men, enjoying travel or finding private practice difficult or undesirable, spent a large part of their careers practicing at sea.[125] These posts could not be a direct introduction to practice in the same sense that an infirmary appointment or a parish medical post might be, since they were literally cut off from the society where private practice was carried on. But as a source of income or capital for later purchase, they were a viable alternative for the man without other assistance.

The diverse patterns of medical men's careers include not only the fortunate men who studied, qualified, and moved directly to a stable and prosperous practice, but also those whose careers are a record of repeated attempts to establish themselves, first in one town and then in another, and repeated acknowledgment of failure. One can trace their progress from London to one, two, or three provincial towns, perhaps back to London, then a sea voyage, only to return to try again. For many of these men, the last resort was emigration.[126] Without connections in England, they went to the colonies, frequently to Australia. In the colonial situation, a man was on a more equal footing with his medical competitors. Social ties in these places were broken for all of them, and for their patients as well, and few could enjoy the advantages of connection at the start. Prospects were thought to be good in colonial practice, but the price was high. Personal values of family, friendship, and home were sacrificed for the sake of a career.[127]

VII

A practitioner built his practice on the same principles by which most careers were begun. The friends and connections that drew him to a town and formed the nucleus of his practice recommended him to others. Chance, a good location, and appointments brought him more. If a man had to rely on medical appointments for a part of his income, he might work to gain other public or contract posts and thus increase his practice. William Martin, the Staine practitioner who had early appointments as a Poor Law Medical Officer and doctor to a variety of clubs, added other clubs to his list: the Royal Oak Sick and Dividend Club, the Sailors' Home Sick and Dividend Club, and the Stanforth Excelsior Sick and Dividend Club employed him in 1890, and in the following years he became the medical man to a number of other provident societies.[128]

Club practice brought a medical man patients from among the working classes. It is likely that club members, when satisfied with their medical man, endorsed him to their friends and brought the doctor practice outside the club. When a man had an appointment at a charitable institution, he might win some of the philanthropic governors of the hospital or infirmary to his practice. William Bousfield Page (1817–1886), FRCS, had no connections but his post when he went to Carlisle to become Surgeon to the Cumberland Infirmary. "He knew no one in the northern cathedral town, . . . but by dint of tact, energy, and skill in surgery he soon made friends."[129] His new "friends" included local elites who were involved in the governance of the infirmary. His work and temperament must have pleased them, for "in a very short time . . . [Page] took the leading place at the Infirmary and was consulted by most of the county families and by the cathedral clergy, who placed implicit confidence in him."[130] Page's infirmary post involved practice among the poor, but it led happily to practice among the more prosperous members of the community and to a successful career.

Advertising by word-of-mouth was an important feature of practice-building, whether among the working classes or the upper ranks of society. Patients like those in Carlisle might be pleased with "tact" or "skill" or with the fact that a medical man was always accessible. H. E. Counsell, in practice in a small southern town in the 1880's, was very aware of the sorts of things he had to do to build his visiting list. He made himself available to patients at all hours but did not find it necessary to make connections on the bowling green, as Stark Munro had had to do. He put all his skills to work, he said, and in the course of practice distinguished himself from other practitioners, and found his name on the lips of the towns-people. First, he used a new drug, cocaine, which had not been previously used in his town. In addition, by success-fully treating a mastoid disorder—which people mistook for an abscess on the brain—he gained a reputation as a medical practitioner of skill. "I sometimes wonder," he commented candidly in his memoirs, "how much of their fame doctors owe to the ignorance of the public." [131]

Beyond the posts a man had, which served as a means of publicity, he could do little in a formal way to build his prac-tice. While a general practitioner was not strictly prohibited from advertising himself in the press or by handbills, it was a risky undertaking, savoring of trade, and generally not fa-vored within the profession.[132] In any event, such practices were of questionable utility and, in the end, a man had to depend on the favor and recommendations of his patients as a source of new practice. Like Stark Munro, many Victorian general practitioners became active in sports, perhaps be-cause of their liking for them; certainly such clubs extended a man's acquaintance in a town. Others joined local literary and scientific societies and musical groups.[133] A few participated in religious and political activities, but many felt that activity in areas of a partisan nature could lose as many patients as it won. To avoid offending any potential patient, many avoided politics, some even to the point of refusing to vote.[134] In a small town, where unconventional or controversial behavior was quickly known to everyone, the medical man was vulner-able to criticism and the loss of practice if he did not conform. John Chapman, a man of distinctly heterodox beliefs and ac-tion, resisted going to a provincial town to practice because he felt he would have to conform to prevailing standards of be-havior and at least "seemingly to acquiesce in all the supersti-tions of the stupidest old ladies with whom I may come in contact." [135] His dependency on lay opinion made him bitter.

The concern for patient opinion that made medical men

avoid controversy in matters of politics or religion also made them careful of their personal style and appearance. With some annoyance, Conan Doyle wrote to his mother about his lack of practice: "These Sheffielders would rather be poisoned by a man with a beard than be saved by a man without one."[136] The favor of women was frequently the target of general practitioners' attention and concern. Such a perspective may reflect the realities of Victorian domestic life and women's role in family health matters. It may also be a reflection of the low status of medical practice that women were left to judge and make decisions. Certainly medical men were frequently urged to attend to their women patients with care. J. H. Aveling, in an address on gynecology to medical students in 1885, explained how women could help or hinder a man's practice:

> [T]he successful management of the diseases of women is the key to general practice and forms a large portion of your work. Women, as you know, enjoy, and always find time for, gossip with one another. . . . Woe to the unhappy practitioner who has failed in his treatment of their troubles; his condemnation will be widely heard. On the other hand he who has been successful will have the trumpet of fame sounded with extravagant force.[137]

As a gynecologist, Aveling was naturally concerned with his special branch of medical practice and its relationship to professional success. Others, who were not so concerned with women's diseases, nevertheless warned ambitious practitioners to avoid behavior that was repugnant to women. Poor grooming, vulgar manners, and bad language would offend female patients and lose practice for the careless doctor.[138] Rather, a medical man should cultivate the social graces and a reputation for tact and sympathy. Robert Waring Darwin, the father of Charles Darwin, may be the classic case of the medical man who built his success on just such traits. He had little of what could be called a "scientific mind," and he disliked much of medical practice. He had, however, the ability to gain his patients' confidence because of his personality and powers of insight into their problems. Women, particularly, found him sympathetic, and much of his notable and rapid success was attributed to his success in winning their trust.[139]

The importance of medical skill in successful general practice is difficult to assess. The patients of eminent and highly qualified physicians and surgeons met untimely deaths despite their doctors' skills, and men with no qualifications at all enjoyed fame from many "cures." Sir Benjamin Brodie, former President of the Royal College of Surgeons, acknowledged in 1861 that, "if the arts of medicine and surgery had never been invented, by far the greater number of those who suffer from bodily illness would have recovered nevertheless."[140] Given the questionable value of much medical treatment, even by the standards of the day, and given the difficulty of judging the quality of medical care, whether the patient lived, recovered, suffered, or died, it is little wonder that patients depended on social criteria in the evaluation of a medical man. If he were a family member or a friend, he could be trusted at the very least to put the patient's welfare above his own monetary gain. If he spoke well, dressed well, and behaved like a gentleman, he was judged to be a man worthy of trust in the treatment of patients. And patients, ignorant, uncaring, and without faith in the character of medical licenses, might finally select their medical man on the basis of his beard or his good looks.

Some general practitioners built their practices with only minimal qualifications. Some held only the Apothecaries' license, others only the qualification of the Royal College of Surgeons. However, many medical men went on to take additional medical licenses after they had been in practice for some years. Some did so for improved status among their professional brethren, but others thought it might improve their practice. The Fellowship of the Royal College of Surgeons or an M.D. degree from one of the universities not requiring residence was typical advanced qualification for the mid-career practitioner. Whether such additional qualifications represented a higher level of skill is open to some question. Some were considered "give-away" doctor's degrees.[141] Some higher qualifications were useful because they opened doors to appointments which demanded more than minimal qualification, but their "chief value" was their attractiveness to patients: "the letters M.D. . . . produce an undoubted impression on the general public, especially upon the ladies."[142]

To produce an impression, to win confidence, to establish and maintain ties of loyalty between doctor and patient— these were the ways to establish a practice. In the absence of professional authority, the general practitioner sought to avoid the taint of trade and profit-making by developing ties of personal connection between himself and his patients. The Victorian ideal was the image portrayed by Luke Fildes in his painting "The Doctor." In the first light of dawn, the medical man sits in a lowly cottage, watching his youthful patient with attention and concern. A prescription bottle, a cup, a pitcher, and a bowl are the only pieces of equipment in sight. The doctor is not primarily scientist or technician but devoted friend. As one medical man said to his students about the painting: "A library of books written in your honour would not do what this picture has done and will do for the medical profession making the hearts of our fellow men warm to us with confidence and affection."[143] He urged his students always to "hold before you the ideal figure of Luke Fildes' picture, and be at once gentle men and gentle doctors."[144]

In a similar vein, Dr. Isaac Ashe, in his Carmichael Prize Essay of 1868, described the professional ideal as one of service and self-sacrifice "regardless of any return . . . by the public."[145] He did not ignore professional skill, but he elevated the personal relationship of doctor and patient to pre-eminence: "True it is that labour, study, and skill have their recognized value, and can be adequately requited; but the sympathy, the tenderness, the patience, the prayers of one who regards his patients as friends, cannot be so requited."[146] Dr. Ashe recognized the unity of self-interest and public welfare: "[O]nly by honestly seeking the interest and welfare of others," he wrote, "can either an individual or a corporate body secure or maintain any real or durable private advantage."[147] Improved professional status would not come to medical men as long as they put income and self-interest above the welfare of their patients and the demands of their medical art. Lacking the authority of socially valued knowledge, they sought to enhance the status of general practice by emphasizing the duty, service, and self-sacrifice that characterized the doctor who was a friend.

The ideal of the general practitioner as the patient's friend was an important counterfoil to the public suspicion that medical practitioners, battling for better pay and higher status in the ranks of public service and in private practice, were motivated primarily by the desire for gain. Medical men were certainly concerned about their incomes, and there is little doubt that many medical reformers saw the injury to the poor that came from foolish economy with public monies. And at some points the interests of the poor and the interests of medical men were one. Those who found themselves in such practice worked to improve the conditions of practice among the poor. At the same time, those who could sought to extend their practice to more prosperous segments of the community. As their practice in these circles grew, they could afford to leave behind the burden of underpaid, overworked salaried posts.

Modern stereotypes notwithstanding, most practitioners did not serve any single class to the exclusion of others. Perhaps in the largest cities, practitioners might draw most of their patients from the working classes or from the middling classes of society. But most general practitioners' visiting lists included a cross-section of society, from the poorest to local elites. William Martin's Yorkshire practice included all classes of the town, from several whom he lists only as "Gentleman" or "Esq." to schoolmasters, a member of the West Riding constabulary, and butchers, postmen, publicans, saddlers, farmers, miners, laborers, and itinerants who received medical care and left town with their doctor's bill unpaid.[148] Perhaps it was as easy to treat a rich patient as a poor one, and, all considerations of service to the suffering aside, the most desirable practices were those that brought higher fees, less onerous labor, association with "good society," and freedom at least from the controls of public or private employers.

The vast majority of men who practiced medicine in nineteenth-century England followed the path of general practice as described here, whether in London or the numberless towns of provincial England. At their best they were "respectable and painstaking medical men,"[149] and in a few instances they were prosperous and successful members of their communities. Most often they were the obscure, underpaid, and "overworked red-lamp practitioners" who carried the burden of the greater part of medical care in Victorian England.[150] According to one Victorian survey of a select group of medical students, less than 10 percent went on to leading practices in large towns or to distinguished medical careers. Fully 50 percent made only an "adequate" living in their practices, while the remaining 28 percent barely survived, or failed.* For most, then, general practice was not the source of any special "esteem or influence in society."[151]

The roots of general practice in the apothecary's trade continued to influence the public image of the G.P. as seller of drugs rather than as diagnostician and prescriber of treatment. The result was public suspicion that medical decisions and advice were self-interested, motivated as much by desire for profit as by the patient's needs. Medical men perpetuated their status as tradesmen by engaging in price competition,

*The data first appear in: James Paget, "What Becomes of Medical Students," *St. Bartholomew's Hospital Reports*, 5 (1869), 238, reprinted in: James Paget, *Selected Essays and Addresses* (London, 1902), p. 27. They are reported again in: C. J. Cullingworth, *On the Importance of Personal Character in the Profession of Medicine. An Address Delivered at . . . Leeds, October 3, 1898* (London, 1898). Cf. S. Squire Sprigge, *Physic and Fiction* (London, 1921), pp. 166 ff., in which a comparison is made between Paget's data for 1839–59 and data for the 1890's and after. Paget found: "Distinguished success," 2.3 percent; "Considerable success," 6.6 percent; "Fair success," 50.7 percent; "Very limited success," 12.4 percent; "Failed entirely," 5.6 percent; "Left the profession," 9.6 percent; "Died during medical training or during the first 12 years of practice," 12.8 percent. He was unable to locate all the students; these data are based on the 1,000 whose careers he could trace. The data may not be typical— Bart's was a very prestigious school and its graduates may have done better than the average.

advertising, submitting to their patients' demands for the "bottle of physic," and by tolerating in many instances the intervention of their employers in the doctor-patient relationship.

It is a sorry portrait, but not a surprising one, when seen in light of the central fact that Victorian general practitioners were not members of a "liberal profession" but of a dependent occupation. Without freedom or authority, their work was defined by laymen, and even in private practice they were judged by the standards of the lay world. They were the servants of their employers and their patients. Their authority, when they had any, came not from their medical knowledge but had its origins in connection, social origins, or social style.

Some medical men, perhaps influenced by the example of their medical school teachers in the London hospitals, began to chafe under the rule of their lay employers, and began to work toward the kind of freedom and authority that the elites seemed to enjoy. Perhaps aware of the destructiveness of competition, they organized pressure groups and professional societies to promote the interests of the profession and to foster cooperation among medical men. Through bureaucratic fiat and parliamentary action, small steps were made in the direction of increasing authority for medical practitioners. It is possible to argue that the monopoly of registered medical practitioners over such matters as birth certificates, death certificates, and service to the state were only public acknowledgment of skill and not, in themselves, public acquiescence to the authority and independence of the medical man and his profession. But these small rights were steps in the improved status of the general practitioner. More important was the slow progress toward medical administration of medical work—the medical inspectorate that supervised the work of public health officers and the medical men who administered the poor law infirmaries and their officers in the last quarter of the nineteenth century.[152]

Besides their important functions as pressure groups, organizations like the British Medical Association, the associations of poor law and public health officers, and the myriad of other local and national associations fostered professional pride and the medical man's belief in his right to authority in medical matters. To the degree that medical associations fostered medical men's belief in the primacy of their achieved status as "registered medical practitioners" and men of science, they were performing an important psychological function that gave medical men the self-confidence to carry on their battle for status and independence. Such self-esteem was a vital component of the medical man's claim to authority, both in the public world of the infirmary, the bureaucracy, and Parliament, and in the private world of the surgery and the sickroom. At the core of it all were the divided values of medical men themselves. As much as they might believe in the worthiness of their medical work, they shared with their lay patients and the rest of Victorian society a belief in the superior virtues of liberal learning and gentlemanliness and the inferiority of technical training and skill. The struggle for the authoritativeness of medical knowledge had to be waged not only in the public arena but within the doctors themselves.

IV

❖

The Formation of a Professional Elite

FAR removed from the grime of the colliery surgeon's life, the gloom of the workhouse infirmary, or the shabby respectability of a struggling urban general practice, the elites of the London medical world lived and practiced among the most prestigious and fashionable members of nineteenth-century English society. A worried nation waited for the physicians' reports when Prince Albert lay dying of typhoid in 1861.[1] Consultation at the bedside of the Prince of Wales a decade later brought instant fame and royal honors to the rising young physician William Withey Gull.[2] Not every successful London consultant could boast royal patients, but many could name earls, marquises, cabinet ministers, and other notables of Victorian political, intellectual, and social life among the patients they treated in the metropolis or the country.[3]

Such practice brought high social connections, prosperity if not wealth, and access to the rewards and pleasures of the upper ranks of Victorian society. Knighthoods or baronetcies, country houses, lavish entertaining, foreign travel, Alpine mountain-climbing, membership at the Athenaeum, art collecting—all were possible for the select few who were numbered among the London medical and surgical elite. They often married well, sent their sons to public school and university; they owned carriages, hired servants, and donned the morning coats and top hats that daily bespoke their elevated status.[4]

Their public visibility was matched by their standing within the professional institutions of London. They held the highest offices in the Royal Colleges. They examined all those who wanted to enter medical practice and judged who were worthy of the higher honors of the profession. They made educational policy for medicine and surgery and laid down rules for the behavior of all medical practitioners. In the hospitals of London, too, they held positions of honor as physicians and surgeons, dispensing charity to the sick poor under the aegis of philanthropic aristocrats and City businessmen. Indeed, early in the century, the hospitals provided a crucial stepping-stone to prestigious medical practice through the visibility and connections hospital posts offered and, increasingly, through the influence of medical and surgical teaching.

While a young man beginning general practice might find a career ready-made in a family "firm" or purchase, the path to the consulting elite could be long, the competition hard, and success rare. Qualifying at age twenty-one, the aspirant to consulting status stayed in London, serving in minor hospital posts, seeking the beginnings of practice, and making what connections and income he could. At age twenty-six, he became a Fellow of his College and, with luck, by age thirty he might be appointed assistant physician or surgeon at one of the London hospitals. For most young men this decade was primarily a time of surviving and waiting for the posts that would secure their future as consultants. Promotion to full physician or surgeon came typically at age forty, and election to Royal College office by age fifty.* If senior status in a London teaching hospital is used as an index of success, then for most of the nineteenth century, the inner circle of elites numbered no more than 180—five percent of all London practitioners and just over one percent of medical practitioners in England and Wales.[5]

*Compiled from information in *Plarr's Lives* and *Munk's Roll*. Of surgeons who earned the MRCS in the decade 1840–49, the median age at Fellowship was 26, the median age at election as an assistant surgeon was 31, and as full surgeon, 41. Among physicians who were elected to the FRCP in the same decade, median ages were: FRCP, age 33; assistant physician, age 34; and full physician, age 40.

Unlike their poorer cousins, the general practitioners, the London consultants did not have to struggle and scrape to make a living. Their connections were prestigious, their patients prosperous when not wealthy. In professional terms, however, the general practitioner and the consultant of the Victorian era shared one crucial condition: both depended on the values, judgment, and power of the lay world. The consultant earned greater rewards for his work, he may have served barons instead of butchers, but his condition of dependence was analogous.

I

The hospital was one of the most significant institutions in the creation of a Victorian consulting career, and its importance grew in the course of the nineteenth century. Despite its primarily medical function, its early nineteenth-century governance was entirely in the hands of laymen. Medical men were the employees of the lay rulers of the great London hospitals. In the days before the new poor law, hospitals had provided a necessary public and philanthropic service to the poor. With the growth of extensive medical provisions under the new poor law, the hospitals offered a respectable alternative to those who needed medical assistance but wanted to avoid the stigma of pauperism. Hospitals owed their existence to the laymen, who created them to bring health care to the sick poor.[6]

Hospital financing came from two sources: ancient landed endowments brought income in the form of rents; and nineteenth-century philanthropists, subscribing a few pounds or many hundreds, supplemented the income of the endowed hospitals (St. Bartholomew's, St. Thomas's, and Guy's) and provided nearly all the operating income for the newly established hospitals of the late eighteenth and early nineteenth centuries.* Like similar corporate institutions, the

---

*See Chapter I, above, for a list of voluntary hospitals in London. Even in 1890 the endowed hospitals drew 75 to 90 percent of their income from land; see: *Select Committee of the House of Lords on Metropolitan Hospitals*, 1890 (392), xvi, p. 214, Q. 3164 (Longley).

hospitals were ruled by boards of governors, who served under the hospitals' charters as trustees of the endowments and overseers of the contributions of their philanthropic fellows. Hospital charters varied in the constitutional details of how governors were chosen, but beyond that their working arrangements were very much alike. Ultimate power rested with the whole board of governors, sometimes called a "Court." The whole board usually met quarterly to receive reports from its committees and its executive officer, to confirm their actions, and to make major fiscal, policy, and personnel decisions. Boards of governors ranged in size from 50 to upwards of 300.[7]

Despite the technical authority of the whole board, most members lacked intimate knowledge of the hospital, and much of their power devolved upon the select group of governors who were elected to the house committee. This governors' committee met monthly, had power over minor hospital appointments, often made inquiries and forwarded recommendations to the whole board on matters of policy and personnel, and in some cases was instrumental in nominating replacements to the hospital board itself. This committee usually had 30 or more members.[8] A committee of almoners or a "weekly committee" of governors admitted and dismissed patients.[9] This group of 4 to 6 governors was sometimes called the "Taking-In Committee."[10]

The duties and powers of the governors covered every aspect of hospital life: the administration of the landed estates, construction and repair of the physical plant, purchase of food and supplies, the appointment of hospital employees of all ranks, and, most important, all aspects of medical life in the hospital. The charity was theirs, and they defined the terms by which it brought relief to the sick poor.

In the early nineteenth century, hospital governors had, individually and collectively, extensive influence over the patients admitted for medical care. One of the perquisites of charitable donations to hospitals and status as a governor was the power to nominate patients. Through the medium of "governors' letters," governors and other subscribers gave "deserving poor" people, sometimes their own employees or servants, entree to the hospital and to medical care. These patients, together with accident and emergency victims and "casual" patients admitted by the governors on "taking-in" day, constituted the objects of the medical man's professional care.[11]

In addition to nominating individual patients, the governors set policy regarding which types of cases should be admitted and which excluded. Some hospitals refused to admit patients considered incurable. Others did not accept maternity cases.[12] The moral objections of some governors and subscribers led the Westminster Hospital board to refuse admission to venereal disease cases.[13] Since the governors paid the piper, they could reasonably expect to be able to call the tune, but their power restricted a doctor's freedom with regard to his patients.

More important, medical men's professional lives, both within and outside the hospital, were subject to the authority of the governors. The board laid down their duties in the hospital in written form, and their obligations were read out to them on their appointment.[14] Governors detailed their hours of attendance, their responsibilities to the governors and other hospital authorities, and specific aspects of their conduct. Governors also ruled some aspects of the staff's extramural professional lives. Medical staff at St. Thomas's Hospital were, for example, prohibited from giving lectures outside the hospital except with the express permission of the governors.[15] Medical men also needed the governors' permission to apply for posts at other hospitals.[16]

The governors of the early nineteenth-century hospitals seem not to have blinked at the idea of interfering directly in the most narrowly medical or surgical aspects of medical men's actions in the hospital.[17] When John Elliotson, a Professor of Medicine at University College London, became involved in research on mesmerism, which he thought to be of scientific value, the college's lay governors stopped him.[18] Hale Thomson, Surgeon to the Westminster Hospital, was attacked in a house committee meeting for his surgical incompetence; the governors held a hearing on the matter, and the judges in the case were all laymen—the hospital treasurer, a lawyer or two, and seven or eight other laymen.* Governors raised questions of medical and surgical procedure frequently enough to indicate that they did not consider the medical man's work beyond their judgment.[19] Their watchfulness and lack of reticence speak well for their attentiveness to the welfare of the sick poor, but they also reveal the limits of medical authority within the walls of the London hospitals.

Finally, governors had complete control over medical and surgical appointments in the hospitals. House committees usually voted on junior appointments, and, following the traditions of private apprenticeship, accepted the nominations of each physician or surgeon for those temporary clerks, dressers, and housemen who would work with him.[20] In the matter of permanent appointments to the senior staff, however, the full board of governors voted; the medical staff of the hospital had no voice whatsoever in the election of their colleagues. This medical impotence came from two basic facts: first, medical men almost never served as hospital governors,[21] and, second, they had no alternative institutional voice through which to exercise influence over the conduct of hospital affairs and over the selection of their peers.

Given the significance of senior hospital appointments as a mark of high professional status, the mechanism of election to these posts deserves close scrutiny. Let there be no question at the outset: scientific and technical standards of expertise and skill were not primary criteria for appointment. The governors' selections were made upon a variety of grounds, most of them unrelated to medical skill. The simplest to deal with were those of educational affiliation and seniority. Simply put, governors nearly always appointed to the senior staff men who had been students to their hospital's surgeons. While the new foundations of the nineteenth century had, by necessity, to appoint medical men trained elsewhere, the old established hospitals tended to limit appointments to their own "old boys." Thus, all surgeons appointed at Bart's Hospital in the first half of the nineteenth century had studied with a sur-

*J. Langdon-Davies, *Westminster Hospital* (London, 1952), p. 186. He was acquitted.

TABLE 8 Educational Background of London Hospital
Appointments to Full Surgeoncies, 1800–1855

Hospital	Total	Education at same hospital	Other London or provincial hospital	Unknown
St. Bartholomew's	6	6	0	0
Guy's	7	7	0	0
St. George's	7	6	0	1
St. Thomas's	7	6	0	1
London	5	4	0	1
Middlesex	5	1	2	2
Westminster	5	2	3	0
University College [a]	5	2	2	1
St. Mary's [a]	5	1	4	0
King's College [a]	2	0	2	0
Charing Cross [a]	3	0	3	0
TOTALS	57	35	16	6

SOURCES: *Plarr's Lives*; H. C. Cameron, *Mr. Guy's Hospital,
1726–1948*; and Norman Moore, *History of St. Bartholomew's Hospital*,
Vol. II.

[a] New foundations in the nineteenth century.

geon at Bart's.[22] The same was true at Guy's. In all, of the
42 surgical appointments to established London hospitals
between 1800 and 1855, five are of unknown educational
background, and of the remaining 37, 32 were in-house appointments[23] (see Table 8). Physicians' ties with the London
hospitals in this period tended to be looser, Oxbridge medical
students migrating to London for a term or more of hospital
training, but most often not doing their full medical work in
London. Nevertheless, physicians' appointments follow the
same pattern of favor to the hospitals' own students.

The governors' preference for their own hospital students might have indicated their supreme confidence in the
teaching skills and professional judgment of their own staff.
Perhaps. But the rule of seniority[24] by which the most advanced student was the first promoted (when other issues
did not intervene) left little room to discriminate among
applicants on the basis of quality performance. The appoint-

ments themselves reveal that professional ability played little part in the hospital appointments system; relationship was everything.

The grossest neglect of merit appointments came in those hospitals where, by contributing a few pounds, persons became governors eligible to vote in staff elections. In such a situation, the candidate and his friends simply "created" governors as long as their money held out. The candidate who could command the most votes was, of course, elected.[25] Most of the London hospitals did not leave their staff elections quite so open to this crass economic influence that took patronage out of their hands. The Westminster, for example, provided that only contributors of £3 with three months' standing could vote in staff elections.[26]

At St. Bartholomew's, sitting governors elected new governors from among those who contributed £100, together with others nominated by the president or treasurer. St. Thomas's Hospital governors were a self-perpetuating body, made up partly of City officials, partly of donors and individuals nominated by the governors in office. At Guy's, new governors were nominated and elected by those sitting.[27] These modes of gubernatorial election precluded virtual purchase of hospital posts, but other sorts of influence over appointments existed that were equally antithetical to merit.

When the Charity Commissioners investigated the finances and administration of the endowed hospitals in the late 1830's, they reported to Parliament on the procedure for appointment of medical staff at St. Thomas's Hospital. They understood that the lay governors found it difficult to judge the competency of candidates for the medical staff. Failing that, the governors made their selections on the recommendations of the hospital treasurer or "some other influential governor, if not by personal favour or connection."[28] What was true of St. Thomas's Hospital was equally true for the other great hospitals of London in the first half of the nineteenth century.

It is nearly impossible to prove that family and friendship provided the primary basis for election to the senior staff of a London hospital. What can be shown is the presence of relatives, as governors, when a candidate was elected to a post. Thus Henry Earle's father, a newly elected governor at St. Bartholomew's Hospital, voted in the election of his son as assistant surgeon in 1815. Similar circumstances attended the election of Peter Mere Latham at Bart's in 1824.[29] Two governors named Powell, presumably relatives of Richard Powell, were present at his election to the post of physician.[30] These random illustrations hint at nepotism in hospital elections. More telling, perhaps, is the failure of governors to rule out the possibilities of nepotism. A member of the board at St. Thomas's Hospital proposed a motion in 1844, "That no Governor be eligible to serve on the Grand or any other Committee who may have near relations occupying places of trust or emolument or being aspirants to such places in the event of vacancies."[31] The motion failed.

Given the size of a governors' board, relatives alone could scarcely guarantee election to a hospital post. Nepotism had to be supplemented by friendly cooperation among the governors. Such cooperation was the predictable outcome of a system in which board members themselves elected new members to the board. The ties of friendship which brought a man into the hospital's governing body would lead to favor to relatives at election time.[32] Some of these affiliative groups were so well defined as to become cliques or parties within the board. At the Westminster Hospital the governors divided between the "old Westminster party" whose members included Anglican clergymen, and the smaller oppositional group headed by two nonconformist preachers. Sectarian issues determined many of the board's decisions and may have been instrumental in the election of Hale Thomson as one of the hospital's surgeons.[33] Perhaps favoritism is best demonstrated through cases of disfavor. Astley Cooper nearly lost in his bid for a surgeoncy at Guy's Hospital in 1800 because of his republican political views—a heritage of his teacher Henry Cline. A timely recantation saved him from defeat. Thomas Hodgkin (1798–1866), now famous for the disease that bears his name, was neither so flexible nor so fortunate. His early scientific promise could not outweigh the unpopularity of his political radicalism. That, and the animosity of the Treasurer of Guy's, led to his defeat.[34]

Hodgkin's case highlights what the Charity Commissioners described as the power of "some influential governor" in decisions about hospital staff.[35] At many of the London hospitals the chief administrative officer was the treasurer. Chosen from among the governors, this officer carried the burden of day-to-day hospital affairs. The treasurer managed funds, chaired nearly all the quarterly, monthly, and weekly governors' meetings, admitted patients, and had power to suspend staff and discipline students. Some even had a large hand in the selection of new members of the board itself. Armed with the authority of the board, he could—and often did—become the single greatest influence in the hospital. His actions were all subject to review by the board, but rarely did a treasurer find himself reversed. By his intimate acquaintance with daily affairs, he could exercise great power in the governors' board rooms as well as the hospital wards. Governors less familiar with the workings of their institution looked to the treasurer for informed advice on policy and, very often indeed, personnel.[36]

The Treasurer of Guy's Hospital, Benjamin Harrison, Jr., is perhaps the archetypal figure of lay authority in the early nineteenth-century medical world. The son of Benjamin senior, Treasurer of Guy's from 1785, the younger Harrison became a governor of the hospital in 1793 and succeeded to his father's post in 1797. Sure of the support of his fellow governors, he ruled the hospital and its staff. He brooked no opposition from the medical staff, considering any resistance a rebellion deserving only to be crushed. Autocratic and arbitrary, Harrison could also be wise; he was devoted to the hospital and it flourished under his fifty-year reign.[37]

Harrison and other treasurers like him lived under no obligation to consult the medical staff. They sometimes did, but only ad hoc; the medical staff was "summoned" when the governors might deign to seek their advice.[38] Harrison, instead, developed a close working relationship with a single member of the medical staff and consulted him when he wished or needed to do so. Sir Astley Cooper, the eminent surgeon, and later Sir William Gull, the physician, were trusted favorites from whom Harrison sought advice.[39]

Harrison exercised monumental powers over the selection of hospital staff. His dislike of Hodgkin has already been mentioned. On the other side of the coin, Thomas Addison, an unknown young physician, found a place on Guy's senior staff despite the fact that he had not been a student there. Harrison's favor overrode this disability and brought to Guy's the discoverer of Addison's disease and one of the hospital's "greatest . . . teachers."[40] Harrison virtually created the career of William Withey Gull, the physician who became his adviser in his later years. Gull, the son of a deceased wharfinger in Essex, lived as a boy on land owned by Guy's Hospital. On one of his visits to the hospital estates, Harrison met the little orphan, "divined in him unusual ability," arranged for his secondary education, brought him into the hospital as a medical student, and saw him eventually ensconced on the senior staff.[41] Gull had a brilliant career outside the hospital as well. He attended the Prince of Wales in 1871, and that case made him famous. Outstandingly successful in private practice, he was a distinguished scientific physician as well, credited with the discovery of myxoedema and many other advances in medical knowledge.[42] Gull's career reveals the excellence of Harrison's judgment of men. It also displays his overriding power in the hospital and in medical men's careers.

Harrison's patronage reached even unto the second generation. Sir Astley Cooper enjoyed influence through his association with Harrison, and his students basked in the light of Cooper's special status, but his surgical colleagues had none, and their students had little or no success when they tried to climb the ladder to the senior staff. None of Thomas Forster's students ever achieved senior rank, nor did those of William Lucas, Jr. In 1840 every full surgeon at Guy's Hospital was one of Cooper's former apprentices: John Morgan, Charles Aston Key, Bransby Cooper, Edward Cock, and Thomas Callaway.[43] Benjamin Brodie at St. George's Hospital and John Abernethy at St. Bartholomew's Hospital seem to have enjoyed the same kind of influence. Their apprentices, private assistants, and junior associates all rose to the senior staff in the first half of the century.[44]

The Cooper monopoly introduces the issue of a different sort of nepotism than that involving governors and candidates directly. In the great tradition of family education, Cooper had two nephews among his students—Bransby Cooper and Edward Cock. Another student, Aston Key, joined the family by marrying Bransby Cooper's sister, Sir Astley's niece.[45] The net effect of Sir Astley's "nepotism" in his choice of apprentices and the net effect of the governors' favor to the hospital's apprentices was extensive familial connection among the surgical staff. Guy's Hospital was not atypical in this respect. Of the 57 full surgeons appointed to London teaching hospitals before 1855, sixteen were related by birth or marriage to senior members of the staff.[46] The habits of apprenticeship fostered hospital nepotism. The positive policy of the governors ensured it. Even when a man had not been a student of the hospital, governors ignored that disability when family relationships existed. Caesar H. Hawkins, without formal ties to St. George's but the grandson of a former surgeon there, made a successful bid for senior staff in 1829.[47] Hale Thomson, eagerly seeking a surgical post at the Westminster in the 1830's, "crowned [his campaign] . . . by marrying the daughter of the hospital treasurer."[48] He won his post in 1834.

Because physicians were educated at the universities and not by apprenticeship, the same extensive ties between family, education, and hospital appointments do not appear. While hospital governors most often selected their physicians from among Oxford and Cambridge graduates, hospital connections still played a role. Governors favored Oxbridge men who had come to their hospital for their practical training, and most students chose the London hospital where they had connections. After completing his baccalaureate at Oxford in 1810, Peter Mere Latham (1788–1875) took up medical studies at Bart's Hospital, where his father John had served as one of the hospital's physicians from 1793 to 1802 and subsequently served as a governor. Awarded the doctorate in medicine at Oxford in 1816, he became a Physician at Bart's in 1824.[49] Fewer sons and nephews of physicians seem to appear in the appointments lists of the hospitals of the early nineteenth century, perhaps because fewer sons of physicians elected medicine as a career. Where such family succession in physic did exist, however, the hospital governors did not hesitate to appoint them to the staff. William Babington's son Benjamin (1794–1866) and his son-in-law Richard Bright (1789–1858) both served Guy's Hospital after him.[50] Other cases included Algernon Frampton (1803–1851) at the London Hospital and Thomas King Chambers (1817–1889) at St. George's Hospital.[51] These successive family appointments rested on the foundation of gubernatorial nepotism, abetted by favoritism.

"Family connexions," writes historian Noel Annan, "are part of the poetry of history."[52] Lord Annan found those connections among England's Victorian intellectual elite. With respect to nineteenth-century medical life, it might be more accurate, however prosaic, to say that family connections were part of the *grammar* of social history. Family and family friends defined the structure, order, and actions of much of Victorian medical life, not only for the general practitioner who went home to practice, but for the elites seeking to climb the ladder to professional success in London. Family status might have served as a clue to character or to political or social allegiance, but it was an unreliable index of occupational performance.

The Charity Commissioners reporting to Parliament in 1840 were careful to avoid evaluating the hospital appointments system in terms of the skills or competence of the appointees,[53] but nepotism and favoritism in their purest forms often flew in the face of considerations of competence. There can be no doubt that many of the physicians and surgeons of early nineteenth-century hospital life were the best men of their era. Sir Astley Cooper had, in addition to his charm, handsome features, and family connections, great skills as a surgeon, and his nephew Aston Key was known for his dexterity and power as an operator. Addison, Gull, Hawkins, and

Richard Bright were all superior in their practical abilities, their science, their teaching, and sometimes all three.[54]

Others could claim only modest abilities: Bransby Cooper, perhaps living too much in his uncle's shadow, lacked self-confidence and sometimes fumbled. Benjamin Guy Babington was "far from outstanding as a physician."[55] John Scott, FRCP (d. 1849), although a Physician at St. Thomas's Hospital, was scarcely known in the profession, his major claim to reputation coming from his work as a scholar of oriental languages.[56]

The nepotism of the London hospital governors led not only to fine or adequate appointments but also to gross incompetence among some who had the care of the sick poor in their hands. At Guy's, the appointment of William Lucas, Jr., to the surgical post vacated by his father brought a likeable but thoroughly incompetent surgeon into the hospital. Best remembered because John Keats was his dresser, the "rash" Billy Lucas made Sir Astley Cooper "shudder" when he took a scalpel in his hand.[57] J. F. South shared Cooper's opinion of the unfortunate Lucas: "[H]is operations were badly performed, and accompanied with much bungling, if not worse. He was a poor anatomist and not a very good diagnoser, which now and then led him into ugly scrapes."[58] Hale Thomson's laziness and incompetence did not keep him from hospital service and promotion, and the governors' friendship protected him from the consequences of his failures.[59]

At the same time, hospitals also lost the services of excellent medical men through the workings of favoritism. Thomas Hodgkin's political views kept him from an appointment at Guy's. Without connections, the talented Richard Grainger never enjoyed a hospital post.[60] Others, careers crippled by their failure in the hospital, may remain unknown, lost in the shuffle of the hundreds of place-seekers who settled in obscure practice for the rest of their lives.

In some instances, governors might have avoided the lazy, the incompetent, and the bungling medical appointees by heeding the voice of the medical staff. Hale Thomson's candidacy aroused a fruitless storm of protest from the Westminster physicians and surgeons.[61] When the Charity

Commissioners asked hospital physicians and surgeons about appointment procedures, they found them "almost unanimous in opinion that an alteration in the mode of election would be a material improvement in hospital administration."[62] Ideas for reform included public examinations, an open application system, or nomination by a committee of the hospital staff. These reforms might have opened the way to appointment by merit. They would certainly have taken patronage out of the hands of the governors or a single favored staff member, distributing power more evenly among hospital physicians and surgeons. But they would also have deprived the governors of their absolute power over appointments. The Charity Commissioners, after their inquiry into the constitutions of the hospitals, concluded that "Such alterations as these, however valuable, are not likely to be adopted voluntarily by the governors."[63] However much influence Sir Astley Cooper or Sir Benjamin Brodie might wield in their respective hospitals, their power was derivative—dependent on the favor and approval of their lords on the board. The ultimate power remained with the governors.

Would-be reformers testifying before the Charity Commissioners may have directed their primary criticism at the favoritism and nepotism of the governors' decisions, but their fellow medical men, by the choice of students and the exercise of indirect influence, cooperated in the system of nepotism and favoritism that ruled promotion in the London medical world. Thomas Wakley, in the pages of the *Lancet*, raised the banner of quality in his war against the nepotism of the hospitals,[64] but the physicians and surgeons of the elite shared with the governors a commitment to social criteria for professional promotion. In the inner circles of the Royal Colleges, where medical men had complete autonomy in the promotion of those they considered the best, the values of professional skill took second place to other considerations.

The rulers of the Royal College of Surgeons, the Councillors, came almost exclusively from among the hospital surgeons of London. A man who enjoyed a surgical appointment by age 30 could expect to join the inner circle of collegiate power when he reached his middle years.* The likelihood of election to the Council without hospital connections was almost nil.† As a consequence, the rolls of the College of Surgeons are replete with the names of sons, nephews, and sons-in-law who followed their senior relatives into the college elite. Whether the Surgeons' nepotism came from their direct selection of relatives, or through the indirect route of honoring those that the hospital governors honored, the result was the same. Benjamin Brodie's niece's husband, Thomas Tatum, found his place on the Council in due course. Sir Astley Cooper followed his uncle William into the Council, and his nephews followed after. Even the wretched Billy Lucas took his place among the surgical elite for seventeen years.[65] He and his fellow Councillors determined the fate of the surgical profession, examined those who sought a surgeon's license, and enjoyed all the perquisites of power in Lincoln's Inn Fields.

Medical education, as contrasted with surgical education, was much less integrated with the hospitals. The power structure of the College of Physicians reflects the hospitals' lesser importance in their eyes. While the surgeons seem to have drawn their leadership almost exclusively from the hospital ranks, physicians did not. For example, of the thirty-two London physicians elected to the Fellowship during the decade 1810–1819, eleven had posts in hospitals. Ten of those went on to hold College office, but nine other College officials from this group never had any affiliation with a hospital.‡ In addition, seven men who held physicians' posts in London

*The median time between qualification and election to the Council of the RCS was 22.5 years. Thus, if a man earned the MRCS in his early twenties, he became a Councillor, typically, in his mid-forties. Calculated from: RCS, *List of Officers, &c. of the Royal College of Surgeons of England, 1800–1895* (London, 1896).

†Of the twenty-four Council members serving in 1843 (the year the FRCS was instituted), twenty-one had London hospital posts. Compiled from RCS, *List of Officers*, passim; and from *Plarr's Lives*.

‡Compiled from *Munk's Roll*. "Officer" in the RCP refers to the President, Vice-President, Censor, Registrar, or Examiner.

hospitals were never elected to the Fellowship, while one man elected to the Fellowship never practiced at all.[66]

Sir Charles Bell, the distinguished anatomist and Surgeon to the Middlesex Hospital, criticized the casual attitude of physicians toward the hospitals. In a letter to the governors of the Middlesex Hospital in 1824, he put forward the view that hospital posts "should be a reward for professional merit," but they were, instead, a training ground and public advertisement for young medical men.[67] "It is unhappily conceived," he wrote, "that young physicians should be introduced to hospitals, that they may there learn their profession, and be prepared for private practice; and that whenever their private patients promise them a livelihood, they should leave the hospital to the next candidate for the notice of the town."[68] According to Bell, hospital physicians took their posts in order to get experience and visibility, but, once achieved, they gave up hospital service and let some new man take his turn in the wards. He justly pointed out that such behavior ignored "the interests of the sick."[69] Since the hospitals did not play the same central role in physicians' education as in that of surgeons, physicians viewed them simply as a stepping-stone to practice, and they played a lesser role than Oxbridge in the calculus of power in the College.*

If hospital status meant little in the endowment of the Fellowship, so did achievement in science—or lack of it. Many early nineteenth-century Fellows were elected between the ages of 30 and 33,† and achievements in medical science did not often weigh in their election. Some Fellows, before or after election, made valuable contributions to medical science, education, or practice.[70] Others made none at all.[71] Moreover, some physicians outside the Fellowship did as much or more scientific work than their counterparts in the senior rank, but they were not, on that ground, elected.[72] The ir-

---

*It should be remembered that hospital surgeons could claim high apprenticeship fees, and their students, in turn, gained access to senior hospital posts in later years. Physicians had no similar monetary stake in the hospital.

†The median age of election to the FRCP in 1840–49 was 33 (range 30–44). Compiled from *Munk's Roll*, IV.

relevance of achievements in science stood out boldly in the testimony of Sir William Macmichael, Physician to the King and former College officer, before the Select Committee on Medical Education in 1834. Committee members, concerned that some Licentiates had been denied the Fellowship, quizzed Macmichael as to the reasons. He defended the College's rejection of one physician on the ground that he had made no contributions to the science of medicine. But when asked how many of the present Fellows had written great works of medicine, he replied: "It is not so necessary to write great works now: the science is advanced so much, that it is not to be expected that we should have very voluminous publications." [73] A cursory examination of the achievements of Macmichael's compeers in the College demonstrates his wisdom in not pressing the point of "great works" of medicine as a standard for election. [74]

The composition of the Royal College of Physicians' elite reveals that they accepted unquestioningly the dominance of non-medical values and judgments over their corporate life. While a man could practice as a physician in London with the License of the College, only Fellows enjoyed voting rights and College offices; and the Fellowship went almost exclusively to Oxford and Cambridge men. In short, physicians were adherents of the Oxbridge mystique.

The restriction of the Fellowship to Oxbridge men was not, by any means, based upon the superiority of medical education in the two universities. When Parliament inquired into medical education in 1834, none of the witnesses from the Royal College of Physicians even tried to claim such a thing. Many willingly admitted that medical education in Edinburgh or London was clearly better. [75] Sir Henry Halford, Bt., President of the College of Physicians, went so far as to declare the quality of Oxbridge medical education irrelevant. He said it "is of very little importance, if they have their preliminary education. They will go and find physic wherever it is to be found, afterwards." [76] According to the physicians, the great strength of an Oxbridge education was that it developed "character" or "moral" superiority, these being inculcated by the Oxbridge residential college system of education.

Others praised the "liberal education" and "good conduct" born of Oxbridge.[77] Behind all the high-minded language, however, the concern of the Royal College of Physicians proved to be "the dignity and respectability of the profession" of physic.[78] The identification of the College and the Fellowship with Oxford and Cambridge assured physicians that their status was on a par with the high class of patients they treated. Sir William Macmichael pointed out that physicians who have studied at Oxbridge "have the same education as those who fill the highest stations in life; they are brought up with those persons and afterwards become physicians."[79]

In view of the irrelevance of science and hospital status and the singular significance of Oxbridge in the selection of Fellows, one might dismiss the Royal College of Physicians as simply a London club for Oxford and Cambridge men who happened to be physicians. But such an explanation trivializes the matter by ignoring the power of the College over the practice of physic, and it ignores the significance of the Oxbridge mystique for understanding the values of the profession. The insistence on a gentleman's education and the indifference to hospital service, medical teaching, scientific contributions, and even practice itself reveal the Physicians' profound commitment to the social values of elite non-medical society. They did not see the College as an institution committed first to medicine. Rather, it was an instrument for the maintenance of physicians' esteem and power among—and by the standards of—the social world they inhabited.

In their hospital duties, physicians and surgeons treated the sick poor of the metropolis. In their private practices, they had as patients the prosperous, the wealthy, and the highest ranks of nineteenth-century society. Such practices grew up in much the same way that general practitioners made theirs, through the fortunate possession of patronage or the adroit recruitment of patients' favor. Hospital posts introduced physicians and surgeons to eminent City officials, merchants, businessmen, and the aristocracy that gave their names, time, and favor to medical philanthropy. Senior medical men in the hospitals and Royal Colleges in turn often helped their young successors build their practices and advance their careers.

They nominated them for travelling posts to the aristocracy, called them in for prestigious consultations, referred new patients to them, and launched them in the elite world.[80]

The career of William Maton, M.D. Oxon., FRCP, illustrates the varieties of assistance that led to a superior private practice. The son of a Salisbury wine merchant, Maton completed his medical studies in 1798 and took the Fellowship in 1802. Although he held a post as Physician to the Westminster Hospital, he had little private practice and tried to build his income by frequenting Weymouth, a fashionable watering place, during the season. He spent his leisure time there pursuing his botanical interests. When one of the royal princesses was there on holiday, she had a botanical question, and Maton was called in to answer. This marked the beginning of royal favor, and his London practice grew to the point that by 1808 he gave up his post at the hospital. In the next decade he served as physician to the Queen and to the Duke of Kent, and later attended the infant Princess Victoria.[81] Maton also inherited the practice of Matthew Baillie and, as a result, had the leading practice in London. In turn, Maton used his high connections to advance the careers of his favorites, William F. Chambers, FRCP, and John Ayrton Paris, FRCP, in London and the country. Chambers' income was reputed to range between seven and nine thousand guineas a year between 1836 and 1851. Favor, whether professional or lay, was as much a matter of chance as quality. Chambers was a very ordinary physician, but he was a sound man of good judgment.[82] Paris was "not the most intelligent of men."[83]

Sir Henry Holland (1787–1873), FRCP, the son of a "respected medical practitioner" in Cheshire, travelled to continental spas and watering places where he learned of the curative powers of the waters and met members of high society, associations that led to a large London practice and royal service. Never a hospital physician, Holland was nevertheless an officer of the College and was said to have earned £5,000 a year. Holland's case illustrates "a remarkable instance of a man rising to eminence in his profession, whilst entirely cut off from all professional interests. . . . Sir Henry was essentially *homme de société*."[84]

Glamorous as it may have been, aristocratic patronage in medical careers only compounded medical men's dependence on lay judgment. No judges of medical quality, the aristocracy often relied on social standards to select their practitioners. Henry Herbert Southey (1783–1865), FRCP, "became a great favorite both as the companion and as the physician of many of the great aristocratic families in the north of England" because he was "remarkably handsome, active, athletic, and fond of the sports of the field."[85] Southey moved to London, and "their favour and support followed him when he . . . settled in practice in the town."[86]

Just as moustaches, good grooming, and personal charm could influence a general practitioner's career, personal characteristics could help or harm aspirants to London consulting careers. Oxbridge education gave a physician the advantages of classical learning and cultivation, and patients of high status were known to "appreciate those advantages."[87] Pelham Warren, FRCP, informed the Select Committee on Medical Education that a physician wouldn't be called upon to practice among the "wealthier classes" unless he had the "manners and morals" of those who mixed with that class.[88] By the same token, a man might lose a Fellowship—and thus status and practice—if he lacked social grace.[89] Medical men of the London elite lived under the rule of laymen, and they judged each other and were judged as much by the standards of social acceptability as by professional education, knowledge, or science.

Sir Benjamin Brodie, distinguished President of the Royal College of Surgeons, accepted the facts of life in his profession. He advised medical students not to "cringe and stoop" in order to gain favor, but he urged them also to avoid "misanthropical independence" in their careers. "Mankind," he said, "are bound to each other by mutually receiving and conferring benefits. . . . As others will lean upon you, you must be content to lean upon them."[90] Sir Charles Bell took a less sanguine view. He condemned the system of advancement which promoted a man "for no merit properly his own. You give him the unfortunate impression . . . that influence is everything; and he becomes a dependant."[91] Under the dominance of lay patronage and control, medical men of early nineteenth-century London looked first to their extra-professional ties: their patrons in the aristocracy, the wealthy classes of society, Oxbridge, and the governors and officials of the hospitals they served. Their first loyalties were non-professional, and as a consequence they lacked a fundamental sense of colleagueship. They fought among themselves, often publicly, and looked to their lay rulers to settle their disputes. They criticized each other in print and in public, seeking first the favor of their lay patrons, even at the price of intra-professional alienation.[92] But developments in the early Victorian medical world brought about profound changes in the values and orientation of medical men that led, by the end of the nineteenth century, to a shift in the sense of identity and the locus of power in the world of medicine. The roots of that change are found in the evolution of the medical school.

II

The eighteenth-century hospital had been the informal site of medical education, with surgeons bringing their hospital apprentices with them to learn at the bedside and in the operating theater. Physicians-in-training had come, paid a fee for hospital practice, and walked the wards, observing patients and physicians at their work. From the late eighteenth century, individual surgeons—and sometimes physicians—began offering courses of lectures within the hospital walls. Out of these casual beginnings came the early Victorian establishment of the medical schools. Sometimes on the initiative of the treasurer, most often at the request of the hospital staff, boards of governors gave their permission for the establishment of a medical school within their hospital.[93] The governors accepted this new role for the hospital because they saw a variety of benefits in such a move. They endorsed the hospital's use as an instrument of education and approved the notion that medical men should supplement their small hospital honoraria with the fees students would bring. Most important, a medical school would bring better medical attendance to patients. Some thought the students would add to the size of the working staff. Others believed that medical students' constant scrutiny of the teaching and hospital staff would lead the hospital's medical officers to treat patients more conscientiously.[94]

The governors, while prepared to endorse the existence of the medical school and allow the use of rooms and wards for teaching, did not intend to lend fiscal support to the school. They had nominal power over the medical schools, but they left their management—curriculum, fees, hours of classes, and personnel—in the hands of the treasurer or, more often, in the control of the teachers themselves.[95] Therein lay the seeds of change, for in their power over students, in the elaboration of auxiliary personnel for teaching, and in the administration of the medical schools, physicians and surgeons had their first sweet taste of power within the precincts of the hospital. The changes began in small ways, but the long-range consequences were great.

The new mass system of Victorian medical education brought changes in the mentality of medical students and in their attitudes toward their teachers. While an apprentice's vision might once have been limited by the horizons of his master's modest surgery or apothecary's shop, now many students saw the highest possibilities of professional success at first hand. With the growth of the lecture system and the increasing centrality of London for the nation's medical education, mid-Victorian students by the hundreds observed the medical and surgical "stars" at the height of their fame and success.[96]

S. T. Taylor, a London medical student in the 1850's, saw many of the great lights of the London hospitals at their work. He was thrilled when he had the chance to see Sir William Fergusson, FRCS, perform a difficult operation brilliantly and in record time. He admired the "tall and majestic" figure of the great surgeon and mused over his fabulous career:

> It is said he came to London with only half a crown in his pocket, which is, of course, a gross exaggeration, although in all probability his pockets were not too well lined. . . . He

is credited with having an income of £20,000 a year, but of course the exact amount is known only to himself, although there cannot be the least doubt it is a very large one.[97]

Behind the myth lay the message that other young men, although poor, could also rise to similar heights. Even when a young man came to London with modest plans for a country practice, the experience of assisting one of the great men fostered a desire to go and do likewise. The son of a poor curate, H. T. Butlin (1845–1912), went to St. Bartholomew's Hospital for his medical studies. He planned to take up general practice in Kent but instead threw himself into the race for a London consulting career. He "felt himself unsuited for a country practice after the stimulus of acting as House Surgeon to Sir James Paget."[98] Dazzlingly successful teachers, the stimulus of student prizes and gold medals, and the ambition of one's fellow students all aroused the ambition of the new generation of medical practitioners in the schools of London.[99]

The early nineteenth-century hospital had provided only rudimentary support staff to the surgeons in the dressers, posts held by the advanced apprentices of individual surgeons. The hospital apothecary served as the resident medical officer. In the effort to provide more extensive service to patients, a variety of student posts began to appear from the 1830's onward. Hospitals continued to appoint dressers, usually three for each surgeon, and clinical clerks were created in like numbers to assist the physicians.[100]

Out of the necessities of teaching and out of new ideas of medical care, record-keeping, and charity administration, the first half of the nineteenth century saw a phenomenal growth in the number of student posts in the hospitals. By 1852, for example, Guy's Hospital had five posts open to second-year students—Medical Ward Clerk, Dresser's Reporter, Dresser in Eye Wards, Dresser in Surgery, and Junior Obstetric Clerk—and four posts open to third-year students—Obstetric Ward Clerk, Clinical Clerk, Dresser, and Resident Obstetric Clerk.[101] A similar growth occurred in the number of temporary junior appointments open to newly qualified medical men. Hospitals created the posts of house surgeon and house physician in the 1840's and 1850's. Housemen were selected from among a surgeon's dressers or a physician's clinical clerks.[102] The resident apothecary, who provided constant attendance on patients, began to be supplemented (and eventually replaced) by resident physicians and surgeons, sometimes attached to special wards. Guy's instituted the post of Resident Obstetric Clerk in 1849, House Surgeon in 1856, Resident House Physician and Assistant House Surgeon in 1865, Assistant House Physician in 1866, and by 1890 there was a resident assistant physician and surgeon attached to each member of the senior staff.* Between 1860 and 1880 many hospitals introduced the post of registrar.[103]

In the medical schools, too, formal regularized teaching and the growth of curriculum led to the elaboration of opportunities for junior medical men interested in London hospital careers. In the early days of the medical schools, the senior physicians and surgeons divided the teaching responsibilities among themselves. The few courses—anatomy and physiology, *materia medica*, and the principles and practice of medicine and surgery—brought students and fees to the senior staff.[104] Auxiliary science courses began to include laboratory work as well as lectures, and the senior lecturer delegated the daily grind of anatomical or pathological demonstrations to one of his former apprentices, later one of his former students. During the period 1840 to 1890, several junior teaching posts of this type appeared: demonstratorships in anatomy first, then morbid anatomy, physiology, and pathology.[105] Support staff in the form of assistant demonstrators for these subjects appeared later in the century.

As licensing bodies added to the number of courses re-

*H. C. Cameron, *Mr. Guy's Hospital, 1726–1948* (London, 1954), pp. 202 and 225. The house physicians took over the clinical duties of the apothecary, and a pharmacist took over his dispensing duties. Thus, the apothecary (as general practitioner) disappeared from the hospital. St. Thomas's Hospital had a Resident Assistant Surgeon from 1847; see: St. Thomas's Hospital Records, Minute Books of the Grand Committee, (H1/ST/A6/12) 10 August 1847, pp. 2–3; and E. M. McInnes, *St. Thomas's Hospital* (London, 1963), pp. 131–133.

quired for qualification and as hospital medical schools began extending the number of optional courses available to students, teaching responsibilities soon grew too heavy for the senior staff to carry unaided. They kept control over the most advanced and prestigious courses, specifically anatomy and the "principles and practice" courses in medicine and surgery, but selected junior men to teach the others. Botany, medical jurisprudence, *materia medica*, obstetrics, and some auxiliary sciences became the domain of junior men.[106] The medical schools developed their own teaching-related agencies—the museum, the library, the collegiate residence—and these, too, provided employment and a small income for junior men and a post in a London medical institution. Curators, librarians, and deans all came from the junior staff.[107]

Student and junior posts had the very practical value of giving young medical men experience in the supervised treatment of patients and of introducing them to teaching. Some men intending general practice took a year or more of postgraduate service as a way of getting further training. For the aspiring consultant, continued service in the hospital and medical school in these posts was the surest line of advancement to the senior staff and, thereby, to prestigious and lucrative careers.[108] As hospital attendance or apprenticeship had been the early nineteenth-century criterion for access to senior staff posts, so study and junior service in the hospital and medical school led to senior status in the latter half of the nineteenth century. Hospitals continued to favor their own.[109]

Because of the assured income and national visibility that went with status as full physician or surgeon at a hospital and as teacher in a medical school, physicians and surgeons alike tended increasingly to hold on to their hospital and medical school positions for as long as possible. In the 1840's, a young surgeon could expect appointment as assistant surgeon at age 31; physicians could expect to reach the analogous position at the median age of 34. Full rank for surgeons came at the median age of 41, for physicians at age 40. By the 1870's, men could expect to spend a similar time waiting for assistant positions but a longer time before they gained promotion to full status. The median age of promotion for full physicians was 42/43 and for full surgeons, 44 years.[110]

Promotion was slow, and the "years of waiting" were hard.[111] Demonstrators spent half the day in the laboratory. Housemen and residents had extensive duties in the hospital, requiring their presence day and night. Neither they nor their seniors, the registrars, had lucrative incomes, and some supplemented their earnings by prizes, private tutoring, or other related work.[112] Study for advanced licenses and degrees also took time and energy. Few had time to build a private practice, and thus most had to live mainly on the small stipends their teaching and hospital posts brought.[113]

Under the circumstances of required hospital residence and relative poverty, most medical men could not afford to marry. John Simon, for example, earned about £200 from his junior posts at King's College and St. Thomas's Hospital in the early 1840's. With financial assistance from his father, he dared to marry at this stage of his career. Even so, the marriage was considered less than prudent.[114] Most aspiring consultants for whom we have data did not marry before age 29 or 30, when they had completed their advanced qualification and secured appointments as assistant physician or surgeon.[115]

Despite the poor pay, the long hours of work, and the long years of waiting for advancement, many young practitioners accepted this difficult and gruelling life on the junior staff because of the greater rewards that lay ahead. Competition was keen. Although the number of junior posts increased in the nineteenth century, the number of senior physicians and surgeons did not grow proportionately. By the end of the century a few hospitals had added a fifth physician or surgeon to their permanent staff, but the average number remained four of each. Openings did not come often. At St. Bartholomew's Hospital, for example, there were ten vacancies in the full surgeons' ranks in the period 1861–1890, an average of one every three years; at St. George's there was a vacancy in those ranks on the average of once every five years.[116] Each hospital surgeon had at least three dressers and each physician three clinical clerks each year, from among whom were chosen the one house surgeon and one house physician that served each senior man. From the house staff were chosen the residents and registrars, along with other junior hospital appointees. When an assistancy came open, many of those who had served as housemen, residents, or registrars sought appointment, but only one could succeed.

Early in the century, before the coming of the medical school, students completed their training and then spent time in private service to the aristocracy, travelling appointments, a bit of study abroad, or junkets to European spas or English resort towns—all in the effort to build practice. Hospital appointments had brought a few men back to the site of their training. By contrast, the creation of the medical school tied young men to the hospital almost continuously from their student days until retirement, if they were among the fortunate few. The sacrifices, the competition, the long hours of labor, and the absence of home and family only bound them more closely to the institutions they served. Stephen Paget thought that junior hospital service was "likely to be one of the happiest times of a doctor's existence. It [gave] . . . him that quiet sense of belonging to the place, that enjoyment of privilege and of near friendships, which make Cambridge and Oxford so delightful."[117] To the prestige of hospital appointment had been added the important role of professional teaching, and students' aspirations to join the select few at the top of the ladder drew them into longer and deeper involvement in the hospitals than most had known in an earlier era.

Extended junior hospital and medical school service also transformed the relationships of students with their seniors in the profession. The permanent senior hospital posts remained firmly in the hands of the lay governors, who also had nominal power in the appointments of junior hospital posts and the medical school staff. However, this latter authority was formal rather than substantive, for the governors relied heavily on the recommendations of the medical staff in these areas. In the early days of the medical schools this was reasonable; while a demonstrator might have been a junior officer of the medical school, he was paid by the senior lecturer and thus the governors would have found it difficult to intervene in appointments.[118] Even after student fees were deposited in a central medical school fund, out of which all teaching staff were paid, the governors continued to leave teaching posts in the hands of the medical and surgical faculty.[119]

Similarly, the governors accepted the nominations of the medical staff regarding the growing number of junior posts in the hospital. Perhaps the traditions of apprenticeship, where dressers and other such officers were drawn from among a surgeon's private students, carried over into the new post-apprenticeship era.* Perhaps the governors reasoned that medical staff would choose those aides who would reflect best on them, thus guaranteeing adequate staffing on the junior level. Governors may have considered it only just that a surgeon or physician have the right to choose those junior staff that made up his "firm." Perhaps, in the end, the governors cared little for the minor patronage of a three- or six-months' appointment. Whatever the reasons, the medical staff's power over junior posts gave them authority over students that they had not hitherto enjoyed. Favor from one's teachers became an avenue to income, however small, and to official status in the hospital. And few could have missed seeing that those who served the hospital and medical school in the early days of their careers formed the pool from which senior staff were drawn. No longer, then, did ambitious young men look only to the lay governors as the source of patronage and profes-

---

*The first step came when dressers no longer paid for their posts, thus removing the appointments from the realm of money influence or "purchase." At St. Thomas's, for example, the governors agreed to pay the surgeons sums equivalent to dressers' fees, and students were selected without regard to their ability to pay. See: McInnes, *St. Thomas' Hospital*, pp. 92, 94, and 96. This change is also reflected in the medical school entries in the *London and Provincial Medical Directory* for various years. McInnes sees this as a shift from money influence to merit, but it is also a shift from student power (through money) to the medical teachers' power. See also: *Select Committee on Metropolitan Hospitals*, 1890, p. 447, Q. 7556 (Fenwick); *2nd Report*, 1890–91 (457), p. 6, Q. 9847 (Lushington); p. 22, Q. 10222 (Perry); and *3rd Report*, 1892 (321), Sess. 1, xiii, p. xii, para. 21 and p. xxii, para. 91.

sional advancement. They also looked to their professional seniors for the advancement of their careers. If they had to "cringe and stoop" to get ahead, they would do so before the physicians and surgeons—as well as before the barons and bankers on the governors' board.

That early Victorian medical staffs gained a degree of influence over appointments through the growth of junior hospital and teaching posts did not transform the promotions system from the patronage of earlier years to the "objective" judgment of medical and surgical talent. When "the hospital surgeons appointed the lecturers to the medical schools . . . they appointed themselves, their relations, and the gentlemen who had paid them large fees to become their apprentices."[120] As apprenticeship declined, and students chose enrollment in the medical school over indenture to an individual surgeon, prior hospital apprenticeship ceased to be the primary criterion for hospital appointment, and appointments to junior and senior staff began to go to former hospital students without this contractual connection.*

However, the traditions of apprenticeship, family education, and connections in medical education died hard. After apprenticeship had disappeared, students continued to choose schools where they had ties of family or friendship, and those ties often smoothed the path through the junior ranks. Medical men, like the governors, were ready to help nephews, sons-in-law, and the sons of their friends. Hence, promotion in the hospitals continued to go to relatives of hospital officers and governors, some with talent, some by mere connection. To mention only a few instances from the latter

---

*The date of this change varies from one hospital to another. At St. George's Hospital, the first surgeon appointed without prior hospital apprenticeship was Caesar Hawkins in 1829; the next such appointment took place in 1843 (Edward Cutler). At Guy's, the first was John Hilton in 1849. However, Bart's named two former apprentices to the senior staff in the 1860's (Thomas Wormald and Holmes Coote). At St. Thomas's, the first non-apprentice appointment was G. Macmurdo in 1843, and the last hospital apprentice to be made full surgeon was John Simon in 1863. All of these cases are drawn from *Plarr's Lives*, s.v.

half of the nineteenth century: Alfred Willett followed his father-in-law Sir George Burrows into the senior staff at Bart's in 1867; W. H. Cripps and J. A. Ormerod at Bart's, and William Howship Dickinson at St. George's, all had relatives on the senior staffs of the hospitals where they were appointed.[121] John Davies-Colley, appointed Surgeon at Guy's in 1880, was the son-in-law of the treasurer of the hospital.[122]

Like family-related appointments in the first half of the century, these varied widely in terms of the skills and abilities of the appointees. Some were excellent medical men. Others could be praised for industry, devotion to the hospital, meticulous attention to detail, or a "business mind."[123] Sometimes the historical record is silent, and, given the praise awarded those who made even small contributions to professional life, the lack of comment suggests lack of any notable skill.[124] Perhaps the most blatant case of family favor defeating talent arose in the case of James Berry and D'Arcy Power. Berry, although physically debilitated, had drive and great talents in surgery. In 1898, after serving in a variety of junior posts, he became a candidate for the post of Assistant Surgeon at St. Bartholomew's Hospital. His opponent, also an experienced junior man, was D'Arcy Power. Power was admittedly less talented than Berry and less interested in surgery than in physiology and medical literature. But Power was the "eldest son of one of the most popular and influential of the hospital's surgeons," Henry Power.[125] The young Power won the post, and the logic behind the appointment is telling: "It was generally felt," one contemporary wrote, "that Berry would make his mark anywhere, but that Power needed the post to give him adequate standing for the development of his talents."[126]

The personal criteria that led hospital physicians and surgeons to act, individually and as a group, to favor relatives in the selection of dressers, housemen, residents, and registrars, sometimes also led to their selection of other favorites. Long-standing friendship and connection could lead a senior man to favor one student over another.[127] Social style could repel or attract a potential patron. Sometimes a senior man might fail to support a young man because he was "academically rather than socially well-bred," and "tactlessness," even with talent, could bar success.[128] By the same token, oratorical skills, courtesy, social grace, good birth, breeding, or dignity attracted the notice of professional seniors.[129] The "well-bred" medical student later became a dignified and cultivated colleague, bringing social if not scientific credit to his patron and to the profession as a whole.[130] John Cooper Forster (1823–1886), FRCS, Guy's Hospital surgeon from 1880 and President of the College in 1884, was noted for his courtesy, gentlemanliness, good looks, and gourmet tastes.[131] Holmes Coote (1815–1872), FRCS, was appointed Surgeon to St. Bartholomew's Hospital in 1864. A man of "good family," his father was a barrister, his brother a Fellow of Trinity Hall, Cambridge, and his wife the daughter of a judge, Coote's surgical career had no distinction. A cautious surgeon, he developed no new ideas in surgery. He had no exceptional success in practice, no special reputation as a teacher, no notable commitment to his profession. In one of his professional publications he "attributed rickets to the dissolution of the monasteries."[132] His rise in the hospital and the profession cannot be explained except in terms of connection or favor.

But if medical men were free to sponsor the mediocre young practitioner for reasons of nepotism or social snobbery, they were also free to reject relatives who had no special skills and lend their support to those of observed talent and ability in medicine.[133] John Bland-Sutton had no connections at the Middlesex when he enrolled there, but his skills in anatomy gained him the favorable notice of the anatomist and surgeon Thomas Cooke, who befriended him and assisted his career.[134] Sydney Ringer, FRCP (1835–1910), the son of a nonconformist tradesman in Norwich, lost his father at an early age and only managed to enter University College, London, through the generosity of a relative. A brilliant student career and early publication of scientific work brought him to the attention of his seniors at University College Hospital where he gained positions on the medical and teaching staff.[135] Similarly, Frederick Akbar Mahomed, FRCP, whose father was the proprietor of a fashionable Turkish bath in

Brighton, became a prize student at Guy's in the early 1870's and distinguished himself by his early experimental work and publications. He was rewarded by an appointment as medical registrar in 1877 and later gained a senior position in the hospital and a teaching post in Guy's Medical School.[136] The medical school offered short-term associations between students and teachers that allowed evaluation of abilities, and they often led to the sponsorship of the talented and the able, as well as the courteous, the gentlemanly, and the well-born.

The impetus toward concern for quality among medical men came from several sources, lay and professional. Hospital governors, despite their tendency to favor relatives, seem to have grown increasingly committed to the idea of professional quality in their appointments. Perhaps the new awareness of Victorians of the desperate social conditions of working men and women made these philanthropists less willing to tolerate the "first-rate indolence" of a man like Anthony White or the incompetence of a Billy Lucas.[137] Whatever their motivation, many governors demonstrated a profound commitment to the welfare of the sick poor in their charge. They took steps to assure themselves and their contributors that medical men attended patients responsibly, that they did not relegate the grimy details of patient care to their juniors, and that they exercised attention to the patients' comfort and well-being.[138]

St. Thomas's Hospital provides an excellent illustration of how governors' charitable motives brought greater attention to the quality of staff appointments. Troubled by reports of neglect, staff squabbling, and declining enrollments in the medical school, the governors made a thorough investigation of their establishment. The result was a resolution, adopted at the General Court of Governors on November 16, 1852:

> That this court being deeply impressed with the necessity of doing everything in their power to maintain and improve the efficiency of the Hospital which can only be maintained by the appointment to the higher Offices of the Medical Department of such parties only as by their talents & acquirements are most calculated to secure these results

by their care of the Patients and their attention to the success of the School, and to the general advancement of the profession they have adopted the Governors are therefore recommended to give their suffrage only to such parties regardless of any supposed claims of seniority or services in a Junior Department unless supported by such paramount and important recommendations.[139]

The St. Thomas's Hospital governors had concluded that nepotism, seniority, and hospital service alone were a bankrupt foundation for the effective functioning of their hospital and medical school, and their resolution served notice that men of talent and acquirements would have first priority. The resolution addressed the voting governors, but there was a message for the medical staff as well: the prestige of hospital appointments and the responsibility of patient care would, in future, be the reward of professional excellence. The medical staff could no longer rest with the knowledge that family ties, seniority, or junior service alone would assure their favorites places on the senior staff. The governors would be seeking quality as well.

As an earnest of their commitment, the governors determined to open hospital appointments to those not attached to St. Thomas's Hospital.[140] Under these circumstances, the medical and teaching staff had good reason to pay close attention to the quality of students they were promoting through the junior ranks. The governors did not always live up to their own resolution, of course, for the habits of favoritism were deeply entrenched, but it was a beginning. In a variety of ways, the governors of various London hospitals in the mid-Victorian years indicated their concern with the quality of hospital practice and teaching that, in their turn, brought pressure on the profession.[141]

Another source of pressure for quality in the selection of junior staff (and therefore, indirectly, senior staff, too) came from those who stood outside the circles of power in the profession. Thomas Wakley, out of his political radicalism and out of his frustration at his own exclusion from the elite, had challenged the nepotism and favoritism of the surgeons in the early issues of the *Lancet*.[142] But his was a voice in the wilderness. When professional men had little influence in the selection of hospital staff, they also had little responsibility for the results. As hospital consultants gained increasing influence in the promotion of students from obscurity to the elite, they had also to account for their choices. In an "age of reform," too, examination systems and the development of professional expertise were becoming notable features of such occupations as pharmacy, engineering, law, and a host of others.[143] Disapproval of the hospital and medical school promotions systems may have originated in reformers' jealousy or disappointment, but the weapon they used to attack a system that had excluded them was one becoming current in Victorian occupational and professional circles—the standard of merit.*

In 1875, William Dale, MRCS, pointed to the growth of competitive examinations in other occupations as a model for the medical profession, not just as a standard for entry but also for promotion: "The conviction has gradually forced itself upon my mind that the competitive principle—which is growing every day, and substituting manly self-reliance for cringing place-hunting—might be applied in determining the relative fitness for junior appointments."[144] Dale's remarks

---

*Harold Perkin, *The Origins of Modern English Society, 1780–1880* (London and Toronto, 1969), pp. 256–258, counterposes "merit" and "patronage" and notes that "merit . . . could be judged only by other professional experts in the same field." Perkin suggests that the "professional ideal" of merit grew out of a commitment to utility and function and was possible because of professional men's relative freedom from economic hardship. Medical men do not fit this model. For similar views see: Charles Newman, *The Evolution of Medical Education in the Nineteenth Century* (London, 1957), pp. 194 ff.; W. J. Reader, *Professional Men. The Rise of the Professional Classes in Nineteenth-Century England* (London, 1966), Chapters 3 and 6; Geoffrey Millerson, *The Qualifying Associations* (London, 1964), Chapter V; and A. M. Carr-Saunders and P. A. Wilson, *The Professions* (Oxford, 1933), pp. 79 ff. Cf. Sheldon Rothblatt, *The Revolution of the Dons. Cambridge and Society in Victorian England* (New York, 1968), pp. 90–93.

reflect the scorn which he attached to those whose success could be credited to their ability to curry favor. Charles Bell Keetley, FRCS, addressed the issue more obliquely in 1885, when he criticized the poor quality of medical teaching in the great London hospitals: "Let us suppose—not a supposition which will appear very outrageous to those who know how hospitals are often governed—let us suppose him [the inadequate lecturer] to owe his whole position to good fortune rather than to merit."[145] Both Dale and Keetley counterposed the servile and the incompetent against the manly, the effective, and the meritorious. Behind these remarks about the system of appointments lies the implication that both junior appointees and the seniors who favored them did not deserve the prestige, respect, and authority which their success should invoke. Medical qualification was no longer enough to justify the advancement of nephews, sons-in-law, or the culturally superior but professionally indifferent favorites of governors and influential medical men. Those outside the circles of power called for the favored ones to demonstrate talents related to the task at hand—medical teaching, hospital service, and professional leadership. By a similar logic students, too, brought pressure on the medical elites. Not bound to any single medical school, they could take their fees where they found teachers that provided them with thorough, if not distinguished, education. When they did not find it, they protested, and sometimes went elsewhere.*

Concern for the effectiveness of the hospital and medical school, for their own role as teachers, and for their credibility as the visible leaders of the profession in the nation—all these eventually led medical men to espouse standards of merit in hospital and medical school appointments. Almost inadvertently, it would seem, medical elites found an avenue to power in the application of standards of medical and surgical ability. When a physician's superior merit was established by his

*See, e.g., H. Hale Bellot, *University College London, 1826–1926* (London, 1929), pp. 195–211 passim. Perhaps centralized education brought a growing number of students to London who, without *social* claims to status in the profession, sought status based on *science*.

knowledge of the classics, lay judgment had as much weight as medical. Medical men could begin to lay exclusive claim to judge their peers and successors when the criteria for medical advancement lay in the arena of skill, medical research, and contributions to science.

The story of the expansion of medico-scientific activities in the nineteenth century would fill a volume by itself. The growth of journal publication, the appearance of medical textbooks to fill the new needs of centralized medical instruction, the prize system in the medical schools, the establishment of students' and practitioners' medical societies devoted to the discussion of medical science and technique, all were forums for the exhibition of medical and scientific achievement.[146] Of course, publication was rarely an avenue for the hard-pressed, struggling, but talented general practitioner to gain scientific eminence. Rather, those who benefited from the efflorescence of medical publications were the men who, by virtue of their hospital posts, had time, income, and access to the laboratories and hospital wards where they could pursue their science systematically.[147] Much of what was published and presented to professional audiences had limited scientific value, even by the standards of the day. One medical man criticized the Pathological Society, for example, for its lack of scientific rigor. The Society, he said, lent itself "too easily to the mere exhibiting of specimens . . . , and some of us, it may be, were tempted to call attention to our specimens for the purpose of calling attention to ourselves."[148] Reputation, built on visibility as well as sound achievement, could be found in the burgeoning industry of professional publication.

One might speculate that new societies, journals, and a certain "prize-mania" were themselves the product of the new populations of the centralized medical schools. As systems of mass education, they brought to the London hospitals the poor, the ill-educated, and the uncultured medical students as well as the more prosperous and well-connected men whose domain they had been in earlier years. Without claim to the culture of the "Latin or Grecian,"[149] their only hope for status came from the possibilities that achievements in medicine, surgery, and the related sciences could offer.

The transformation from scientific indifference to scientific primacy did not take place quickly. The medical profession during the mid-Victorian years served two masters, the values of the lay public and its own science. Expertise in teaching, publication, or science marked the careers of such men as Sydney Ringer, Sir Frederick Taylor, Samuel Fenwick, Sir William Hale-White, Sir Samuel Wilks, and Sir William Jenner.[150] Other successful consultants of the mid-Victorian years published little and left no scientific mark.[151] Sir Hermann Weber (1823–1918), FRCP, published minor works on climatology and health resorts, but he was "a man of extraordinary charm" and "quickly obtained a large and distinguished practice."[152] He counted among his patients five prime ministers—Derby, Russell, Salisbury, Rosebery, and Campbell-Bannerman—and many of his most distinguished fellow-medical men.[153] As late as 1892, the Royal College of Physicians still included among its official criteria for election to the Fellowship not only "Professional Eminence" and "Distinction in . . . Science," but also "Distinction in Literature" and "Social Position."[154]

Victorian medical and surgical elites continued to measure their colleagues and successors by the standards of lay culture, social distinction, and other non-professional criteria. But as their power over hospital and medical school personnel grew, they began to take serious account of those qualities directly related to their professional work. Most important, medical men were gaining the power over promotion in the hospital and medical school that made the application of scientific and medical criteria possible. Power over junior posts accrued to medical men because of the hospital's traditions and because of the surgeons' traditional role in medical education. But the governors, by allowing medical men power over medical students and education in the hospitals, had opened the door to medical men's growing assertion, first of interest and then of authority, in all aspects of the hospital.

III

It is not a little ironic that the creation of the medical school, a measure designed to improve the work of charity, brought, instead, division, conflict, and ultimately new power relations within the hospital. Early nineteenth-century governors and hospital staff had shared a view of the patient as the object of medical charity. The governors intended that the medical school should simply improve the quality of patient care. However, in the hands of medical and surgical teachers, patients became instruments of education. They were "audio-visual aids" in the task of teaching. One medical man, praising the resources of a teaching hospital, could scarcely avoid the poetic as he described the patients and their diseases:

> The clinical material is simply overflowing, especially in the surgical and gynaecological departments, and there is any amount of opportunity for men to work clinically at dresserships and clerkships, if they will only come and finger the material for themselves. It is a perfect paradise for every kind of tumour known, and the accidents are numerous.[155]

This new vision of the hospital patient as the bearer of some disease, the treatment of which was an educational experience for student and teacher, brought physicians and surgeons into direct conflict with the lay governors of the hospitals. Governors continued to hold the "ease and comfort" of the patients as the standard of hospital care and the primacy of poverty as the criteria for admission to the hospital, while the teaching staff increasingly ignored such matters when they interfered with what they considered effective teaching.[156]

Obstetric and fever cases exemplified the tension between benign charity and medical education. Governors feared the violation of female patients' modesty and comfort if numerous medical students attended a delivery, but efficient teaching demanded student experience with maternity care.[157] The question of fever patients also demonstrated the divergence between philanthropy and teaching. At St. Bartholomew's Hospital in 1885, a special committee of governors recommended the closing of fever wards for fear of infecting the rest of the hospital. The medical staff, however, wanted the wards open for teaching. The governors, thinking that these wards' teaching value was "more apparent than real," closed the wards until separate buildings could be allocated to fever patients.[158]

At the level of day-to-day hospital life, governors and medical staff lived with the tension between the intention of the laymen to bring health care to "deserving" persons, i.e., the truly poor, and the physicians' and surgeons' desire to accept "interesting cases" of value in their teaching, regardless of their economic status.[159] Early in the century the selection of patients had rested almost entirely with the governors, through the use of "governors' letters" and the decisions of almoners or taking-in committees. But with the growth of hospital teaching, a "trivial" case with a governor's endorsement posed a problem for the medical staff, who were primarily interested in patients whose illnesses illustrated important medical or surgical problems.[160] A prosperous artisan with a rare disease might be a particularly useful subject for clinical teaching, but he might be entirely unsuitable as a hospital patient from the standpoint of wise charity.

The one place where the medical staff had virtually complete freedom in selecting cases was in casualty. A small unit, casualty was primarily intended as a receiving department for accident and emergency cases as they arose, and no governors' letters were required for admission. The medical officers of the hospital began to admit cases other than emergencies in casualty, and thus found the freedom over selection of patients that gave them independence from the governors' letters and the taking-in committee. Patients found casualty more convenient, since they could seek treatment there on any day of the week, while the admission of patients for in-patient and out-patient care by the taking-in committee took place only one day each week.[161] By 1890, when a parliamentary committee investigated patterns of treatment in the metropolitan hospitals, the power of governors' letters had taken second place to the decisions of the medical officers in the selection of patients. At some hospitals the letters continued to be used, but at many the casualty medical officer had become the chief admitting officer, and governors' letters were irrelevant.[162] Hospitals in the last decades of the century began to employ laymen to investigate the patients' ability to pay, but the numbers of patients were so large and the time of the officer so limited, that medical staffs had relative freedom to select those patients for treatment that they judged medically most needy and pedagogically most useful.[163] As long as the great hospitals continued to be purely private charitable endeavors, the uneasy coalition between the needs of medical education and the goals of philanthropy continued to create tension between the laymen who held the purse and the medical men who treated the patients; but professional men had quietly asserted their power over admissions and thus extended their freedom over their professional practice.*

The Pandora's box of medical intervention in hospital administration did not stop with the selection of patients. The governors of the early nineteenth-century hospitals had occasionally sought the advice of the medical staff on matters they considered relevant to medical and surgical concerns, but such consultation was always initiated by the governors or the treasurer. The staff had no committees, no formal voice, no corporate existence.† The governors' attitude toward their professional staff was perhaps best exemplified by the statement of the University College Council in response to an address from the medical teachers in 1828: "Where the Council

*Governors worried about wise charity and their power over the hospital (see: *Select Committee on Metropolitan Hospitals*, 1890, p. 87, Q. 1316 and 1347 [Bousfield]) but saw danger in ignoring medical opinion (ibid., 1890, p. 521, Q. 8986, 8989 [Nixon]). At the same time, medical men tried to avoid offending governors by appearing to attend to cases they sent in (ibid., 1890, p. 83, Q. 1256 and p. 89, Q. 1347 [Bousfield]; and p. 25, Q. 228 [Montefiore]).

†*Select Committee on Metropolitan Hospitals*, 1890, pp. 137–138, Q. 2138–9 (Mackenzie); and p. 505, Q. 8716, 8720 (Buxton). Medical men were sometimes involved in the foundation of hospitals in the nineteenth century, and in those hospitals there was a tendency for them to have more influence in governance (ibid., p. 84, Q. 1261 [Bousfield]; and pp. 138–140, Q. 2139, 2168–70 [Mackenzie]). At St. George's, medical men became governors on the same footing as laymen by the payment of £5 subscription. Thus, they had a voice, albeit not *ex officio*, in the governance of the hospital (ibid., 1890–91, p. 100, Q. 12018 [Todd]; and the *Times*, July 27, 1880, p. 4).

think a collective opinion desirable the professors will be expressly summoned for the purpose."[164] There was a world of difference between summoning the staff for an opinion, or seeking advice through a friendly chat between the treasurer and a favored physician or surgeon, and systematic formalized consultation with the medical staff on hospital affairs. As long as the initiative came from the governors, authority over hospital affairs remained in their own hands.

From time to time, hospital staffs proposed that they be formally represented on the governors' committees, to participate in their deliberations on hospital matters. The St. Mary's Hospital staff proposed such an arrangement in 1863. The governors vetoed their request but allowed, instead, the creation of a separate committee composed solely of medical men.[165] At St. Bartholomew's Hospital, the Medical Council had been established in 1843. Composed of all senior members of the hospital staff, it met intermittently to consider matters of hospital policy. It was purely advisory to the treasurer and almoners "upon all matters submitted to it."[166] These separate medical staff committees did not initiate change, and their views came to the governors through the treasurer.

The formal establishment of the medical schools, however, introduced medical men to a new view of themselves and their relationship to the hospital, the governors, and the decision-making processes of their institution. Nominally under the governors and treasurer, the medical school committees had authority and responsibilities independent of the governors. At Bart's, the Medical School Committee was created in 1834 to carry on the business of the school.[167] The London Hospital Medical School had a College Board, composed of six governors from the House Committee and six members of the medical staff.[168] The Medical School Committee at the Westminster Hospital, created in 1840, included one governor together with the medical staff.[169]

Unlike the ad hoc meetings of hospital staff, these medical school committees met regularly and kept minutes of their meetings. They had an official existence and formal liaison with the governors. They had duties to perform and powers to exercise. They were responsible for curriculum, course arrangements, the distribution of fees for teaching, and other purely medical school matters, together with the nomination of junior hospital staff, their assistants. At first they continued their passive role of responding only to requests for advice from the governors' committees.[170] The hospital, as the instrument of medical education, became increasingly important to the medical staff in their role as lecturers, and the distinction between medical school affairs and hospital matters blurred. In the interests of improved medical education, the teaching staff initiated proposals for changes in the hospitals' policies, conduct, and staff. For example, in 1847 the Committee of Lecturers at St. Thomas's Hospital recommended the creation of a new hospital post, that of Resident Assistant Surgeon. They argued that such an officer would "increase the usefulness of the hospital and . . . promote the welfare of the school."[171] The lecturers did not stop with the suggestion of a new officer; they also recommended what qualifications he should have and how he should be appointed. They urged that preference be given to St. Thomas's students, based upon "distinction" in their student careers, and they proposed that the hospital's surgeons have the responsibility for verifying to the Grand Committee the "talent and good conduct" of candidates.[172] Medical men, in their committees, also proposed the institution of new wards in the hospitals for special types of cases (ophthalmic wards, maternity wards, children's wards, and the like).[173] Such proposed elaboration of staff not only improved the quality of patient care and provided posts and experience for junior men, but also extended the patronage powers of the medical staff and extended their formal influence over the conduct of the hospital as well as the medical school.

Reasonably amicable working relations between the staff and the governors seem to have emerged from this set of parallel committees for the first generation of the medical schools' existence. From the 1840's through the 1860's the senior hospital staffs were largely made up of men who had been educated and spent their early careers under the aegis of strong gubernatorial authority. By the decade of the 1870's, however, a new generation of medical men had come into senior positions on the staffs, and eruptions within the hospitals marked a turning point in the relations of medical men and their lay rulers.[174] The trigger for medical-gubernatorial conflict in many of the hospitals proved to be the reforms in nursing which came in the wake of efforts by Florence Nightingale and others to improve the quality, education, and status of this sector of medical personnel.

Florence Nightingale established the first training school for nurses at St. Thomas's Hospital in 1860. She intended, among other things, to recruit women of character and intelligence into nursing, as well as to improve the training of all those who served the hospitals.[175] Negotiations between Miss Nightingale and the treasurer and almoners of St. Thomas's set the terms of the nursing school's existence. The medical staff was not consulted. Nightingale received her strongest support from the governors and the influential apothecary, Richard Gullett Whitfield, who took charge of instruction in the new school. The response of the staff was mixed. Some favored the changes, some were indifferent, and some openly hostile. Most vocal in his objections, senior surgeon John Flint South addressed a protest to the governors in which he indicated his fear that "lady nurses" would seek to "take over" the teaching hospitals as they had the military ones, resulting in "collisions" and "annoyance to the Medical and Surgical Officers."[176]

At first, South's fears seemed baseless, but crises arose in the next decades that indicated his prescience. At St. Thomas's the trouble came over what seemed a very small issue. The medical staff had, since 1858, made their hospital rounds between 8:00 and 9:00 A.M. They found those hours increasingly unsatisfactory, since they interfered with both teaching and private practice. In the 1870's the staff proposed to return to afternoon ward visiting, from 1:30 to 2:00, the hours that had prevailed before 1858. Strong opposition to the change came from Florence Nightingale, on the ground that morning visits better served the nurses' convenience and the patients' welfare. After much consultation and debate, the governors' Grand Committee settled on a compromise schedule of hours that gave victory neither to the nurses nor to the medical staff.[177] Behind the issue of the time of ward rounds was the issue of authority in the hospital wards, the independence of the medical staff, and the lack of medical consultation in the deliberations and decisions of the governors.

At Guy's Hospital similar problems arose, but with greater heat. In December, 1879, the new matron, Miss Burt, in consultation with the treasurer, put forward a plan for changes in the system of nursing at Guy's. Two important features of the plan involved the introduction of a nursing sisterhood and the institution of a program of nurses' training, including a rotation system of ward nursing to give nurses experience of all kinds of medical and surgical cases. The governors' adoption of the plan brought a storm of protest from the medical staff. In a letter to the governors and treasurer on December 29, 1879, a united staff raised their objections to the reforms.[178] They warned of the dangers to the patients' well-being which such instability in the nursing staff would bring about, but the fundamental issue was the authority of the medical officers.

The new system threatened to undermine medical authority in the wards in several respects. First, the reforms introduced an Anglican sisterhood among the nurses. The medical staff attacked the introduction of religious affiliation and services in the hospital as mere sentimentality, related to benevolence but undermining freedom of religion and contributing nothing to the quality of medical care in the wards.[179] More important, they feared that the sisterhood would be a "guild," uniting the nurses outside the framework of the hospital and placing religious observance and the Church above their allegiance to the medical staff and their commitment to medical care.[180] For the medical staff, the only acceptable order of nursing was medical supremacy. As Sir William Gull, Consulting Physician to Guy's Hospital, wrote: "[L]et it be laid down, as a first principle, that the nursing system is to be under the auspices and regulated by the advice of the medical officers."[181]

The reform of ward service also threatened medical dominance. Under the old system of nursing, each sister had been attached to a single ward, where she learned as she worked and developed a long-standing relationship of service to the medical staff in charge of that ward.[182] The medical staff opposed the program of rotating the nurses from ward to ward, intended as a training device for the sisters, because it would disrupt the work of the wards and do injury to the patients.[183] Equally important, rotation fostered a centralized system in which ward sisters owed their allegiance only to the matron and to no single member of the medical staff; these senior nurses no longer studied the needs and ways of individual medical men. In effect, ward rotation made the nurses independent of the medical staff in a way impossible under the old system.[184]

The rotation system constituted only one aspect of the larger plan for nursing reform and for making Guy's an institution for the training of "lady nurses," who would afterwards work at Guy's or go out to other hospitals and into private nursing practice.[185] Advocates of reform urged that the new system would remove women of low character from places of authority in the wards and replace them with women of breeding, refinement, education, and skill.[186] As Margaret Lonsdale, a former lady-pupil and publicist of the "new nursing" argued, "The presence of refined, intelligent women in the wards imposes a kind of moral restraint upon the words and ways of both doctors and students."[187] The medical staff, in defending the old nursing system against charges of drunkenness and immorality, and in affirming the kindly, skilled, and attentive care which their unreformed staff had provided, expressed their unwillingness to deal with nurses whose claims to high social rank had "an alloy of self-assertion."[188] Medical men feared that the new nurses' claims of social equality with (if not superiority to) themselves might undermine respect for the medical staff and lead to nurses becoming "agents of a system of espionage" and "meddlesome busybodies" in their attempts to serve as watchdogs over the "tone" of the hospital and the behavior of the staff.[189]

The potential independence of the new nurses, born of social rank, was only compounded by the training which they received. Even Lonsdale admitted that "It is a real . . . danger, that highly-trained nurses are more likely to be tempted to overstep the true limits of their position than were the old-fashioned charwomen."[190] Medical men saw that even brief training led not only to unauthorized treatment of patients in the wards, but to a "supposed supreme knowledge of lady-nurses for nursing," and, as a consequence, "the fancied independence of their position and work."* Lonsdale argued for the separation of nursing from medical knowledge and for the autonomy of the nurse when she insisted that "A doctor is no more necessarily a judge of the details of nursing than a nurse is acquainted with the properties and effects of the administration of certain drugs."[191] In the attempt to carve out a sphere of independent activity in the hospitals, the nurses confronted directly the medical staff's claims to power in the treatment of patients, and medical men responded forcefully. "The profession," wrote William Gull, "can never sanction a nursing system which claims for itself not to be under their control and direction. . . . There must be no 'divine right' assumed for nurses."[192]

The crisis at Guy's Hospital drew wide attention in the press, and medical interest and discussion indicated that the problem of medical authority in the wards was not unique to Guy's. The matter of doctor-nurse relations, a Westminster physician admitted, "is still in controversy."[193] Medical counterclaims in the debate over nurses' independence sometimes took the form of questioning the gentility of the new nurses, charging them with "fine-ladyism," social snobbery, and lack of true refinement.[194] At the same time, they defended the medical staff's status by pointing out the fame of senior men and the distinguished social origins of the "young gentlemen" in the wards.[195] The great weight of the doctors' rebuttal of the nurses' attacks on their authority and their attempt to

---

*William W. Gull, "On the Nursing Crisis at Guy's Hospital" (No. I), *Nineteenth Century*, 7 (May, 1880), 887. It appears that the nurses were attempting to "professionalize," i.e., to escape the domination of the doctors and establish their own authority in the wards. Brian Abel-Smith uses the term without exploring the authority question (*A History of the Nursing Profession in Great Britain* [New York, 1960], pp. 25 and 27–29).

maintain their own supremacy in the wards rested, however, on their claims to superior knowledge. Samuel Habershon, senior Physician at Guy's, urged that harmonious and successful work could only come about if medical men ruled: "The physician must lead, while the nurse must be content to follow and to learn. . . ."[196] This order of medical care would, he insisted, prove that "long experience and professional science are of more value than sentimental theories."[197] Gull concurred in the notion that the superior knowledge of medical men gave them authority over every aspect of patient care: "In fact, there is no proper duty which the nurse has to perform, even to the placing of a pillow, which does not or may not involve a principle, and a principle which can be only properly met by one who has had the advantage of medical instruction. It is a fundamental and dangerous error to maintain that any system of nursing has sources of knowledge not derived from the profession. . . ."[198]

That medical men in 1880 had to spend nine months in debate over, and protest against, the claims of nurses to autonomy in the wards indicates, in part, the fragility of their professional authority. That they could be effectively challenged by women with minimal medical knowledge but extended social prestige bears witness to their lack of supremacy in the sphere of their expertise. They were unhappy that the governors had introduced a system at Guy's *where medical men are ignored,*" and the wards governed by rules introduced by "self-taught nurses."[199] The threat from the ladies was, however, a symptom of a more profound problem of medical status in the hospitals.

The protests of the medical men had begun in the narrow sphere of nursing: they called for a return to the old order in the wards and for the resignation of the troublesome new matron, Miss Burt.[200] As the discussions and debates went on, however, the nursing issue became the trigger which set off discussion over the larger issue of the constitutional structure of the hospital. An early hint of staff dissatisfaction appeared in their first letter to the Guy's governors in December, 1879: "[W]e feel," they wrote, "that important changes should not have been introduced on this or on other occasions without consultation with the Physicians and Surgeons, who have for many years faithfully served the Hospital. . . ."[201]

In their public statements during the spring of 1880, medical men restricted their discussion to the issues of nursing and only hinted at this deeper question. Walter Moxon, a Guy's physician, assessed the negative results of nursing reforms and remarked, obliquely, that "if the above considerations had been duly weighed before committing anybody to an impracticable course, there would have been no crisis at Guy's."[202] Without quite saying so, Moxon laid the blame for the crisis on the shoulders of the governors, who should have consulted the experts before deciding on reform. Samuel Habershon, too, touched at the heart of staff concern, but without elaborating the point, when he pointed out that the rules for the new nursing system were laid down *without any consultation with the staff*."[203]

At this point, the staff fixed on the treasurer as the source of trouble, and some identified the difficulties as a "struggle between the Treasurer and the medical staff."[204] Apparently attempting to win the sympathy of the governors by appealing to them while pointedly ignoring their treasurer, the medical staff neglected to address their correspondence and petitions to the executive officer. But the governors were not to be divided from their man, and they warned the medical staff of "their determination, while admitting with gratitude the great services of the Medical Staff, to maintain without any diminution the authority and position of the Treasurer of the Hospital."[205] The treasurer, himself a governor, embodied lay authority in the hospital, and the staff's challenge to his authority met with failure.

The medical men's anger over nursing reform at Guy's had led them to hint that there were "other occasions" when the hospital administration had acted without due regard for medical opinion. By the summer of 1880, the debate had expanded beyond Miss Burt and her new nursing system, beyond the treasurer's authority alone, to the whole issue of medical power in the hospitals. Not surprisingly, it was an anonymous correspondent to the *Times* who dared to be most explicit and most critical and who took the issue beyond nursing and beyond Guy's Hospital to all the hospitals of London. He described the governance of most London hospitals as irrational. They are controlled, he asserted, by a treasurer who is "an autocrat," and who is "supported at all hazards" by the whole board because he is "their representative." With heavy sarcasm, he indicted hospital governors for their resistance to "any interference from those whose sole claim to interfere rests upon such trivial grounds as knowledge or responsibility." The anonymous author explained the governors' unwillingness to consult the medical men: "[T]hey are jealous of what they call their 'authority' in the hospital."[206]

In the medical men's early challenge to unilateral rule by the governors, they had claimed a voice on the basis of their faithful service to the hospital. The unnamed *Times* correspondent, however, laid the governors' social claims to power over against the knowledge and responsibility of the medical staff. While the governors, he noted, were "persons mostly of good social position," they had "no necessary knowledge of hospital management," and, in the nursing crisis at Guy's, decisions were made "with the most utter and absolute ignorance" while medical opinion went unheard. He argued at length that sound decisions about hospitals had to come from deliberations informed by "medical knowledge." To exercise authority without due regard for the "knowledge and experience of . . . physicians and surgeons" was to court disaster. "They forget, or they never knew, that a beneficial authority can only be founded upon knowledge."[207]

In search of a solution to the conflict at Guy's, the governors established a special committee to make a full inquiry into the charges and countercharges that had come to surround nursing reform.[208] The committee sat for fourteen days in the spring of 1880 and heard testimony from the treasurer, the medical staff, and the matron and sisters. The solutions proposed by the committee indicate the governors' desire to conciliate all parties, to maintain their continued authority in the hospitals, and to prevent the possibility of similar crises in the future. The governors granted that everyone had the best interests of the hospital in mind in the conflict, insisted that none had "connived" to undermine the authority of the medical staff, and acknowledged that the new matron and her reforms had been introduced without due attention to the medical officers.[209]

The crux of the committee's recommendations addressed itself to medical influence in the hospital: they proposed the establishment of a joint committee of governors and staff representatives, to meet monthly "with the view of deliberating on any matters relating to the medical and nursing arrangements; that regular minutes be kept of the proceedings . . . , and that such minutes be brought for confirmation before the next court of Governors . . . ; and that in any difference of opinion the views of the medical staff, as well as those of the Governors, be recorded on the minutes."[210] While reminding all concerned that the governors were "the sole executive body authorized by Act of Parliament" to rule the hospital, the investigating committee called for formal, regular medical representation in the governance of the hospital.[211]

By this time, Guy's medical men were so embittered by the debate that they were unwilling to accept the compromise solution so long as the specter of Miss Burt was to haunt their lives in the wards. Some at first saw the joint medical-gubernatorial committee as mere trickery, designed to soothe the medical officers without giving them any real influence.[212] After further public bickering, calls for staff resignations, and apologies, the storm died down. Whatever their initial feelings, the staff accepted their consultative role, and by 1881 they had extended their power in the hospital to areas they had never influenced before. In addition to their direct regular access to the governors through the joint committee, they gained the power to nominate senior permanent staff. While the formal vote came from the governors, Guy's physicians and surgeons had the practical power of appointment in their own hands.[213]

The conflict at Guy's Hospital was exceptional, in that most difficulties between laymen and medical men in the hospitals did not receive such wide publicity nor provoke such long and embittered conflict. But throughout London, changes like those at Guy's were occurring, transforming the relations of governors and medical men.[214] New medical committees were created where none had been. Established medical committees gained new powers. By 1880, for example, the Medical Council at St. Bartholomew's Hospital screened all candidates for senior staff. Unlike Guy's staff, they did not make the final choice but, in closed session with the treasurer, presented their "informal recommendation" of their first choice. The treasurer, in turn, passed their recommendation on to any interested governors.[215] After the turn of the century, Bart's medical men gained full voice in the selection of their colleagues on the senior staff.[216]

Where early Victorian governors had placated their medical officers by offering them the opportunity to establish their own separate-and-hardly-equal medical committees, joint committees began to appear in the 1880's and after. Westminster Hospital established its "Hybrid Committee" in 1893. Composed of medical staff and members of the governors' house committee, this composite group conferred on matters of hospital regulation and policy.[217] At many hospitals medical men took seats on major governors' committees, and regular consultation with the medical staff became a feature of hospital life.[218]

Medical men claimed—and the lay world began to accept—their right to power based on their special knowledge. The *Times* in 1880 acknowledged the basis of medical authority in "skill and knowledge."[219] By 1890, when the House of Lords' select committee inquired into hospital governance, many of their lay witnesses testified to the growing influence of the medical men. Sir Sidney Waterlow, Treasurer at Bart's Hospital, noted that the hospital governors "are guided, and I think I may say they are always anxious to be guided by . . . the view of the medical council."[220] Another witness claimed that "In the large hospitals associated with medical schools the medical element has a tendency to have an overpowering influence upon the executive."[221]

In staff appointments as well as hospital policy, the physicians' and surgeons' knowledge was coming to be seen as the source of wise decision-making. Sir E. H. Currie, a governor of the London Hospital, advocated an end to the system of canvassing in the hospital's elections for the senior staff. Indifferent to the career concerns of junior medical men, he cared only for his responsibility to the poor. In view of that duty, he considered the canvassing system an avenue to favoritism and an inadequate system for finding the ablest men to serve the hospital: "I would like some one much better qualified than I am to judge who is the best man to look after these sick poor. . . . I would have a system which would bring trained men to bear, who would be able to know who the best man was."[222] The system of gubernatorial control died slowly, but the demands of the hospitals for skilled staff, the growing certainty among laymen that training was a prerequisite for medical judgment, and medical men's assertion of authority based on medical knowledge—all these opened the door to professional power in the hospitals.

IV

The nursing crisis at Guy's exemplifies not only the transformation of authority relations between laymen and medical men, but also the changing relations among medical men themselves. Early in the century, hospital consultants had relied on their individual relations with governors as a source of private influence—often at the expense of their fellow medical men. The atomistic character of medical power was well described in the pages of the *BMJ*: "Few persons, unless they have lived in London, could form any idea of the power of the ruling body of these [Royal] Colleges," Dr. Lankester wrote, "not so much in their corporate capacity, as in that of individuals. They were the medical attendants of nearly every member of both Houses of Parliament, and they were frequently consulted by those members with regard to particular Bills which came before them."[223] Individual relations of influence between medical men and hospital or government authorities had fostered an individualism and lack of collegiality that also found expression in the personal attacks, professional disagreements, and medico-political debates which medical men aired in the lay press.[224]

Public discussions of professional affairs implied that medical men looked to the lay world for support in their debates, and relied on non-medical judgment in professional affairs. The nursing crisis at Guy's, despite its public character, reveals medical men's growing abilities to act in concert, to unite in the defense of their corporate interests. The medical corporations at the same time discouraged public criticism of medical men by other medical men, and labored to settle intraprofessional disputes internally. The evolution of the etiquette of consultations, ostensibly to protect patients from distress, further discouraged the airing of medical men's differences in public and promoted the appearance of professional unity and mutual support.[225] Medical men who conducted themselves with courtesy toward their colleagues received the highest praise from their fellows, for such behavior fostered public esteem for all professional men. Dr. Thomas Watson, FRCP, was such a man, "courteous to his Colleagues and willing to listen respectfully to the opinions of the youngest, avoiding in tone and words all that could wound their feelings, lower their self-respect, or lessen the esteem in which they were held by their patients."[226] To the degree that medical men could contain their disagreements and settle them within their own ranks, they could begin to establish their independence of lay judgment and lay power.

Perhaps medical men found public unity most difficult in matters of personnel. As long as governors ruled appointments to the hospitals' senior staffs, medical men had no power and therefore had no quarrels on those matters. Once the powers of nomination or recommendation came into their hands, they had the choice of disagreeing and leaving the final choice to the lay governors, or coming to a joint recommendation and bringing the weight of a united medical staff to bear on the governors in the choice of their senior colleagues. Torn between their commitments to their own protégés and friends and the knowledge that medical disagreements relinquished power to laymen, the staffs of hospitals moved haltingly toward effective unity in their committee nominations.[227]

Out of a consciousness of their shared interests, the corporate leadership of London worked toward the integration of teaching, hospital, and College elites. Early in the nineteenth century, hospital senior staffs had been an amalgam of men from Oxbridge, the Scottish universities, and those holding licenses from medical corporations throughout the kingdom. By mid-century, hospitals had adopted regulations that hospital posts be filled only with holders of advanced qualifications from the London Colleges of Physicians and Surgeons, ensuring those two corporations a monopoly of appointments in the metropolis.[228] Soon after the introduction of medical schools in the hospitals, the physicians and surgeons began to insist on the integration of the hospital and medical school staffs—their goal being "to avoid any separation of interests between the Teachers and the Medical Officers."[229] And interests indeed there were. The effectiveness of the teachers bore directly on the reputation of the school, which, in turn, influenced the number of students, the fees they paid, and the total income of all the medical teachers.[230] Lack of "interest" in the hospital and the medical school could lead to neglect of duties, student discontent, and declining enrollments and income. Corporate interest in the welfare of the hospital went beyond reputation and *esprit* to the livelihood of every member of the staff.

While creating the medical staff's teaching monopoly, the elites also extended the integration of senior hospital officers with the Royal College leadership. While only half of the officers of the Royal College of Physicians had hospital affiliations in the 1830's, by the 1890's the integration was nearly total. Both the physicians' and surgeons' Colleges drew their leadership exclusively from among those who held senior hospital rank.* The interlocking directorate of College and

---

*Of those elected FRCP in the decade 1880–89, nineteen went on to hold College office. All nineteen also held hospital posts. The College of Surgeons followed the same pattern. A survey of the whole century reveals the following: of those who were elected

hospital elites protected their interests in both institutions. With power to define the curriculum required for medical qualification, the Royal Colleges held the key to the structure of the hospital medical school and the protection of their established interests. Required courses drew students, while optional courses could lead to pecuniary and professional failure for the teacher.[231] By excluding from College power those men whose interests lay outside the medical schools or the established curriculum, the physicians and surgeons gained a firmer hand over power and patronage in the profession.*

Finally, through the establishment of the Conjoint Board Examinations in 1884, the Royal Colleges of Physicians and Surgeons joined forces in the licensing of general practitioners, and in so doing won the field for themselves. The early nineteenth-century isolation of the two Colleges had begun to break down with the establishment of the General Medical Council and the liaison that organization provided. Not long after the passage of the Medical Act in 1858, discussion of the "single portal of entry" to general practice was taken up, with the Colleges, the universities, and the Apothecaries' Society all taking part. After twenty-five years of debate and discussion, and the withdrawal of the universities and the Apothecaries, the Royal College of Physicians and the Royal College of Surgeons settled the regulations under which they would jointly offer their MRCS and LRCP to medical practitioners.[232] The new conjoint examinations gave the two Colleges near hegem-

---

FRCP, 1800–49, and went on to officialdom in the College, 63 percent also held hospital posts; for the period 1850–89 the proportion was 84 percent. In the Royal College of Surgeons (calculated by the date of the MRCS), the figures are: 1800–49, 77 percent; and 1850–89, 90 percent.

*Men whose hospital posts tied them to such "specialties" as obstetrics, ophthalmology, or dermatology commonly did not gain College office; as a result, when attempts were made to expand the teaching of these subjects in the medical curriculum, specialties found little support in the College councils. See, e.g., Royal College of Physicians, Annals, Vol. XXXIII (28 April 1881), p. 20; and (23 May 1882), pp. 128–131.

ony in the licensing of general practitioners and relegated the Apothecaries to a separate and inferior position in corporate professional circles.[233] As the Apothecaries had lost their place in the hospitals in the 1860's and 1870's, so in 1884 they lost their supremacy in the licensing of general practitioners as well.*

The elites of the two Colleges, while consolidating and extending their influence over the institutions of medical life, also grew cognizant of their "responsibilities and obligations toward the profession" whose rank and file provided the "broader basis of support" for the Colleges.[234] As Sir George Burrows told the Physicians in 1875, "We can never again attempt to wrap ourselves up in proud isolation, and rest contented with the prestige of former days." He called on the College Fellows to exercise their leadership and to commit themselves to "uphold[ing] the status of the profession" by "their learning, their scientific attainments, and their honourable bearing."[235] When the elites of London medicine and surgery turned their gaze toward the rank and file, however, they faced a complex problem. The elites, who as individuals had enjoyed connection and sometimes influence with the upper orders of society, had begun to carve out for themselves a place of institutionalized, corporate, professional power, while their brethren, the general practitioners, struggled on without power, without professional respect, and

---

*The incomes of the three corporations reflect their relative status. Before 1855, the Royal College of Physicians' income never rose above £2,500 a year; during the period 1882–90, its average annual income was £13,234 (compiled from: RCP, *List of the Fellows* . . . [London, various years]). The College of Surgeons' income almost doubled, from £14,000 in 1858 to £27,000 in 1890 (from: RCS, *List of the Fellows* . . . [London, various years]). The Apothecaries' Society's income averaged just under £3,000 a year during 1856–62; and £6,341 per year in 1882–90 (from: Society of Apothecaries, Minutes, various years). For the Apothecaries' attitudes toward competition from the Physicians, see: Society of Apothecaries, Minutes, 1 June 1860, pp. 67–68; 28 June 1861, pp. 132–133; 4 August 1863, p. 258; 14 October 1863, pp. 279–280; 30 October 1863, p. 284; 26 June 1867, p. 468; and 30 June 1875, p. 296.

often without the economic resources for survival. In order to end the "proud isolation" of the elites from their own rank and file, the Royal Colleges had to do more than say the word, for the estrangement that Wakley and others had criticized in the 1840's had been compounded, in the intervening years, by the growing fame, solidarity, visible wealth, and power of the exclusive London elite. The consolidation of the elite had been won at the expense of continued alienation between the heads of the profession and ordinary medical men.

V

The Struggle for Status and Income

THE elites of the London medical establishment could make effective claims to status in the upper ranks of Victorian society, not because of their profession but by virtue of their prestigious associations, university education, prosperity, and the "paraphernalia of gentility."[1] Their successful claims to status should not, however, disguise the fact that the profession of medicine, *qua* profession, did not enjoy great prestige in the mid-Victorian years. Anthony Trollope, that keen-eyed observer of Victorian society, recognized the problem of medical status. In *The Vicar of Bullhampton*, his Miss Marrable endorsed the Church, the law, and the army and navy as suitable occupations for a gentleman: "She would not absolutely say that a physician was not a gentleman, or even a surgeon; but she would not allow to physic the same absolute privilege which, in her eyes, belonged to the law and the church."[2] Medical men, in full understanding of their position in the social hierarchy, tried to explain their status in terms of the natural order of human life. Dr. William Stokes, in an address to the British Medical Association in 1869, pointed out that man's first priority was spiritual, his second his "worldly interests," and third, his health. Hence the professions drew their ranking—divinity first, law or government second, and medicine last.[3]

When not offering a philosophical rationale, medical men tried to circumvent the issue of occupational status by invoking their claims to gentle birth. Sir George Turner, son and grandson of medical men, began his memoir of Victorian medical life with a discourse describing his descent from an old Devonshire family, Lords of the Manor of Shobroke in the seventeenth century. He apologized for including this part of his family history:

> Details of one's family are not of much, if any, public inter-
> est, but the fact that one has had a few ancestors has before
> now helped me to "bear my burden" when I have had to
> deal with either the *nouveaux-riches* or snobs among the
> well-born themselves, those who imagine that no doctor
> can be born a gentleman. That such people exist was
> artlessly shown by a little girl who, when her mother said
> she must see a doctor (my father), said "Oh, but Mr.
> Turner is a gentleman, not a doctor." [4]

Turner had a further reminder of the low social status ascribed to medical practitioners during his school days. At the
dame school, he reported, "My gentility was tested . . . by a
question as to whether my father had gone to Epsom [a school
for medical men's sons]. If he had gone, he was not a gentleman." [5] Turner could escape the equation of medical practice
and social inferiority by pointing to illustrious ancestors.
Others relied on their academic and social connections, their
cultivated "graces," and their life style as a counterfoil to the
status medicine alone gave them. [6]

Below the ranks of the well-born, prosperous, and well-
placed few, the great mass of medical men had no such alternative claims to social esteem. Sir George Turner recalled
that the image of the Victorian medical man was one of
"humility," of "charity" toward the poor, and "submission" to
the lay governors of medical institutions. [7] A country surgeon
recalled with some pain his inferior position in his community, where he was "looked down upon with humiliating condescension by the rector and the squire of the village." [8] A
medical journalist complained that "Aspersions are frequently cast both upon medical men and the art which they
practice." [9]

While the fictional Miss Marrable was kind, Marie Louise

de la Ramée (Ouida), the novelist and fervent anti-vivisectionist, was vicious. In her battle against the use of animals in
medical research, she attacked medical men at their weakest
point, their claim to social prestige. She placed medical men
"socially on the same grade with the merchant, the shipowner,
the attorney, the manufacturer, the master builder, the con-
tractor, the engineer, the banker," all of whom, she claimed,
were distinguished for their grasping dishonesty and insincer-
ity. She damned as "vain" and "pretentious" medical men's
claims to social honor.[10] In a more moderate tone, another
anti-vivisectionist denied the prestige of medicine: "In no invidious sense, but as a simple matter of fact, they should be
understood to be a *parvenu* profession, with the merits and
defects of the class."[11]

The inferior status of medicine as a profession came
partly from its connections with the "craft" of surgery and the
"apothecary's trade." Medicine's all too recent associations
with the occupations of artisan and shopkeeper tied the profession to the world of competition and profit, both of which
were antithetical to status as a gentleman.[12] Victorian medical
men continued to have the image of trade-competitors, and
laymen used their competitiveness as justification for not allowing medical men to govern medical affairs.[13] Medical men
themselves admitted that their "sense of professional honour
and rectitude is liable to be blunted by the often degrading
character of the competition to which they are exposed."[14]
Competition, moreover, implied a man's dependence on public approval rather than reliance on his professional authority.

Medical education, however infused with the developing
sciences of anatomy, physiology, and pathology, could not
compete with a classical education in the race for social prestige. It was "that worst of all educations—a technical one,"[15]
and it had no power to elevate a man or to bring him the
cultivation of a gentleman. While a liberal education suited
both the freedom of mind and social autonomy of the ideal
gentleman, the medical profession, both in its technical training and its subsequent occupational subservience, had only
marginal appeal to those who valued gentlemanly independence and liberty.[16]

I

Observers of the mid-Victorian profession had the impression that it did not attract those born to the "higher ranks" of society.[17] One author pointed out that most medical men were sons of "men of the secondary professional classes or of tradesmen," of "intelligent artisans," and sometimes of humble tradesmen or domestic servants' families.[18] If this writer's assessment is correct, medical men were caught in a dilemma of circularity. Their social origins gave them no claim to gentlemanly status; their professional activities were inimical to such claims; and the inferior status of the profession discouraged sons of gentlemen from entering and thus raising the social standing of the whole group.

Systematic data on the social origins of medical men of all ranks are not available. Records of varying completeness exist only for three groups: Fellows of the Royal Colleges of Physicians and Surgeons and those apothecaries who registered their apprenticeships at the London Society of Apothecaries. These data tend to reflect the social origins only of the upper-ranking members of each corporation. Moreover, the data for surgical Fellows include a large number of men of unknown origin, requiring a certain tentativeness as to the conclusions that can be drawn. Nevertheless, the evidence indicates that the casual impressions of Victorian observers were correct: medical men in nineteenth-century England did not, as a rule, come from the upper ranks of society. The data (Table 9) suggest that men from the upper professions, the landed classes, and the aristocracy comprised only a small portion of the profession, but the only legitimate analysis comes from a comparison with the social origins of other professional groups.[19] (See Appendix B for a breakdown of the various categories.)

Sheldon Rothblatt has compiled data on the social origins of students matriculated at Sidney Sussex College, Cambridge, 1843–1914.[20] They are not entirely comparable with data on medical men, in that (except for apprentice apothecaries) the medical men were all established in careers, while the Cambridge students are not defined by profession

TABLE 9 Social Origins of Physicians (FRCP),
Surgeons (FRCS), and Registered Apothecaries' Apprentices
in the Nineteenth Century

Father's occupation	Physicians Percent	Surgeons Percent	Apothecaries Percent
Medical profession	22.4	11.7	35.2
Clergy	8.9	3.4	6.3
Dissenting minister	0.3	0.3	0.1
Schoolmaster	0.1	0.3	0.6
Legal profession	2.6	1.1	2.7
Services	2.5	1.5	4.1
Scholar, university professor	0.9	0.2	—
Miscellaneous new professions and para-professionals	2.1	0.9	2.5
Civil service and local government	2.5	0.8	1.4
Business and manufacturers	7.1	3.5	6.7
Trade, craft, and labor	3.2	1.1	6.8
Gentleman, esquire	2.2	1.1	17.2
Landowner	1.1	0.1	—
Kt., Bart., MP (and no other occupation known)	0.7	0.1	0.1
Planter	—	0.1	0.4
Farmer, yeoman	0.8	0.8	1.8
Miscellaneous occupations	0.1	0.2	0.8
Unknown	42.5	72.8	13.3
TOTALS	100.0 (756)	100.0 (2452)	100.0 (1241)

SOURCES: *Munk's Roll*, *Plarr's Lives*, and Society of Apothecaries,
Minutes. See Appendix B for a breakdown of these statistics and a
description of their scope.

but by the fact that they were enrolled in the university, beginning studies which in most cases led to professional
careers. The largest group of Sidney Sussex students came
from clerical families, and many later followed clerical
careers, paralleling the father-son succession in medicine. Despite the fact that Sidney Sussex was known as a "poor boys'"

college, these university men came from higher social strata than men in the medical profession, even in its highest ranks. While 4.1 percent of Rothblatt's Cambridge students came from legal families, the physicians drew 1.1 percent and surgeons 2.6 percent of their Fellows from that rank, and most of those were solicitors' sons. Sons of landed gentlemen, knights, and baronets appear at least four times as often in the university statistics as they do in those of the medical profession.

At the other extreme, men of unknown origins constitute a large proportion of the medical profession (13.3 percent of the apothecaries, 72.8 percent of the surgeons, and 42.5 percent of the physicians), while those of Sidney Sussex College men amount to 19 percent, and this figure includes "gentlemen" of unknown occupation. This "unknown" group may simply be a problem of random lost information, not reflecting in any way on the social standing of medical men. However, since information loss is more likely in the lower ranks of the social scale, a large "unknown" group may indicate a large number of men in the profession whose social origins were inferior by Victorian standards.*

British Army officers offer a second comparison with the medical elites. C. B. Otley has gathered data on the social origins of entrants to Woolwich and Sandhurst in the nineteenth century which he presents as evidence for the social rank of British Army officers. His findings indicate that there were almost no cadets from "lower middle-class backgrounds" at either academy before 1910.[21] In the period from 1810–1869, 33.7 percent of cadets came from families of "gentlemen" (including landed families, peers, baronets, and the like), while 4 percent of physicians, 1.3 percent of surgeons, and 17 percent of apprenticed apothecaries came from this social stratum.† During the same period, 57.2 percent came

---

*Perhaps official biographers avoided mentioning the modest origins of many of their subjects out of a sense of "delicacy" or a (perhaps unconscious) desire to underplay the modest social origins of men in the profession.

† The Apothecaries' data are based on the registration of indentures of apprenticeship, in which the apprentice's father was presumably responsible for identifying himself. The other data are

from "military professionals" families—the largest single group, just as the largest group of medical men came from medical families. Thus, both professions follow a pattern of internal recruitment, of sons following their fathers' professions. Among military cadets, 9.4 percent come from civilian professional families, a larger proportion than are represented among surgeons and apothecaries (if the medical profession is excluded) and a slightly lower proportion than among physicians. The most notable difference is the larger number of medical men drawn from the "lower orders" of society. Military cadets were, with the exception of two businessmen's sons, all drawn from families of military men, professional men, or "gentlemen."[22] Trade, craft, labor, farming, yeomanry, and miscellaneous occupations contributed at least 4.1 percent of physicians, 2.1 percent of surgeons, and 9.4 percent of apothecaries, while business and manufactures represent 7.1 percent of physicians' fathers, 3.5 percent of surgeons', and 6.7 percent of apothecaries'.

D. H. J. Morgan's data on the social backgrounds of Anglican bishops[23] in the nineteenth and twentieth centuries are not entirely congruent temporally with the statistics here presented on medical men. In addition, the bishops represent a more distinct elite than do surgical Fellows and registered apothecaries' apprentices. Some features of his data are, however, worth noting. Among bishops holding office between 1860 and 1899, 20 percent came from clerical families, showing a pattern of father-son succession similar to that of medical men. More significantly, 60 percent of bishops came from professional families (including clergy) in the same period, a far larger proportion than among medical men.

The data on Army officers and bishops suggest two conclusions about the medical profession: first, that in father-son succession medicine was similar to other professions; second, if the profession is to be judged as to its status on the basis of the social origins of its members, these data indicate that

---

based on biographical sketches in which social origins were judged by a third party.

medicine was indeed of lower social rank than the Army or the Church.

Aristocratic connections provide another clue to the social position of Victorian medicine. First, the notion that younger sons of the aristocracy entered the professions deserves to be tested against information available on the medical profession. While there are no sons of aristocrats anywhere in the medical groups analyzed, it is suggestive to examine all known aristocratic connections for what they reveal about the relationship of medical men to the upper ranks of society. While such connections are too rare among Fellows of the College of Surgeons to merit mention, those among Physicians are more extensive. These are tabulated in Table 10. Between 1800 and 1849, a total of four physicians could claim any connection at all with aristocracy, and in the latter half of the century, to 1889, seven have some traceable connection with aristocratic families. When these connections are examined more closely, however, it is clear that they are slim threads indeed. One physician's maternal grandfather was a "relation" of a viscount; another was the son of a man who could claim "descent" from a cadet branch of a noble family.[24] Several were affiliated with the aristocracy through the new titles granted to relatives: Sir John Sanderson's nephew was created first Lord Haldane; Peter Latham's wife was the niece of the first Lord Laurence; similarly, William Playfair's wife was the sister of the first Lord Airedale, and his brother was the first Lord Playfair. Montague Lubbock's older brother, Sir John, became the first Lord Avebury. Thus, most medical-aristocratic connections were new; they came by marriage or other relationship to recent arrivals in the ranks of the peerage. Alexander Patrick Stewart, whose maternal grandfather was the tenth Lord Blantyre, constitutes the single exception.[25]

Connections with the ranks of baronets and knights are more common, but scarcely plentiful. Sixteen physicians had relatives who held the title of baronet, and fourteen who held the title of knight. Of these thirty, eleven are connections by marriage (knights and baronets in the physician's wife's family), four are lateral connections (cousins or brothers), and fif-

TABLE 10 Physicians' Connections with Aristocrats, Baronets, and Knights, 1800–1890, by Date of Fellowship, RCP

Decade	Aristocrat		Baronet		Knight	
	n	Degree of relationship	n	Degree of relationship	n	Degree of relationship
1800–09	2	m, no details mgf, "lord"				
1810–19	1	fa, "descent" no details				
1820–29			2	gf mgf	1	fa-in-law
1830–39					2	fa(med) m-uncle
1840–49	1	co(wi) = da 2nd earl	2	fa-in-law fa	2	ggf mgf
1850–59	1	mgf 10th lord (Scot)	1	fa	2	co(med) fa-in-law
1860–69	2	ne, 1st lord wi uncle = 1st lord	3	fa-in-law mgf (2)	2	br fa-in-law

1870–79	2	wi = si, 1st lord *and* br = 1st lord wi = da 2nd marquess	2	br uncle(med)	4	fa fa-in-law br-in-law br
1880–89	2	br = 1st lord wi = da 3rd baron	6	fa (2) fa(med) fa-in-law (2) br-in-law(med)	1	fa-in-law
TOTAL	11		16		14	
Summary	senior	5	senior	10	senior	5
	lateral	2(+1)	lateral	1	lateral	3
	junior	1	junior	0	junior	0
	marriage	3(+1)	marriage	5	marriage	6

KEY: m = maternal   da = daughter   gf = grandfather
fa = father   co = cousin   (med) = knight or baronet in
br = brother   ne = nephew   medical profession
si = sister   wi = wife

SOURCE: *Munk's Roll.*

teen are senior connections (i.e., fathers, uncles, and grand-fathers). The number of new peers that appear in these data and the physicians who marry into families with some title signifies relatively rapid and recent social mobility either for the physician or for a member of his family.*

By contrast, D. H. J. Morgan's study of bishops' landed and aristocratic connections reveals that, among those holding office between 1860 and 1899, there were as many landed and peerage connections as there were bishops.[26] By the most generous interpretation of data on physicians presented here, this elite of the profession could be said to have a rate of landed and peerage connection of no more than 6 percent (compared with the 100 percent of bishops).

A number of medical men were granted knighthoods and baronetcies, the former most often for military service, the latter for medical service to the Queen and the royal family. A total of 47 physicians and surgeons received baronetcies for such royal service in the Victorian period.[27] No apothecaries received such honors.† While one-third of all new peers created between 1886 and 1914 were professional men, only one was a medical man: in 1893, Joseph Lister became a baron.[28] All in all, the connections between the medical profession and the titled orders of Victorian society were slim indeed.

More telling, perhaps, than its paucity of aristocratic connections is the failure of the medical profession to draw into its ranks the sons of high-ranking professional men in the law and the Church. Although medicine did attract sons of lawyers and clerics, they were typically from the more modest ranks of the professions. Sons of clergymen above the rank of

---

*Marriage between medical men and aristocratic families increased slightly in the last half of the century, suggesting that the status of the profession (or at least of physicians) improved. The numbers are too small to draw any firm conclusion. Cf. Seymour M. Lipset and Reinhard Bendix, *Social Mobility in Industrial Society* (Berkeley and Los Angeles, 1967), pp. 42–43.

†Society of Apothecaries, Minutes, 12 August 1881, pp. 636–638, records that the apothecaries were prepared to lodge a protest with the Crown because of this neglect.

curate number less than ten, and barristers' sons who entered the profession, only nineteen.[29]

In families, as in professions, the patterns of career choice provide evidence of the inferior status of the profession. It is highly likely that first-born sons in a family had the choice of the best profession a family could afford for him and that younger sons had the less advantageous choices of occupation. If prestigious families left medicine for younger sons, such a phenomenon would support the notion that the medical profession held inferior rank to other professions. Unfortunately, the data on ordinal positions of medical men are sparse. The best information available pertains to the Fellows of the Royal College of Physicians. A survey of sibling positions of physicians whose fathers came from clearly superior social occupations is, however, suggestive. Of eighteen physicians whose fathers were highly placed clergy (3), masters of public schools (1), barristers (2), baronets (including medical baronets) (5), landowners (3), and Navy officers (4), only one is a first son; seventeen are younger sons. Among manufacturers, merchants, and bankers whose sons entered the profession of physic and whose family positions are known, four are first sons and fifteen are younger sons. Even minor clerics tended to send younger sons into medicine rather than first-born sons, four older and eleven younger sons in the sample. At the other end of the social scale a reverse pattern of birth order and medical careers occurs. We know the sibling positions of thirteen sons of non-professional, marginal, and trade families (druggists, ironmongers, yeomen, innkeepers, carriage builders, and the like). Of these, seven are first-born sons and six are younger sons.[30]

Even within *medical* families, this pattern of ordinal position and career choice appears. Medical men holding prestigious qualifications (FRCP or MD) tended to send younger sons rather than first-born sons into medicine: of the twelve for whom birth information is available, four are older and eight are younger sons. Among ordinary practitioners, medical sons come almost equally from the ranks of the first-born and younger sons (in a sample of twenty). Moreover, impressionistic evidence regarding the occupational choices of sons of the members of the medical elite supports this small numerical sample. Despite the fact that relatives of well-placed physicians and surgeons tended to find success in the medical profession, sons of Royal College Fellows tended to choose professions other than medicine.* They seem to have preferred the risk of a new professional environment to the established groove of medical careers.

Sir Benjamin Brodie, the younger son of a clergyman, rose to the Presidency of the Royal College of Surgeons and was created a baronet. He brought up two sons, neither of whom entered the medical profession. The elder son became Regius Professor of Chemistry at Oxford and the younger son a clergyman.[31] Similarly, Borradaile Savory, the grandson of an East End London medical man, and son of William Scovell Savory, Surgeon at Bart's and President of the Royal College of Surgeons, went to Cambridge and into a clerical career.[32] Cases of this sort could be multiplied and suggest a pattern (untestable because of the limited data) of sons of very successful physicians and surgeons leaving medicine entirely and moving into other professions—not the newer professions such as architecture, engineering, and the like, but the older and more prestigious professions of the law, the Church, and the university. Medicine seems to have served as a stepping-stone profession; it stood on the margins between respectable trades and crafts and the securer status of the "higher" professions of the law and the Church.

II

A few medical men could avoid the dilemma of membership in a marginal profession by virtue of their social origins; others, coming from socially rising families, hid their modest origins beneath the veneer of a public school and university education purchased by a father's success in business or craftsmanship.[33] Many had to rely on their profession alone

---

*Exceptions include: Peter Mere Latham (*Munk's Roll*, III), Henry Earle (*Plarr's Lives*), and Stephen Paget (*Plarr's Lives*). This is not meant as a denial of nepotism, but it should, rather, emphasize that uncles and nephews (and in-laws) were the significant relationships.

to provide the items of conspicuous consumption that might provide some appearance of gentility[34]—or, at the very least, to supply the next generation with an education and a profession suitable to gentlemen. Successful medical men could afford servants, carriages, country homes, fashionable holidays, advantageous education for their sons, and accomplishments and dowries for their daughters.

Scattered evidence regarding the highest-ranking London consultants indicates that many earned upwards of £1,500 a year. Sir Benjamin Brodie, for example, earned between eight and ten thousand pounds a year as a consultant surgeon during the period 1824 to 1846.[35] Sir Astley Cooper's annual income ranged, according to contemporary reports, between £15,000 and £21,000 a year.[36] Even lesser-known consultants in London earned substantial incomes in medical or surgical practice. Buxton Shillitoe, FRCS, earned only a modest income in his early years, but by the time he was forty years old, in 1866, his income reached £1,700 a year, and in 1881 he earned £4,755.[37] In the 1880's the provincial consultant, Sir Thomas Allbutt, FRCP, earned £4,000 to £5,000 a year in his Leeds practice.[38]

The only systematic information available on the wealth of medical elites consists of data on the value of their estates at the time of their death. Table 11 shows the distribution of estate values among leaders of the three London medical corporations who died between 1856 and 1928. Because real property values were not included in the total estate assessment, the total wealth of medical men does not appear in these data. The value of an estate could also be influenced by marriage settlements, trusts, inherited wealth, income from investments, and reductions through gifts and other alienations of wealth during the testator's lifetime, and thus the data are of little value for evaluating lifetime income. Such assessment is further complicated by differences in family size, savings, investment, consumption, and other expenditures which would influence the size of a man's estate. It is sufficient here to suggest some rough gauges of range.

Buxton Shillitoe, whose income ranged between £1,700 and £4,700 during the middle years of his career, left an es-

TABLE 11 Estate Values of Heads of Medical Corporations
Who Died between 1856 and 1928

	RCP: Presidents and censors	RCS: Presidents and vice presidents	Society of Apothecaries: Masters and wardens
Highest decile	£118,122	£110,289	£27,104
Q3	£ 50,000	£ 78,886	£14,469
Median	£ 17,478	£ 45,000	£ 8,500
Q1	£ 7,711	£ 30,000	£ 2,000
Range	£385,084–195	£264,789–1,500	£58,292–378
N	(71)	(32)	(24)

SOURCE: *Calendar of the Grants of Probate and Letters of Administration made in the Probate Registers of the High Court of Justice in England . . .* (Hastings, var. years). Data on office-holders from *Munk's Roll, Plarr's Lives* and Society of Apothecaries, Minutes.

tate valued at £28,900.[39] Given the precision with which Shillitoe kept his income records and attended to the details of his will, he was probably a cautious and careful spender.* Sir Benjamin Brodie, whose annual income was more than double Shillitoe's, left an estate of comparable size, valued at under £30,000.[40] But Brodie was more lavish in his style of life, even to investing in a country estate in his later years.[41] The country house and its 450 acres of land would not be included in his estate assessment, but the costs of maintaining such an establishment would reduce absolutely the net value of his personalty.

These data on the Shillitoe and Brodie estates suggest that the largest fortunes were most liable to underrepresent annual income by virtue of a more expansive style of consumption and expenditure. However qualified our conclusions must be, the survey of medical elites' estates shown in

*Shillitoe counted literally every sixpence of his income until he was earning well over £1,000 a year. See: Buxton Shillitoe, Visiting Lists, Mss. 4519 and 4520. His will, *P.C.C.*, Folio 703 (proved March 14, 1917), paid meticulous attention to details of bequests.

Table 11 indicates that medical men in the consulting ranks had, in a few instances, sizable fortunes, and in a number of cases substantial financial resources.* These data also indicate that the fortunes of Apothecaries' Society officials—who were, of course, an elite of general practitioners—fell, even at their maximum, well below those of surgeons and physicians.

With fortunes such as these, medical men in the upper ranks lived comfortably, when not truly lavishly. J. A. Spencer Wells, the London surgeon, wore a flower in the buttonhole of his grey frock coat and a tall white hat on his head and rode through the London streets in a phaeton behind a fine pair of horses. His large medical income allowed him the luxury of a house in Upper Grosvenor Street and another, with noteworthy gardens, in a suburb of Golder's Green.[42] S. H. Snell's practice provided the £25,000 that he spent on the secondary and university education of his four sons and two daughters.[43]

If evidence on elite incomes is partial or indirect, it is almost nonexistent for the ordinary medical man. Records of private income are exceedingly rare, and these, even with supplementary information, do not provide any substantial clues to the distribution of medical incomes in the nineteenth century.[44] While advertisements in the Victorian medical journals offering practices for sale do not establish any basis for assessing the distribution of income in the medical population, they do suggest something of the range of income in general practice and the level of income considered superior. Among practices offered for sale in the *British Medical Journal* in 1876, for example, those with "good middle class" patients and minimum midwifery fees of a guinea promised income of £500 a year.[45] A prestigious general practice, calling for a purchaser with "high qualifications" who was "accustomed to good society," proffered an income of £1,100 a year.† Such

*High college office might have cut income by taking time away from practice, but officers also earned money as examiners, and their offices served as a form of advertising and probably also justified higher fees.

†*BMJ*, 1876, i (February 12), "Advertiser," no pagination. These advertisements were liable to inflate income, since that raised the selling price.

standards—and such income—appeared only infrequently in *BMJ* advertisements.

Schedules of medical fees appeared from time to time in the pages of the medical press (see Tables 12 and 13). Such schedules often came with proposals for raising or standardizing fees in order to end price competition and improve medical incomes, and thus they do not necessarily reflect current practice so much as hope.[46] Their usefulness in assessing income is also limited because medical men did not receive the same fee from all their patients. Costs varied both according to the type of service rendered—from a simple call to midwifery or minor surgery—and the socioeconomic status of the patient. A very poor patient might pay sixpence for the same services that cost a prosperous shopkeeper five shillings.[47] Furthermore, a variety of factors beyond the fee itself influenced the income of a practitioner: the number of patients in a community, the number of other practitioners, the class composition of the community, the local economy, the existence of hospitals and "sick clubs," the population density of the region (which determined time spent in travel from one home to another), and the professional qualifications and fee-setting practices of a practitioner's rivals—all these circumstances affected both individual fees and total annual income. Finally, expenditures for drugs dispensed by those practitioners who not only prescribed but supplied a "bottle of physic," the salaries of assistants, and the loss of income from bad debts all took their toll in the practitioner's final accounting.

While fee schedules, in the absence of other indicators, do not lead far in the search for income information on the whole medical population, they do suggest that medical men might have had to work very hard to make a living. If a medical man made ten calls a day, six days a week, at an average fee of two shillings a call, his annual income would amount to a little more than £300. A man might see two or three times as many patients if he kept an open surgery, where patients came to him, but only poorer patients were willing to call at the medical man's address, and they paid lower fees and most often expected drugs to be supplied.

TABLE 12 Tariffs of Medical Fees for General Practitioners
(Sydenham Medical District, 1867, and Shropshire, 1870),
Based on House Rental (i.e., "Class of Patient")

| | | Annual house rental | Fee for ordinary visit (at home or in doctor's surgery) | |
			Inclusive of drugs	Exclusive of drugs
Sydenham				
	Class I	Under £50	2/6–3/6	a
	Class II	£50–£100	3/6–5	a
	Class III	Over £100	5–10/6	a
Shropshire				
	Class I	£10–£25	2/6–5	1–2/6
	Class II	£25–£50	3/6–7	1/6–3/6
	Class III	£50–£100	5–10/6	2/6–5

Night visits: double ordinary fee.
Midwifery: range 15s to 5 gns and up.
Consultation with another practitioner: double ordinary fee.
General practitioner called in as consultant: one guinea.

SOURCES: "A Tariff of Medical Fees adopted by the Sydenham District Medical Society," *BMJ*, 1867, ii, 554; and BMA, *A Tariff of Medical Fees Recommended by the Shropshire Ethical Branch of the British Medical Association*, prepared by J. De Styrap (Shrewsbury, 1870), pp. 5 and 7.

[a] Fees not given.

Another source of partial information about medical income derives from information on the incomes of salaried general practitioners, such as Medical Officers of Health, Poor Law Medical Officers, and military medical men.[48] Local variation in public health and poor law posts, part-time versus full-time status, and the extramonetary perquisites of some salaried service such as housing or meals, make generalization difficult. More important, some salaries were likely to be set in order to compete with private practice. Other agencies set salaries on the understanding that they could be low as long as they were immediate and regular, features not to be expected in private medical practice. On the whole, salaries for full-

TABLE 13 A Fee Schedule Based on Practitioners' Qualifications, 1880

Grade	Qualification	Style of practice	Fees
I	Fellowship: RCS England, Edin.,[a] Ireland RCP London Mast. Surg. (var. univ.) MD (var. univ.)	Consultants: Physicians and Surgeons ("May do non-dispensing general practice and charge accordingly.")	1–5 guineas
II	Membership: RCS England RCP London, Edinburgh Fellowship: KQCP Ireland FPS Glasgow RCS Edinburgh, Ireland Bachelor of Medicine, Surg. (var. univ.)	Non-dispensing general practitioners	5s, 7/6, 10/6, 1/1/0 for visits 1, 2, and 5 guineas for midwifery 1 or 2 guineas for consultation

III	Licentiate: RCP London, Edinburgh KQCP Ireland RCS Edin., Glasgow, Ireland Membership, RCS England (and var. corporate and univ. licenses in med. and midwifery)	General practitioners dispensing their own medicines (May keep "open surgeries" but to be discouraged from doing so.)	2/6, 5, 7/6, 10/6 for visits[b] 1s—visits to paupers[b] 4s per member for clubs 1/6, 15s, 1–2 guineas for midwifery 1 guinea for consultation
IV	Licentiate: Soc. Apo., London Apo. Hall, Dublin	Open surgeries	1s, 2/6 for visits 4s per member for clubs 10/6 for midwifery 10/6 for consultation

SOURCE: W. E. Steavenson, *The Medical Act (1858) Amendment Bill and Medical Reform; a paper read before the Abernethian Society at St. Bartholomew's Hospital* (London, 1880), pp. 30–31. The chart is drawn from a proposal for "Grades in the Medical Profession."
[a]"Not to be bought."
[b]Except when practitioner holds poor law appointment.

time salaried service in poor law, public health, or military medicine rarely rose above £250 a year for those without some administrative rank.[49]

In the late 1870's, government concern over the quality of recruitment in the Army Medical Department stimulated an investigation into such matters as conditions of work and pay in military and civilian practice. The report of the Secretary of State's committee constitutes a rare attempt on the part of the government to assess medical incomes. The data are inconclusive, partly because the committee found itself unable to extract data on the "net earnings of civil practitioners" from "medical schools and other sources"[50] and thus had to rely on guesses and estimates from their professional witnesses. Moreover, the desire of medical witnesses to encourage the government to raise military surgeons' salaries may have provoked them to inflate, perhaps unconsciously, their estimates of civilian income. Not surprisingly, the estimates of income from civil practice varied. All agreed that medical incomes had risen between 1851 and 1871, but they had to admit that a younger man in the first year or two of practice could not hope to earn much more than £100 a year.[51] After eight to ten years, however, when a man could consider himself established, most could expect to earn, by conservative estimates, £500 a year. However, some estimated that deductions for horses, drugs, and other professional equipage required an expenditure of one-third to three-fifths of a man's gross income.[52] Less conservative witnesses thought only the "unlucky" man had an income of less than £500 a year after ten years' practice, and considered £800 to £1,000 a year an average income for the established medical man. Some mentioned a figure of £1,500 a year for men with some postgraduate training.[53]

Medical men testifying before the House of Lords' Select Committee on Metropolitan Hospitals in 1890–1893 offered their impressions of the levels of medical earnings in the capital. As eager as witnesses in 1878 may have been to verify high earnings among medical men, those testifying in the 1890's had every reason to deflate them. Nearly every general practitioner who came before the committee urged the necessity of greater control over charity medical care. They insisted that many received treatment in hospitals who could well afford the fees of private practitioners, and the hospitals' lack of rigor in screening applicants in order to exclude those who could pay resulted, they argued, in loss of income to London private practitioners. As a consequence, they said, it was "not unusual" for a London practitioner to earn only £3 a week, or little more than £150 a year. One witness testified to his own difficulties in earning a satisfactory living in the shadow of London medical charity. He noted that, with thirteen years' experience, he earned £7 to £10 a week.[54]

Medical men considered their income crucial to their status. They believed higher income and the "respect" of the public were tied together.[55] The marginal status of their profession made them feel acutely the need to "keep up appearances" in their efforts to gain recognition as gentlemen.[56] Perhaps most important, medical incomes offer a clue to the degree of autonomy the individual practitioner felt. If medical incomes were, for the majority of medical men, adequate to provide a gentlemanly standard of living, then earnings might have bolstered medical men's sense of psychological independence vis-à-vis their patients, even in the face of lay authority in many medical institutions. The Victorians themselves were well aware of the liberating influence of unearned or sufficient income, and it was no accident that they called income from inheritance or investments an "independence." An adequate income allowed a practitioner some freedom from the need to please every patient, while a marginal or substandard income perpetuated and compounded the inferiority and dependency that the social status of the profession bred. For these reasons it is important to make every effort to establish what incomes medical men had.

Given the partial and impressionistic data available for Victorian medical incomes, it is necessary to turn to some twentieth-century data to find information on the distribution of income within the whole medical population. On the basis of Inland Revenue records for 1913–14, Guy Routh has calculated the distribution of medical incomes for those years. He found the following:

MEDICAL MEN'S EARNINGS, 1913–1914*

Highest decile	£1,200	
Q₃	700	Average of
		median and
Median	370	quartiles: £422
Q₁	195	

According to Routh's calculations, 25 percent of all medical men were earning £195 per annum or less in 1913–14, and fully 75 percent were earning £700 or less. The lowest quartile would include both new practitioners, not yet established in practice, and medical men of advanced age whose incomes tend to drop, but it would necessarily also include a large proportion of medical men whose practices were, in some sense, established. The lowest quartile aside, fully 50 percent of medical men earned between £195 and £700 a year in this period. The interquartile differences indicate, further, that medical incomes were clustered well below the upper quartile limit of £700.

A clue to the relation of these twentieth-century statistics to Victorian professional earnings may be found in a contemporary account of medical incomes. In 1911, Sir William Plender prepared a report on the remuneration of medical men in selected towns as part of the government's plans for National Insurance; the report came before Parliament in 1912. For his study, Plender examined the books of all medical practitioners in Darlington, Darwen, Dundee, Norwich, and St. Albans.[57] (See Table 14 for a summary of the report.) His report includes no details regarding individual incomes, range of income, distribution by town, or the status of doctors whose books were examined; all his data are aggregate. However, the employment of forty-two assistants, dispensers, and nurses by these practitioners in 1910 indicates that many of the subjects of the study were medical men in the upper in-

*Guy Routh, *Occupation and Pay in Great Britain, 1906–1960* (Cambridge, 1965), Table 29, p. 62; also pp. 63 and 172. The tax exemption limit was £160, but Routh extended his calculations to cover the whole population of practitioners.

TABLE 14 Income of Medical Men in Five Selected Provincial
Towns, 1910 and 1911

	1910	1911
Total Gross Income[a]	£139,012	£143,329
Bad debts	£7,322	£7,128
Salaries of assistants, dispensers, and nurses	£3,547	£3,565
Drugs and other materials supplied to patients	£6,989[b]	£7,263[b]
Collection fees	£1,443	£1,458
Total deductions	£ 19,301	£ 19,414
Total net income before rent, rates, taxes, and transportation expenses	£119,711	£123,915
Total number of medical men	(167)	(171)
Average gross income	£832	£838
Average net income	£717	£725

SOURCE: *Report of Sir William Plender to the Chancellor of the Exchequer on the Result of his Investigation into Existing Conditions in respect of Medical Attendance and Remuneration in Certain Towns*, 1912–13 [Cd. 6305], lxxviii, 679.

[a] Gross income includes fees for visits, surgery attendances, medicines supplied (except for Dundee, where practitioners did not supply drugs to their patients), operations, maternity and other services, certificates, public and other medical appointments, fees for inquests, and contract practice, both in and out of town.

[b] Except Dundee.

come range (consultants and general practitioners with large practices), since only these could afford such assistance.

While Plender may have assumed that the five towns chosen presented conditions typical of medical practice in Britain as a whole, there is clear evidence that they were exceptional. While the doctor-patient ratio for Britain as a whole was 1/1568 in 1911, the ratio in Plender's five towns was 1/2420.[58] The probable effect of the differences in doctor-patient ratios would be to drive medical incomes in these five towns well above the national average. The arithmetic mean (gross) income in these towns was £832 in 1910 and £838 in 1911. The average net income in these years (with deductions for bad debts, salaries of assistants, drug costs, and collection fees) was £717 and £725 respectively. Both gross and net income stand well above Routh's median figure of £370 for 1913–14.

Assuming no radical change in medical incomes between 1910–11 and 1913–14, the difference between income figures derived from Plender and those from Routh are in part explained by the atypical nature of Plender's sample towns. The other source of difference lies in the nature of the statistics themselves—arithmetic mean in the one case and median in the other. Economists Milton Friedman and Simon Kuznets, in their study of professional income, have shown that the pattern of income distribution and average income is such that the arithmetic mean income is always higher than the median.[59] Thus, the fact that Plender's average net income falls close to Routh's upper quartile figure is predictable in view of the advantageous doctor-patient ratio and represents a typical pattern of professional income distribution.

In spite of the atypically high incomes of Plender's medical men, his data allow the calculation of an average fee for each visit. The average fee (excluding contract practice, operations, and midwifery) for an ordinary visit in 1910 was just under three shillings (2.99s.).* Scattered evidence from the

---

*£80,766 total fees divided by 539,616 visits = 2.99s. per visit (*Report of Sir William Plender to the Chancellor of the Exchequer on the Result of His Investigation into Existing Conditions in Respect of Medical Attendance and Remuneration in Certain Towns*, 1912–13 [Cd. 6305],

1870's and 1880's indicates that many, if not most, medical men received three shillings or less for ordinary visits. The penny-conscious Conan Doyle described Stark Munro's father's practice as a busy one, with a typical fee of 3s.6d. for an ordinary visit, and an income of £700 a year.[60] Fee schedules appearing in 1870 and 1880 show fees as low as one shilling for ordinary visits (Tables 12 and 13). Practitioners appearing before the Lords' committee in 1890 indicated that fees of one shilling to 2s.6d. were common and that most general practitioners did not expect to get as much as 3s.6d. a visit.[61]

A further indication of the similarity of fees in the mid-Victorian period and 1910 may be found in the rates for contract or "club" practice. Plender found that practitioners in his selected towns earned 3s.11d. per year, per patient, from medical clubs. In 1880, W. E. Stevenson proposed a minimum fee of four shillings for clubs (Table 13), and scattered evidence indicates that club practitioners were charging as little as 2s.9d. per annum premiums to club members in the mid-Victorian years.[62]

If typical fees were roughly equivalent in 1870 and 1910, and if fee ranges were similar in those two sample years, then it is possible to hypothesize that there is some comparability in the distribution of medical incomes in those two time periods as well—i.e., that Routh's statistics present a picture of medical incomes in 1870 as well as in 1913–14. If this were the case, then most medical men in 1870 made less than £370 a year, and perhaps as many as three-fourths made less than £700 a year. Real difficulty would only arise if medical incomes were higher in 1870 than in 1910 and in 1913–14.

Based upon knowledge of the profession and of the British economy as a whole, there is no reason to believe that

---

lxxviii, 4–5). For 1911 the figure was just over 3s. per visit (£82,432 fees/537,185 visits). No deductions have been made for bad debts. Visits outside town boundaries brought an average fee of 8s.9½d. The higher fees came through mileage charges for out-of-town visits; it is also likely that well-to-do patients lived out of town and paid higher fees for both care and travel costs. Cf. Isaac Ashe, *Medical Education and Medical Interests* (Dublin, 1868), pp. 107 and 157.

medical incomes could have been higher in 1870 than they were in 1913–14.* First, the ratio of medical men to population was about the same at those two dates, i.e., about one medical man to 1,500 persons.† Further, our best knowledge of price indices at these two dates suggests that prices were, overall, at about the same level in 1870 as in 1913–14.[63] Finally, per capita income in Britain doubled in the period between 1870 and 1914, indicating that money expended on medical care would, if anything, have been greater in 1913–14 than in 1870, given an equivalent doctor-population ratio.‡ If medical incomes were, on the whole, lower than these figures, such a fact will only serve to reinforce the

*This is not meant to suggest any conclusions one way or another about *trends* in medical income during the period from 1870 to 1914, but only their comparability at those two points in time.

†Brian Abel-Smith, *The Hospitals, 1800–1948* (London, 1964), p. 101n, indicates the following doctor-population ratios in the latter half of the nineteenth century: 1861—1/1400; 1871—1/1550; 1881—1/1700; 1891—1/1500. For twentieth-century data, see: W. J. Reader, *Professional Men* (London, 1966), p. 208, Table 1.

‡Phyllis Deane and W. A. Cole, *British Economic Growth, 1688–1959* (Cambridge, 1964), pp. 284 and 329. On the basis of rising per capita income (and an equal doctor-population ratio), one can argue—even assuming similar fees—that medical incomes were *higher* in 1913–14 than in 1870 (i.e., that individuals had more money to spend for medical care in 1913–14 and might have used medical services more frequently than they had at the earlier date). Such a finding would only strengthen the case being made here for sub-standard incomes of medical men in 1870. Of course, doctor-*population* ratios do not necessarily reflect doctor-*patient* ratios. Conceivably, a greater proportion of the population came under medical care in the period 1870–1914. Relative increases in the number of patients and in the number of visits per patient both imply a higher proportion of (a growing) per capita income being spent for medical services in 1913–14. Under such circumstances, doctors practicing in the same doctor-population ratio and under the same fee structure in 1913–14 as in 1870 would have earned more money in 1913–14. The price index alone shows nothing about medical fees. Prices of other goods or services comprising the index may have dropped while medical costs rose.

argument that medical men were earning less than a "gentleman's" living and that there was a large discrepancy between the incomes of the bulk of general practitioners and the elites of the profession.

On the basis of this admittedly tenuous argument and impressionistic data on medical income in mid-Victorian England, it is possible to suggest that most medical men, more particularly the rank and file of general practitioners, were attempting to live as "professional gentlemen" on incomes that were at best marginal and most often well below the income of £700 defined by Banks as required in order to sustain the "paraphernalia of gentility."* Conceivably, a majority of all medical men in Britain in the 1870's were trying to maintain a gentleman's household on half that amount.

One can only suggest how these nationwide statistics apply to London, the central focus of this study. According to one estimate, there were about six thousand medical men in London, serving a population of four and one-half million, a ratio of 1/750 and a very competitive situation compared with the overall national ratio.[64] This competition would in all probability depress incomes of London medical practitioners: there were simply fewer patients to go around, and the competition for these patients would lead practitioners to lower their fees. These pressures would only apply, of course, to general practitioners, who were competing for a localized London practice. The prestigious London consultants' incomes, on the other hand, were likely to be inflated by their national and international reputations and practices. They practiced not only in the metropolis, but also made visits to wealthy patients all over the country—and some even went abroad for medical consultations.

Moreover, the pattern of income distribution common to urban populations supports the argument that London medi-

*J. A. Banks, *Prosperity and Parenthood* (London, 1954), pp. 71–76, 88, 102, and 123–124, sets a *minimum* gentleman's income in 1870 (for a married man with children) at around £600 to £750 a year. W. J. Reader, *Professional Men*, p. 192, puts medical incomes somewhere between £200 and £600 a year; see also p. 200.

cal incomes would tend toward the extremes. Economists have found that professional incomes tend to be distributed across a broader range in highly populated urban centers than in communities of smaller size.* In sum, then, it is reasonable to argue that the distribution of medical incomes in London was, if anything, more extreme than in the provinces—that poor medical practitioners were, on the average, poorer, and wealthy consultants, much wealthier, than their provincial colleagues.

Impressionistic evidence suggests that J. A. Banks' figure of £700 a year as a minimum income for a gentlemanly standard of living was congruent with medical men's experience of the cost of living in 1870 and after. Felix Semon, with a promising career ahead of him, contemplated marriage in the late 1870's but records that "I knew we could not marry until I was making at least £600 a year."[65] Semon could consider this figure a minimum and expected, and rightly, that his consulting practice and income would grow as his family expenses increased. By 1882, Semon was earning over £1,000, and "For the first time," he writes, "I was independent."[66] Stark Munro's father was less fortunate. The senior Munro did not live lavishly, or even comfortably, on his £700 a year: the household employed only one charwoman, and Mrs. Munro did the cooking, scrubbing, and other household labor.[67]

Medical men in the 1870's felt acutely the pressures of attempting to maintain a gentlemanly life style on their professional earnings. Their near-obsession with income and fees offers further substantiation of the discrepancy between their

* Milton Friedman and Simon Kuznets, *Income from Independent Professional Practice* (New York, 1945), Chapter 5, especially pp. 188 and 199–212. Non-medical incomes in the population of London as a whole probably followed this same pattern of extreme distribution. The results of such a pattern would be a larger number of very poor people who either went to charity hospitals for care or had no medical care at all. For the general practitioner this would mean a reduction in the number of potential patients (already below the national average). Such a situation might also induce medical men in London to reduce their fees, resulting in a further reduction of income.

financial resources and the status they wanted to claim. Provoked by a rising standard of living in the mid-Victorian years, and perhaps by their own rising aspirations, medical men discussed at length their crippled financial condition. One author believed the medical profession suffered greater hardships than other groups in society: "The exigencies of the professional standard of attainment, early education, social habits, and private expenditure, have been increased of late years, and are increasing in a ratio even more rapid than the ordinary increase which is observed in the general expenditure of all classes."[68] While rising expenses put greater demands on the practitioner's budget, his income lagged behind:

> It is difficult to say why the medical profession alone should consent to pay nearly fifty per cent more for all the necessaries of life than they did a generation ago; should concur in enforcing on their body a larger and more costly education, and the rejection of all trade-profits from the sale of drugs, a general law of gratuitous service to necessitous persons, and habits of generosity—all of which well become and fitly adorn their character; and should yet approve of an arrest of honoraria at the standard fixed long years ago when different rates of value were current.*

However accurate this writer's assessment of the economic facts, his view of the plight of medical men is clear: their income fell far short of their needs and aspirations.

As mid-Victorian medical men looked around them, they saw others enjoying "the increase of wealth among the several classes of the community," and at the same time felt "the diminished value of money" when they tried to meet the costs of "drugs, of medical education, of servants, of equipage, of

*BMJ, 1872, ii, 170; cf. p. 169; and Robson Roose, *The Wear and Tear of London Life* (London, 1886), p. 19. The cost of living did not rise by 50 percent, but there was a marked increase in prices from 1850 to 1870, and, as J. A. Banks has shown, the standards of middle-class expenditure rose in that period (*Prosperity and Parenthood*, p. 112 and passim).

house rent, and of living."* The medical man, "like all persons with fixed incomes, loses at both ends."[69] The difficulties of maintaining a gentlemanly standard of living led some medical men to gloomy forecasts about prospects in medical careers. One noted that "Only a very few [medical men] become rich, and many have to keep up an appearance that drains profits to the dregs."[70] Medical careers did not live up to the glittering promise apparent in a man's student days. After observing the difficulties of his medical colleagues, this medical man could draw a single lesson: "I write it with all honesty and sincerity, the profession is not worth all the trouble and expense to get into it. . . . [M]y advice to those who think of entering into it is—think twice."† Professional pride, self-esteem, and independence grew dim when practitioners had to struggle for bread.

III

Medical men and medical associations during the mid-Victorian years put forward a variety of proposals for solving the problem of medical income, and they saw these as part of a larger effort to improve the status of the profession. When the *British Medical Journal* published proposals for standardized fees, their editors admitted that adoption of the new schedules would not necessarily provide incomes adequate to "the maintenance of the proper status of the profession."[71] The fee schedules published by local chapters of the British Medical Association publicized existing practice and encour-

*BMA, *A Tariff of Medical Fees . . .* (Shrewsbury, 1870), p. 3 (for a summary of which, see Table 12, above).

†*Confessions of an English Doctor* (London, 1904), pp. 28–29; see also p. 27. S. W. F. Holloway argues that there was a direct relation between the high cost of medical education and licensing and the economic prospects of a man in practice ("Medical Education in England, 1830–1858: A Sociological Analysis," *History*, 49 [1964], 299–324). Friedman and Kuznets, on the other hand, suggest that the chance of a high income is more important than the fact of a lower average income in influencing the choice of medicine over other professions (*Income*, pp. 128–130).

aged medical men to increase their charges when they fell below the norm.

Implicit in the discussion of standard fees was the problem of price-competition and undercutting. During the early Victorian years, competition among medical men had been considered the source of low salaries in the poor law medical service. In the 1870's medical spokesmen saw fee-cutting as the source of low medical incomes in private practice as well. Hard pressed to make a living, the poor practitioner reduced his fees and took on "club practice" (another form of bargain medical care), in order to attract patients. Others, fearing the loss of patients to their competitors, cut their fees as well.[72]

The matter of price-competition went beyond the important question of income. Competition was "degrading,"[73] for it put medical men in the same category as shopkeepers and businessmen, a status all too close to the truth of their historic past. Linked to medical efforts to end fee-cutting, there were also attempts to divorce medicine from its tradesmanlike mentality and practices. Medical men heard the exhortation to remember that they had "entered an honourable and dignified *profession* and not a *trade*."* Medical associations encouraged medical men to forego the itemized annual bill which "savour[ed] of the custom of tradesmen" and lowered their status.[74]

Nowhere did medical men find themselves more tradesmanlike than in their continued practice of drug dispensing. While consulting elites, by definition, never provided drugs to their patients,† leaving that task to the chemists and druggists,

*BMJ, 1857, i, 529 (emphasis in the original). Cf. William Dale, The State of the Medical Profession in Great Britain (Dublin, 1875), p. 34, on the "degrading" and "disreputable" nature of drug sales except to one's own patients. In William Makepeace Thackeray's The History of Pendennis [1850] (New York, 1917), Chapter 2, the senior Pendennis, an apothecary, enjoyed "the odour of genteel life" only after he left off working as a medical man.

†RCP, Charter ..., pp. 66 ff.; and RCS, Bye-Laws ..., pp. 5 and 21–22. The physician further avoided the appearance of trade by not sending bills to patients, by calling the fee an "honorarium" or

general practitioners often found it necessary to engage in compounding and dispensing as well as diagnosis. Dispensing, together with the itemized bill, allowed patients to continue to see the medical man as a tradesman rather than as the source of medical advice based on scientific knowledge and resulted in the derogation of medical men's status.[75] Professional associations made repeated attempts to discourage dispensing practice, but they found little success. Patients, especially of the poorer classes, expected drugs as part of their fee, and medical men feared that their refusal to provide them would drive the patient to another practitioner or to the druggist who would sell them what they wanted. To maintain a practice in what seemed to Victorian medical men a highly competitive market, practitioners could afford neither to raise their fees nor to refuse patients the prescriptions they expected.[76] While it is impossible to say how many general practitioners provided drugs to their patients, it seems likely that many, probably most, did so until the twentieth century.*

In their search for solutions to the problem of low income, general practitioners recognized the injury they did to themselves and each other by their competitive practices, but they also had a sense of sympathy for those among them who were driven to such practices by the exigencies of an overcrowded profession and the needs of life. While they may have had only dim hopes for cooperation among the hard-pressed rank and file, they looked to the upper ranks of the profession for support in their efforts—and they found none. The sense of alienation that had found earlier expression in

---

"gratuity," and by prohibiting partnerships and suits for unpaid fees. See: Charles Newman, *The Evolution of Medical Education in the Nineteenth Century* (London, 1957), p. 1; Sir Peter Eade, *Autobiography* (London, 1916), p. 34; and BMA, *A Tariff of Medical Fees . . .* , p. 4.

*Norman G. Horner, *The Growth of the General Practitioner of Medicine in England* (London, 1922), p. 25. Cecil Wall, *The London Apothecaries* (London, 1932), p. 8, writes that the Society of Apothecaries "finally and totally severed its connection with trade and became a purely professional body" in 1922. The National Health Insurance Act of 1911 separated drug provision from medical care for those insured.

Thomas Wakley's diatribes against the exclusiveness of the consulting elites, now appeared in the general practitioners' anxieties about their economic troubles.

The *British Medical Journal* in 1872 laid the blame for the stagnation of general practitioners' fees squarely on the elites of the profession: "[T]he indifference and the traditions of the successful and eminent practitioners at the head of consulting practice are among the chief causes which combine to stereotype, and therefore relatively to depreciate, the remuneration of practitioners in general."[77] The "great consultants" enjoyed the bounty that came from service to distinguished patients: "A thousand guineas for a visit to Paris, four thousand guineas for an operation on a monarch, baronetcies and great honoraria for repeated country visits."[78] But this wealth, the *BMJ* asserted, was built on the foundations of "the guinea and two-guinea consultations which are still tolerated by the highest and most experienced consultants, both for these accessories and because they form the staple of a large income, and allow a man of great reputation to acquire a large income by incessant and destructive labour."[79]

As the *BMJ* saw it, general practitioners could not raise their fees as long as consultants continued to accept fees in the lower ranges; no patient would pay a guinea to a general practitioner when he could seek advice from an eminent consultant for the same fee. Consultants sacrificed their own health and the well-being of the medical rank and file in their greedy pursuit of income and fame. The problem would be solved if those with "seniority" or "high professional status" would charge higher fees whenever circumstances permitted.[80] Such an escalation of consultants' fees would allow ordinary practitioners to charge more without fear of bringing themselves into obviously unsuccessful competition with their professional superiors.

At times, medical men voiced their dissatisfaction with considerable desperation. They suspected consultants of the lowest forms of competition with the poor general practitioner: when consultants were found to be "charging for bottles of medicine, attending low midwifery and taking clubs at the lowest possible scale," one publicist wrote, "I think it is time for the profession to cry out."[81] General practitioners' fears of competition with the consultants led them to view with ambivalence the proposal that the medical profession adopt the kind of referral relationship that existed between barristers and solicitors. However attractive such a scheme sounded in theory, general practitioners feared that any patients they sent to a consulting physician or surgeon could be stolen away from their general practice.* The superior charm, skill, and authority of the consultant allowed him to lure away just those well-to-do patients on whom the general practitioner relied to raise his income above the survival level.†

Medical charity only compounded the problem of medical income and brought the conflicting interests of consultant and general practitioner once again to the fore. With the growth in the number of general hospitals and the expansion of out-patient departments, one observer estimated that one-fifth of the population of London had received charity treatment in the year 1887.[82] From the 1850's on, medical practitioners showed increasing concern that many whom the consultants treated without charge in the hospitals could well afford to seek private medical care.[83] Free care to those who could afford to pay constituted not only an "abuse" of charity but also deprived the private practitioner of the shilling or half-crown fee he could have earned. The medical press urged that hospitals screen patients carefully as to their socioeconomic status and refuse treatment to those who could afford private care. Since the medical staff had control over

* Abel-Smith, *The Hospitals*, pp. 109–117. Patient-stealing was an old fear in the profession. See: Lester S. King, *The Medical World of the Eighteenth Century* (Chicago, 1958), p. 232. The fear was expressed widely in the nineteenth century, but there is no evidence of its extent. At the very least, such fears indicate the competitiveness of medical men and the lack of group solidarity that could counteract the temptation to profit at the expense of colleagues.

† *BMJ*, 1894, i, 977 and 983. Whether consultants actually engaged extensively in such practices is less important than the fact of such suspicion among general practitioners toward their professional superiors.

admission of patients, the responsibility of judicious medical charity would seem to belong to them. But hospital staffs steadfastly refused to inquire into the ability of patients to pay, insisting that their sole task was the diagnosis and treatment of disease.[84] Moreover, the hospital consultants' best interests as teachers lay not in the economic status of patients but in the medical and surgical character of their cases.[85] Frustrated, the general practitioners protested that charity care to those who could pay resulted in "great injury and robbery of the medical profession."[86]

Declining income from land in the agricultural depression of the 1880's and the new desirability of hospital care in the wake of antisepsis led a number of London hospitals to introduce pay wards, where non-charity patients could find hospital treatment.* The attempt to avoid "charity abuse" through paying wards only aggravated the problem of private practitioners and added to the already serious dilemma of "competition from both the hospital and consultant for the clientage of the public."[87] Medical charity, private practice, and the new pay wards all brought general practitioners into competition with their own professional elite.

Robert Rentoul, writing in the *BMJ*, thought that "The whole struggle between the general practitioner and consultant is one of bread."[88] Conflicting economic interests certainly brought general practitioners into opposition with consultants. The fiscal questions were, however, tied to the whole question of social differences within the profession and the alienation of the rank and file from their own leadership. Some attributed the consultants' lack of cooperation in the matter of fee increases to their greed; but they also believed that the "indifference . . . of . . . successful and eminent practitioners" lay at the bottom of their non-cooperation.[89] Economic difficulties exacerbated and brought to the level of consciousness the more deep-seated differences of prestige, power, interest, professional style, culture, and class.

* Sir Henry Burdett, *Hospitals and Asylums of the World* (London, 1891–93), iv, 846. By 1893, five of the eleven teaching hospitals were accepting paying patients.

The "indifference" of the elite toward the rank and file of their own profession masked what general practitioners believed to be deeper feelings of superiority and condescension. As one general practitioner wrote:

> The holders of medical and surgical degrees, with few exceptions, speak so contemptuously in public as well as in medical circles, of their professional brethren who hold the diplomas of the Medical Corporations that a practitioner who has not graduated at a University is, all other things being equal, seriously handicapped in the practice of his profession.*

The contempt of the elites found a response in the distrust and hostility of general practitioners: the officials of the Royal Colleges, they said, "never did anything for us, and never will."† The new medical man watched his five-pound registration fee disappear into the coffers of the General Medical Council, "money extorted from young men just at their entrance to life" which made no contribution to the well-being of the ordinary practitioner but simply made its way into the pockets of elites on the Council.[90] Professional elites recognized the distinctions between themselves and general practitioners without acrimony but with no less clarity. Sir James Paget, President of the Royal College of Surgeons, divided

---

*The General Practitioner, i (1900), 553–554. Cf. BMJ, 1857, i, 14. The BMJ, after carrying discussion for some time, refused to publish any more letters in which the problem of G.P.-consultant relations were "acrimoniously" discussed. The BMJ acknowledged that "there exists a feeling of grievance in this, . . . pretty generally felt, and the cause lies deeply" (BMJ, 1886, i, 1114—quoted in Abel-Smith, The Hospitals, p. 114)

†BMJ, 1889, ii, 286. Walter Rivington, The Medical Profession (Dublin, 1879), p. 17, speaks scornfully of the physicians' fear of "contamination" from association with the general practitioners. Sampson Gamgee, Medical Reform: The Present Crisis (London, 1870), p. 10 [in Sir John Simon's Papers, File Box marked "Medical Profession: Bills," RCS Library Ms.], speaks of the injustice and exclusiveness of the corporations toward the G.P. See also: BMJ, 1857, i, 549, and ii, 612.

the medical profession into ranks of "officers and men," thereby distinguishing those who followed from those who led.[91]

General practitioners, finding no adequate leadership in the collegiate elites, took matters into their own hands. They created new organizations to serve the specific needs of men in general practice. One such society, the Medical Defence Association, was created to do what the General Medical Council had not done—to enforce the Medical Act of 1858 by prosecuting unqualified practitioners, thereby protecting general practitioners from economic competition from that quarter.[92] The Association of General Practitioners, established in 1886, had the specific aim of regulating professional relations between consultants and general practitioners.[93] While the AGP denied any conflict between itself and the medical corporations, its own words belie such a denial:

> The Association has been formed in no spirit of hostility towards any corporate body, or to any existing organization in the profession; but self-help lies at the base of independence, freedom and just principles, and it is only by the combination that GPs can relieve themselves of having their most momentous interests dealt with by small or irresponsible councils, self-elected or elected by small constituencies of which the general practitioners, who form the immense majority of the profession, and who are its backbone, have no share.[94]

The Medical Act of 1858 had done little to ameliorate the problem of professional disunity. Ironically, the superficial unity symbolized by the General Medical Council and the integrated medical schools made the distinctions between the London elites and the mass of medical practitioners more obvious. Corporate indifference and grand discrepancies of social status became the source of greater rancor in those who had come to expect improvements in their status as a result of medical reform.

The most important voluntary organization in the swelling demand for change was the British Medical Association. Born of disaffection with the inaction of the London corporations, the BMA grew only slowly in the first generation of its existence. In the latter decades of the nineteenth century, however, its membership grew from one-ninth of all registered practitioners to more than half of the profession—from 2,000 in 1867 to over 17,000 in the 1890's.* On a variety of fronts, the BMA waged an aggressive war to improve the status of the general practitioner.

Some of the BMA's efforts grew out of a continuing belief in the validity of the ideal of the gentleman. The *BMJ* called for improvements in the general education of medical men, for it "raises a man's status in the eyes of the lay world" and "enables him to ask for and get, not only more social privileges, but also a higher fee." [95] The President of the East Anglian Branch of the BMA called for "such a standard of general education as shall ensure that every aspirant to medical practice has the education, and therefore the chances of acquiring the feelings, or I might say the *instincts* of a gentleman." [96] Some believed a strong preprofessional liberal education to be particularly important because of the practical and technical character of medical training. Even in the process of arguing that "the claims of medicine and of general culture are not incompatible," medical men betrayed their awareness of the tension between Victorian cultural values and the demands of medical knowledge. [97]

Nevertheless, the Association fostered the improvement of practitioners' medical knowledge—both through the scientific articles in the *BMJ* and in the commitment to presenting scientific subjects at the Association's annual meetings from 1865 on. The meetings and the journal promoted medical men's sense of solidarity with their fellow practitioners and encouraged cooperation on such matters as fee schedules, local medical politics, and concerted lobbying on the national level. Active in discussions of medical reform from the 1840's on, the BMA established a Parliamentary Bills Committee to watch over and promote the interests of general practitioners in the houses of Parliament. When legislation on any subject

*Paul Vaughan, *Doctors' Commons* (London, 1959), pp. 53 and 131, cites figures of 2,000 (1867), 11,600 (1886), and 17,000 (1898).

relevant to the concerns of general practitioners came before Parliament—from notification of infectious diseases to lunacy legislation, the registration of midwives, the eyesight of railway employees, and the suppression of baby farms—the BMA committee labored to promote those measures which fostered the public good,[98] and in the process advanced the authority and responsibility of the medical practitioner.

When intramedical issues arose, the BMA labored on behalf of general practitioners' interests. Their efforts to suppress unlicensed practice—a source of further competition to general practitioners and a detriment to their economic well-being—had no direct success. But they rejoiced when the Royal Commission recommended the representation of general practitioners on the General Medical Council and the Medical Act Amendment Act of 1886 adopted their recommendation as law.[99] Representation on the General Medical Council marked one aspect of medical men's attempts to gain some degree of power in medical institutions and to achieve thereby greater parity of status with the consultants of the Royal Colleges. The BMA stood aside from much of the conflict that went on *within* the corporations during the mid-Victorian years; they left it to the members themselves to advance their interests within the bastions of ancient privilege.

Licentiates in the Royal College of Physicians took up the issue of their inferior status by raising the question of whether they had the right to the title "Doctor." The early nineteenth-century practice of the College had been "to regard in the same light" all those who held any college diploma and thus had addressed all as "Doctor."[100] In 1859, before introducing their new general practitioners' license (the LRCP), the College reversed its stand and limited the title "Doctor" to those holding the M.D.* When the Licentiates raised the issue in 1875, some saw the move as an attempt to raise the status of

---

*RCP, Annals, XXXI (20 December 1875), 247–249. The College decision of 1859 resulted in "considerable dissatisfaction" among the old Licentiates and Extra-Licentiates, and in 1864 the action was amended to allow the *old* Licentiates to continue to use the title "Doctor."

the general practitioners in the College. The Council referred the inquiry to a committee, enlisted legal counsel, and, in all, spent five months considering the matter. Tempted at first to reserve the courtesy title "Doctor" to Members and Fellows only, the Physicians finally took the more cautious line of denying that any College license, whether LRCP, MRCP, or FRCP, entitled the holder to use the designation "Doctor."* The right to this superior designation was left, by the Council's default, to those who held the M.D. degree, and those were, in large measure, Fellows and Members. In a seemingly small issue, the decision of the College rulers denied symbolic equality to their rank and file. There was great bitterness among medical men over the question.[101]

The governing body of the Royal College of Surgeons, like their peers in the College of Physicians, guarded jealously their status as a "professional aristocracy,"[102] and resisted as far as they could any general practitioners' attempts to encroach on their authority and blur the distinctions between the rank and file and themselves. General practitioners had long been critical of the College policy of excluding those who "practiced generally" from voting rights, office, and power in the College.† In the late 1870's and 1880's two unofficial surgeons' organizations—the Association of Members of the College and the Association of Fellows of the College—put forward several proposals designed to increase the influence of ordinary practitioners over the powerful College Council. They advocated such measures as the election of the Presi-

*RCP, Annals, XXXI (20 December 1875), 249; (27 January 1876), 262–263. On the basis of a ruling of the Court of Exchequer, the College concluded that it had no right to *prohibit* any Licentiate, Member, or Fellow from using "Doctor," since the court had ruled that "If a man is registered he may call himself what he pleases" (ibid. [20 December 1875], 247–248). See also: (10 April 1876), 276–277, where the College made it a regulation that registered titles be used in official correspondence.

† RCS, *Bye-Laws. . . ,* p. 5. Holders of the FRCS could, of course, engage in general practice, but candidates for the Council had to prove they were "pure surgeons" by offering testimonials that they had not practiced "the apothecary's trade."

dent and Councillors by the membership at large, self-nomination of candidates for the Council (rather than by the endorsement of Fellows only), and the modest proposal of an annual meeting of all members of the corporation to discuss the business of the College. This last proposal was rejected out of the conviction that it would "breed discord instead of harmony" in the College.[103] Other proposals met a similar fate.

General practitioners took a single symbolic step forward when the College of Surgeons changed its regulations for membership on the Council. Under great pressure from general practitioners in the 1880's, the Council decided to allow a general practitioner to sit on the Council, and the first, S. W. Sibley, took his seat in 1886.* A token general practitioner on the Council was, however, no substitute for the regular participation of ordinary medical men in the decision-making processes and day-to-day life of the corporation. The frustration of would-be reformers led them to rash action which resulted in public hostilities and near-confrontation.

In February 1889, the Association of Members of the College requested that a meeting of Fellows and Members be held in the College hall. The College President refused the request on the ground that such a meeting was "illegal and contrary to the Bye-Laws" of the College.[104] Brashly ignoring the Council's refusal, the Association proceeded with plans for the meeting and published notices in the medical press that the meeting would be held at the College. When called to account for their unauthorized actions, the Secretaries of the Association, W. C. Steele and W. A. Ellis, declared that their actions, "including the advertisement, were designed to maintain what the Association believed were 'ancient and indisputable rights of the College.'"[105] In a classic rhetorical move, they denied that they were attacking the College; rather, they

---

*Plarr's Lives, s.v. The first *provincial* consultant to be elected to the Council of the RCS was Thomas Paget, who served from 1862 to 1870. The Medical Act of 1886 (49 & 50 Vict. c. 48) provided for the election at large of one GMC representative. In effect, this gave G.P.'s a representative on that body.

equated the totality of the corporation not with the small governing elite but with the rank and file of members whom they represented. The College Council responded with all due speed and notified the medical press that the meeting was illegal. Fearing that their prohibition alone would not serve to stop the meeting, the Council decided to lock the building, forestalling any possible trouble. The Association sought an injunction from the Court of Chancery but were refused, and, on the day of the meeting, the buildings were duly closed.*

This modest but ill-conceived effort on the part of College members to claim broader rights in the College indicates the sharp divisions which continued to exist between professional elites and their rank and file. General practitioners experienced frustration in their various attempts to gain greater influence in their profession, and their attempt at unilateral action to hold a simple meeting in the College hall indicates the elites' failure of leadership. Lack of an effective voice and lack of confidence in their leadership led the ordinary practitioners of the College to try to usurp, by their own action, the Council's control over the corporation—its buildings and its business. In order to keep power in their own hands, the College Council could not afford to give way on even the smallest point, and both sides knew what issues were at stake.

IV

Various general practitioners' groups took matters into their own hands because they had little faith that the College elites would act in their behalf. Corporate inaction sometimes stemmed from a sense of complete detachment from general practitioners' concerns. At other times, it grew out of their failure to understand the professional consequences of their decisions. On still other occasions, their behavior suggests that they had no confidence in their own power to influence government authorities in medical affairs. Insecurity about their

---

*"President's Report to the Council," in RCS, *Minutes*, 14 March 1889, pp. 268–269; and 11 April 1889, p. 277. A further effort to obtain an injunction also failed.

own status led the elites to work first for their own advancement and the increased advantages of their own corporation—sometimes to the detriment, sometimes to the indirect advantage of the rank and file.

The Royal College of Physicians displayed its lack of involvement in the plight of the general practitioners when the matter of fees arose. The Shropshire Ethical Branch of the BMA presented its proposed new schedule of fees to the Royal College of Physicians in 1875. The President, Sir George Burrows, noted its receipt but informed the Fellows that "This document did not require any particular notice by this college, because it related . . . to . . . members of a different order in the profession than our own."[106] Burrows did use the general practitioners' document as a point of departure for discussing the unsatisfactory state of the London physicians' compensation. He bemoaned the difficulties of inflation which, combined with stable fee levels, produced a "great pecuniary disadvantage" for the physicians who had to meet the costs of houses "in suitable localities," carriages and horses, and the rising wages of servants.[107] While the necessaries of life continued to plague the struggling general practitioner, the physicians talked of the rising cost of servants.

Uncertainty about their authority certainly made the Physicians hesitate to act in the 1860's, when the plight of the Army and Navy medical officers came before them. Somewhat unwillingly, and after lengthy discussion, the Council presented the officers' grievances to the Secretary of State for War and the First Lord of the Admiralty in a "Memorial" couched in delicate language and phrased with great deference.[108] They argued not for the interests of the profession but for the welfare of the services: the Army and Navy did not attract the best medical men, they said, and such a state of affairs worked to the disadvantage of the "well-being of the British Soldier."[109] The Physicians' memorial and consultations with government officials brought what the College President termed a "happy settlement."[110] Sir Thomas Watson later admitted that the Council had been reluctant to act, but had proceeded because a small group of Fellows "who had formed a more sanguine and, as it turned out, a more just estimate of the weight and efficacy of our influence with the authorities" had pressed the matter on their colleagues.[111] The Royal Colleges acted with alacrity when called upon by the government to give opinions on medical affairs, drugs, diseases, and the like.[112] But perhaps out of fear that their status would be tainted by too close an identification of rank and file interests with their own, perhaps out of a desire to ingratiate themselves with government officials, and perhaps out of fear that complaints, criticism, and pressure might alienate their friends in high places—the Royal Colleges did not take the lead in fighting for the improved status, working conditions, and remuneration of the rank and file of medical practitioners.

The corporate rulers of the profession sometimes did not act in the interests of general practitioners because they failed to understand the professional consequences of their decisions. One obvious long-term solution to the problem of overcrowding in the profession, with concomitant competition and low fees, would have been to limit enrollments in the medical schools and increase the standards for passing licensing examinations and thus control entry to the profession. None of these possibilities was considered by either of the Royal Colleges during the mid-Victorian years. Even when the governors of St. Bartholomew's Hospital proposed limiting medical school enrollments in their institution in the 1880's in the interests of the greater comfort of patients, the medical faculty brushed the proposal aside as unnecessary.* Meanwhile, enrollments in the medical schools of London and the country at large rose steadily until the last decade of the century.† Since the prestige and income of the medical

---

*St. Bartholomew's Hospital Mss., Minutes of the House Committee (Ha 1/25), 14 June 1883, pp. 373–375. The medical staff indicated that no other medical schools limited enrollments.

†William Hunter finds enrollments increasing until, in the quinquennium 1890–94, an average of over 1,000 students per year registered for study in England (*Historical Account of Charing Cross Hospital and Medical School* [London, 1914], pp. 160 ff. and Charts 1 and 2).

teachers depended directly on the numbers enrolled in medical courses, it is difficult not to conclude that the elites of the
profession acted in their own economic interests, even when it
flew in the face of general practitioners' critical needs.

The Physicians' discussions of laws on poisons present
another instance of professional lack of vision. In the early
1880's it was still possible for a prescription containing a
poisonous substance to be written by a person without any
legal medical qualification. A chemist or druggist could, with
equal legality, fill such a prescription or could compound and
sell such medicines at the request of the consumer. At the
invitation of the Home Office, the Royal College of Physicians
discussed the possibilities of new legislation to control the sale
of poisonous substances. A committee of the College reported
to the Council of Fellows on their findings. They agreed that
stricter controls should apply to the wholesale vending of
poisons and to the sale of patent medicines containing
poisons. However, the committee was completely divided
over the matter of laws on prescriptions. Half of the committee felt it "advisable to . . . restrict the right of prescribing
poisonous substances to legally qualified medical practitioners, and to make it unlawful for a person not medically qualified to prescribe, or of his own initiative to ordain medicines
containing poisons."[113] Proponents of control also urged that
prescriptions should only be renewed by a medical man.

Passage of such legislation would have brought to all
medical practitioners increased authority over drug-taking
and the physical welfare of the public. Physicians who opposed
prescription laws argued, however, that it was impractical and
injurious to pass such laws. Legitimate prescriptions could not
be distinguished from false ones, and legal restraint might
cause hardship to veterinarians, drug dispensers, and suffering individuals.[114] The Physicians forwarded a recommendation to the Home Office regarding wholesale distribution of
poisons, but excluded any reference to restrictions on prescribing and dispensing. The opportunity to increase the authority of medical men in this sphere was lost. The Physicians'
failure of foresight was perhaps compounded by their fear

that their influence would be no match against the ideals of laissez faire and the interests of the animal doctors, the chemical shopkeepers, and private citizens.

Occasionally the corporate elites did attempt to support the efforts of general practitioners to improve their status. In 1870 the College of Physicians supported the Poor Law Medical Officers' Association in their struggle for passage of a superannuation bill.[115] In small ways they gave general practitioners, individually and collectively, greater access to the grand buildings that had once been the exclusive preserve of the elites. When the BMA held its annual meeting in London in 1869, officials of the two Royal Colleges, in a new departure, held a social evening for BMA members.[116] And in 1870, Licentiates of the Royal College of Physicians for the first time gained access to the College reading room.* College rulers attended more often to their own interests, however, and frequently entertained laymen in Pall Mall or Lincoln's Inn Fields.

Through the medium of the *soirée* or the *conversazione*, the Physicians attempted to establish and extend their liaisons with distinguished laymen. Sir George Burrows noted that men "distinguished in the Legislature, the Church, in the Law, in Science, Literature, and Art" came to the College's festivities and mingled with the Fellows there. He endorsed such activities, believing "that the position of the College in relation to the surrounding world is much improved by these acts of hospitality and social intercourse."[117]

In more serious matters of professional policy, the Colleges successfully withstood those measures which would have diluted their status and undermined their corporate authority and independence. The negotiations over the proposed conjoint board examinations[118] illustrate well the Colleges' insistence on making professional policy on their own terms. Not long after the Medical Reform Act of 1858, discussions on the possibility of a single examination in medicine, surgery, and midwifery began. Ideally, all of the licensing bodies in Eng-

---

*[Sir James Alderson], *Address* [1870] (RCP Library), p. 3. Members, however, could use the library.

land should have organized a single examination system for licensing all medical practitioners. Such an examination, with the endorsement of the corporations and the universities, would have been more than a convenience to medical students; it would have undermined some of the hierarchical ranking that came from the differential status of the various universities, the Colleges, and the Apothecaries' Hall. More uniform qualifications might have led to more uniform status among practitioners.

The government fostered such cooperation by passing further enabling legislation in the mid-1870's. The real difficulties were not legal but social and professional. The negotiations dragged on for over two decades, during which the universities withdrew their intended participation, and the two Royal Colleges and the Apothecaries' Society battled over their respective rights to examine candidates in the various subjects of the curriculum. The Physicians and Surgeons refused to grant the Apothecaries parity in such subjects as the principles and practice of medicine and surgery, and tried to limit their role in the examinations to the minor subjects of the curriculum.[119] Unwilling to share their authority—and perhaps their status—with the "inferior" order of apothecaries, the Royal Colleges resisted any compromise and finally succeeded in excluding the apothecaries and establishing the conjoint boards by themselves.[120] The establishment of the Conjoint Board Examinations in 1884 placed the two Royal Colleges at the center of the profession in the matter of licensing general practitioners, and it probably improved the status of general practitioners to have ready access to the licenses of these august bodies.[121] But the Colleges had accomplished their ends without giving way to the competing authority of the universities, without concessions to the Apothecaries, and without loss of corporate identity or privilege. Successful examinees at the conjoint boards received the MRCS and the LRCP.

In the wake of the negotiations over the conjoint examination, the London Colleges received a petition signed by more than six hundred "Teachers, Practitioners, and Students in Medicine" urging the amalgamation of the two corporations into a "Royal College of Medicine" for the purpose of granting the M.D. degree to those who passed the conjoint examinations.[122] Not a new idea, it grew out of practitioners' dissatisfaction with existing arrangements in the University of London and their conviction that the M.D. degree offered greater status to its holders as an escape from the second-class citizenship of mere licentiates.* The Royal Colleges favored the scheme, but the idea of tying the M.D. degree to the conjoint examinations was buried beneath a variety of proposals which were put forward—some to create a new university in London, others to reform the existing university. Some involved not only the university and Royal Colleges but the medical schools as well. The argument over university education in London lasted for decades, involving a series of parliamentary and royal commissions, endless debates, objections from the provincial universities, Oxbridge, the Royal Colleges, the hospital medical schools, and one or another medical association.[123] The delays and failures in the attempt to unify and upgrade medical qualification in London under the aegis of the Royal Colleges and the university reflect, as Dr. Alexander Cooke has so gently stated it, "an overdeveloped sense of loyalty to institutions."[124]

The general practitioners' agitation bore fruit in the long run, however, for in the twentieth century the London hospital medical schools and the University of London joined forces in medical education, and many more medical students had access to university medical degrees.[125]

The elites of the mid-Victorian medical profession in London had to deal with a complex and difficult situation. They faced, on the one hand, the insecurities of their own professional position—their knowledge that to be a medical

---

*It should be remembered that, aside from King's College Hospital and University College Hospital, no other medical schools in London had any university affiliation. According to the committee report presented to the RCS Council, of 16,192 medical men in practice in 1886, 5,219 had medical degrees, only 622 of which were granted by the University of London.

man, even a prosperous one, involved questionable status and limited authority. On the other hand, their own rank and file members were clamoring for assistance in raising their standing in the eyes of the world—assistance which, if given, might lead to the dissolution of the hierarchy which the elites so jealously guarded. They succeeded in protecting their elevated status and their identities as corporate elites, with all the traditional privilege accruing thereto, but the price they paid was the continued division of the profession. For general practitioners, corporate distinctions between physicians, surgeons, and apothecaries had lost much of their meaning. What now divided them from their own professional elite was their powerlessness in the face of growing elite authority, their ignoble status in the face of the consultants' high prestige, their poverty in the face of wealth, and their dependency in the face of the consultants' growing independence. Invidious comparisons between the rank and file and the elites made it clear that, while they all belonged to one profession, they did not belong to the same social class.

VI

Medical Entrepreneurship and Professional Order

ROBERT Abercrombie, MRCS, spent the early years of his medical career in obscurity. He practiced in West Bromwich for nine years, in Manchester for five, and then moved to London in 1861.[1] His financial condition was precarious; the purchaser of his Manchester practice paid him none of the half-yearly installments agreed upon and finally declared bankruptcy, ending all hope of a return on the sale. Abercrombie fared badly in London and family troubles brought him to the brink of despair. He scarcely saw how he could support his invalid wife, child, and aging mother. In 1864 he published a book entitled *A Popular Treatise on the Anatomy and Physiology, Pathology and New Treatment of Specific Diseases of the Genital Organs in Males*. Written for lay readers, Abercrombie's book outlined the character of "spermatorrhoea" and offered readers "a system of treatment in many respects . . . original, and only practised by the author."*

*Robert Abercrombie, *A Popular Treatise on the Anatomy and Physiology, Pathology and New Treatment of Specific Diseases of the Genital Organs in Males* (London, 1864), pp. v and vi. Spermatorrhea was a disease characterized by any involuntary loss of semen: nocturnal emissions and traces of semen in the urine were considered symptomatic (Abercrombie, *Popular Treatise*, pp. 31 and 33). The disease was a fiction of Victorian medical quackery. Cf. Samuel La'Mert, *Self-Preservation: A Medical Treatise on the Secret Infirmities and Disorders of the Generative Organs, Resulting from Solitary Habits, Youthful Excess,*

Perhaps as a result of his *Popular Treatise*, Abercrombie received an invitation in December, 1864, to affiliate himself with the Strand Museum and to lend his name to the institution. The museum, owned by one Mr. Lowe, was a profit-making venture. Beneath a thin veneer of appeal to popular interest in science, the museum's anatomical displays and publications were designed to entrap and terrorize those who believed they were suffering from venereal disease and who, as a consequence, were prepared to pay high fees for treatment.[2] Abercrombie set up a consulting room next to the museum and took up "the practice of seeing, as patients, persons . . . attracted into that Museum."[3]

By the summer of 1865, Abercrombie's financial circumstances had improved, but difficulties came to him from another quarter. His employer, Mr. Lowe, found himself with three suits for fraudulent malpractice. One claimant charged that Lowe had represented himself as a qualified medical man, treated him with bichloride of mercury, and collected a total of £37 for the course of treatment.[4] When the patient's condition worsened and his health seemed to decline, he turned to a qualified practitioner for assistance and brought the unscrupulous Lowe to court. Reports of Lowe's trial came to the notice of the Council of the Royal College of Surgeons, and Abercrombie's affiliation with Lowe and his publication of the *Popular Treatise* became the subjects of an official College inquiry. The Council offered Abercrombie an opportunity to explain his behavior and informed him that he was in danger of losing his qualification to practice because of professional misconduct. Abercrombie tried to justify his actions

---

or *Infection; With Practical Observations on the Premature Failure of Sexual Power*, 47th ed. (London, 1852); and A. F. Henery, *Cure Yourself! A Textbook of Practical and Effective Instruction* . . . (London, 1863). Harry Lobb described similar symptoms but called the disease "hypogastria"; see the advertisement for his book, *Hypogastria in the Male*, in the *Times* (London), February 11, 1873, p. 12. For a treatment of the subject in the American context, see: John S. Haller, "Bachelor's Disease: Etiology, Pathology, and Treatment of Spermatorrhea in the Nineteenth Century," *New York State Journal of Medicine*, 73 (1973), 2076–2082.

on the ground that "ruin was staring me in the face." He insisted that he had reformed his professional ways and begged the Council not to revoke his license: "I crave your leniency and forbearance. Oh! I beseech you to censure me, but do retain my name...."[5] His pleas and promises availed him nothing: the Council found his book "disgraceful" and his conduct unprofessional and voted to remove him from Membership.[6]

Abercrombie's case illustrates the problem created by the centralization of medical education, the technical unification of the profession, and the emergence of a bipartite status structure within the profession. While the new medical schools fostered competitiveness, ambition, and rising expectations among professional men, the overcrowding of the profession undermined medical incomes, especially in the lower ranks, and dashed the hopes of aspirants to professional success. The invidious distinction between the visible and successful consultants and the struggling general practitioners drew a sharp line between the two ranks and made the inferior condition of the latter all the more odious. Institutional affiliation with a hospital, medical school, or other agency of professional visibility had become the outward sign of inward grace, and medical men who could not find a place in the London teaching hospitals accepted consulting positions in agencies outside the establishment or created institutions of their own. Medical publication was also a mark of elite achievement and a source of visibility and practice. Some ambitious or desperate practitioners combined these techniques of professional reputation-making with the promotion of special remedies; in so doing, they fell back upon that traditional source of general practitioners' income, the drug trade. Medical profiteers and the new medical specialists were entrepreneurs in the world of medicine. Their activities brought into sharp focus the dangers to the profession of nonconformity, competition, and medical individualism.

I

Medical entrepreneurs offered a number of public statements regarding their motives for engaging in exceptional medical behavior. Chief among these was humanitarianism. Abercrombie hinted in his *Popular Treatise* that he intended to rescue his patients from "illegal practitioners" who engaged in everything from deception to extortion in order to collect "extravagant fees."[7] Harry Lobb, MRCS, author of *Hypogastria in the Male*, directed his book advertisements to all those "interested in the welfare of youths."[8] Such protestations of sympathy for the victims of unlicensed quackery do nothing to hide the fact that real humanitarian concern, undiluted by the profit motive, would have led the inventor of a new cure to make its properties known to all practitioners and hence available to all "suffering humanity" and not only his own patients.

Some medical innovators waved the banner of medical science in their attempts to justify their deviance from professionally acceptable practices. Lobb claimed to have devoted himself to the study and practice of the new science of "Medical Electricity" and informed the public of the extensive research he had done. He justified publication of *Nervous Diseases and Their Successful Treatment* and its sale to the lay public on the ground that he had "no wish to see my labours of the last 15 years entirely thrown away."[9] Abraham La'Mert, too, claimed to be advocating "rational treatment" in the face of widespread professional ignorance, when he published his work, *Self-Preservation: A Medical Treatise on the Secret Infirmities and Disorders of the Generative Organs, resulting from Solitary Habits, Youthful Excess, or Infection; With Practical Observations on the Premature Failure of Sexual Power.*[10]

Assertions about love of humanity and science from the vendors of patent medicines have little credibility. They are more difficult to assess in connection with the new medical specialists who appeared in the mid-Victorian years. Clearly, those young men who wanted to pursue medical research in one special area of disease or a single organ of the body would have found themselves frustrated by slow progress from the servitude of junior hospital rank to the relative freedom of senior status and independent authority over a hospital ward.[11] Perhaps, too, the activities of German and French medical men in the area of medical specialism provided a model of medical practice and research that they admired and desired to emulate.[12]

The new specialists and their supporters all claimed that love of humanity and the advancement of science motivated them to establish the special hospitals and infirmaries that appeared in the mid-Victorian years. The specialist institutions, like the general hospitals, devoted themselves to the "relief of distress—alleviation of suffering poverty."[13] Some of the founders of these institutions received praise for their devotion to their scientific "spécialité."[14] In some cases, however, their actions did not live up to their public claims. The laryngologist Morrell Mackenzie failed to keep case notes on the patients he treated[15]—a rather poor practice for anyone seeking to advance laryngological science.

Granting the possibility that ways of thinking about disease and new techniques in gynecology, laryngology, or urology stimulated medical men to engage in specialized research, such innovations in medical science and practice are not enough to explain why a host of medical practitioners would abandon the medical establishment to set up institutions of their own. The general hospitals of London had superior supplies of "clinical materials" in the thousands of patients who sought attention and help at Bart's, Guy's, and the other London hospitals. Moreover, these hospitals, through their policies of mandatory retirement and the introduction of special departments, were opening up the possibilities for advancement and special research within their own walls. Between 1855 and 1875 the number of special departments in the London teaching hospitals had grown from 23 to 52—an increase of over 125 percent (see Appendix D, Items B and C). Neither technical invention nor medical men's desire for research explains, in itself, the efflorescence of specialist institutions in the mid-Victorian years.

Men's motives for engaging in medical profiteering and medical specialism often grew out of a desperate search for economic survival or ambition. Abercrombie and Lobb both claimed that their economic circumstances, inadequate to the needs of their families, drove them to the adoption of secret remedies and advertising.[16] They may have been telling the truth. Medical men's complaints that their incomes were stagnating while the cost of living and the demands of a genteel style of life were rising support the notion that economic pressure was one factor driving men to take exceptional measures to bring in patients. Moreover, worries about the overcrowding of the profession may not reflect statistical realities so much as they reveal medical men's sense of the difficulties of competing in the professional world.[17]

Sympathetic observers of the new specialism were ready to admit that self-interested motives stood behind the foundation of special hospitals: "The underlying motive of the founders of our hospitals does not the least concern us. It might have been pious inspiration, love of fame, ambition, even self-interest, or self-advertisement, distinguishing characteristics which enter into various concerns of human life and guide all human action."[18] Medical practitioners shared with their fellow men the capacity for self-interested behavior.

Changes in the structure of medical education in the early Victorian years contributed to the young medical man's ambitions while increasing the number of those who tried and failed. The medical schools and the elaboration of junior staff posts gave students a sustained look at the glamour and rewards of hospital status, and many sought the same path to success. Some succeeded. Some voluntarily withdrew from the race, finding the demands of hospital life and the small remuneration uncongenial or unsuited to their private circumstances. Some held out until they realized that they would never advance beyond the position of houseman or demonstrator. Their failure was the natural result of the pyramidal structure of the hospital and medical school hierarchy— where many were called but few were chosen—and most went off to establish themselves in private practice as physicians, surgeons, or general practitioners in London or the provinces. For a few, however, nothing would satisfy but the limelight and lifestyle enjoyed by the elites. Unable to succeed within the establishment, they created institutions of their own. One specialist freely admitted that the special hospital and practice was a "short-cut to fame."[19]

Natural attrition in the ranks of the hospital hierarchy

was not the only reason for the failure of some to achieve status as hospital consultants in London. Medical education fostered ambition not only among the select few who enjoyed the favor and aid of the "great men" of London, but also among the sons of small farmers, petty tradesmen, and others of non-genteel origins. Sometimes able, sometimes no more than ordinary, these socially rising men had to stand up under the scrutiny of an elite that cared as much—perhaps more—about the social graces of their hospital colleagues as they did about their medical or surgical skills. Sherard Freeman Statham illustrates the problem well. At University College, London, in the 1840's, he won gold and silver medals for his work as a student before obtaining the MRCS in 1848 and the MB in 1849. After brief service as a medical assistant in Buckinghamshire and study in Paris, he gained the FRCS and was appointed Assistant Surgeon at University College Hospital in 1851. Between 1848 and 1852 he carried on medical research on cholera and inflammation. Despite his respectable social origins as the son of a curate, Statham lacked social grace. He was considered "brusque and even uncouth" and often aroused antagonism among his associates.[20] His bad manners extended even into the operating theater. One patient, awaiting surgery for *fistula-in-ano*, suffered the indignity of a slap on the buttocks from Statham. The medical students were amused, but his colleagues considered his actions offensive. On many occasions Statham used harsh language, his speech liberally punctuated with terms such as "bloody." His rudeness and his obvious professional jealousy led to a request for his resignation from the hospital staff. He proceeded to establish a general hospital of his own.[21]

For some, medical qualification marked their upward mobility into the lower reaches of the "professional classes." Unprepared by their upbringing for the demands of polite medical society, they misjudged the character of their new social role. Some displayed "oversensitiveness," "affectations of humility," or "snobbishness"[22] in their attempt to find a modus vivendi for themselves. Social pretensions, eccentricities, and personality quirks sometimes marked the parvenus of the profession.[23]

Even for those, like Statham, whose social origins might have prepared them for graceful participation in professional life, the pressures to succeed may have taken their toll. Indeed, the very personality traits which often accompanied ambition—aggressiveness, self-assurance, independence— could be the source of conflict between the aspirant and his colleagues. Tense social relations, psychosomatic illness, and emotional disorders often characterized the ambitious and mobile men of the medical profession.[24] Among medical entrepreneurs such problems were commonplace. Julius Althaus, founder of a hospital for nervous diseases, was known as a "bit of a dictator," not an easy colleague with whom to work.[25] Armstrong Todd was such a "difficult colleague" that he was asked to resign from the hospital he himself had founded.[26]

The leaders of the medical profession had no margin for tolerating those whose ambition or social background led to ungentlemanly behavior and social embarrassment. Concerned for the image of the profession, the hospital and medical school elites paid special attention to the social reputations of those whose careers they helped promote:

> In the breast of the ordinary middle-class John Bull no emotion is stronger than the desire to appear "respectable"; in the heart of the medical body corporate this feeling is intensified almost into a passion. The truth is that in this country at least we are just a little doubtful as to our position in the social scale, and we are naturally therefore somewhat ticklish about the matter.[27]

Specialist Greville MacDonald put the matter more strongly: in "the professions . . . it is a law of nature that the eccentric shall not survive, they starve him."[28]

A sensitive elite, guarding the status and dignity of the profession, excluded some from advancement in the hospital and medical school ranks. Ambition and the need for economic security, as well as the desire to serve humanity or science, impelled some Victorian practitioners to seek alternative avenues to pecuniary and professional success.

II

The medical profiteers of the Victorian era were those who transformed the practice of medicine into a business. A few, like Abercrombie, affiliated themselves with laymen's entrepreneurial ventures in the pursuit of income, but most were "loners" who set themselves up in competition with both lay and professional men. They used advertising, the criticism of their colleagues, and secret remedies or exclusive modes of treatment as a means for gaining a competitive advantage in the medical marketplace.

Advertising, the most obvious form of commercial practice, was not absolutely prohibited by the by-laws of the London Colleges. The College of Physicians' By-Laws of 1862 made no mention of advertising but simply prohibited "dishonourable or unprofessional" behavior. Members and Fellows of the Royal College of Surgeons had only to avoid advertising or publishing anything which might be "prejudicial to the interest or derogatory to the Honour" of the College or "disgraceful to the profession."[29]

It is impossible to say how many Victorian medical men engaged in some form of advertising, and the line between a "professional notice" or public announcement and an advertisement was then, as now, often unclear. Harry Lobb, MRCS, LSA, certainly took advantage of the public press in promoting his practice. The *Times* carried advertisements of Lobb's practice in 1869, and, while some members of the profession objected, the Council of the Royal College of Surgeons did nothing.[30] Lobb continued to advertise, knowing that he risked collegiate censure for his self-publicizing activities. The issue came to a head in the winter of 1872–73, when Lobb used the pages of the *Times* to publicize his books, *Nervous Diseases, and Their Successful Treatment* and *Hypogastria in the Male*. His advertisement included a description of his fifteen years of labor in the study of nervous diseases and their treatment, and hinted that his electrical treatments would help those suffering from sexual impotence and venereal disease.[31] Lobb patterned his advertisement on the format used by J. & A. Churchill, the noted firm that published the works of many London hospital consultants and also advertised in the *Times*.[32] While the Churchills' advertisements carried the institutional affiliations of their authors, Lobb provided his readers and potential patients with the address of his private surgery. The Council of the College found Lobb's advertisements "objectionable," but they found themselves unable to act against him under the terms of the by-laws.[33]

Lobb's case made clear the difficulty of distinguishing book advertising from self-advertising, and the Royal College of Surgeons attempted to solve the problem by encouraging all medical men to separate their professional activities from the public sphere. In January, 1873, the College Council adopted a motion expressing the view "That the practice of frequently advertising Medical Works in the 'Non Medical Press' is in the opinion of the Council . . . not conducive to the honour or dignity of the Medical Profession."[34] The College of Physicians, in adopting a similar motion in June, 1873, particularly discouraged "the addition of laudatory extracts from reviews" and insisted that such advertising was "derogatory to the authors themselves" as well as "injurious to the higher interests of the Profession."[35] These condemnations of medical self-promotion in the public press had no legal force, but they made clear to medical men the leadership's disapproval of publicity. Tradesmanlike practices injured the social status of the profession. By encouraging the men of the profession to limit medical book advertising to the *medical* press, the leadership endorsed the notion that medical publications and medical knowledge belonged to the profession alone and were no business of laymen.

Medical entrepreneurs took a more serious step in the direction of trade when they affiliated themselves with lay entrepreneurial ventures. Such action was not absolutely prohibited by corporate rules, and Robert Abercrombie's affiliation with the Strand Museum was not an isolated case of medical connection with such activities. The popular medical museum seems to have been a fairly commonplace phenomenon of the mid-Victorian era. As a medical student in 1860, S. T. Taylor amused himself by going to "Dr. Kahn's Museum." He found it a "decidedly indecent pseudo-scientific affair, founded by a quack doctor, bent on filling his pockets by trading on the ignorance and pruriency of his fellow creatures." Taylor considered the lecture he heard at the museum "disgusting."[36] While "Dr. Kahn" may have been a fraud, other museums had the services of licensed medical men. R. J. Jordan, MRCS, was connected with the London Anatomical Museum, and a Birmingham practitioner joined the staff of a medical museum there.[37]

In some quarters, feeling ran strong with regard to these profit-making ventures. The Church of England Purity Society, the Society for the Suppression of Vice, and the National Vigilance Association all campaigned against what they considered vicious and obscene businesses.[38] Little wonder, then, that the medical corporations frowned on those medical practitioners who, in offending Victorian ideals of gentility, brought discredit to the profession to which they belonged. But the museums were also "money-yielding agencies" where "high-priced questionable books, professedly of a scientific or philosophic character" were offered for sale.[39] Medical men affiliating themselves with these institutions lent their professional names and titles to the service of trade and in so doing invited collegiate censure. Moreover, by affiliating themselves with popular museums, these medical men ceased to rely on their licenses alone as sources of professional endorsement. They brought themselves under the aegis of lay business for the sake of professional advancement.

That trade and profit were sensitive issues is clear in the case of F. Robertson Haward, MRCS, and Byron Blewitt, MRCS. Their names appeared in a prospectus for a new drug firm, Sutherland's "Rheumaticon" Manufacturing Company, as members of the firm's board of directors. The Surgeons' Council could not take direct action against these men under existing by-laws but expressed clearly its disapproval of medical men becoming shareholders and "thus deriving benefit from the sale of a quack Medicine."[40] It was unseemly, if not illegal, for medical men to profit from a business whose interests conflicted with those of the profession.

While there were no rules to cover shareholding in pharmaceutical concerns, there were prohibitions against other sorts of trade affiliations. In the College of Physicians, medical men were forbidden from entering into profit-sharing agreements with retail chemists or druggists, and general practitioners who held a License of the College could not, under their by-laws, engage in trade by keeping an open shop and selling drugs to persons other than their own patients.[41] Through such measures, the Royal Colleges sought to elevate general practice above the status of retail drug-selling—to lift the profession out of the mire of trade.

Medical men resorted to business alliances in the hope of increased visibility and increased practice. Implicit in such activities was the distancing of the professional man from his medical colleagues. Some medical entrepreneurs opened the breach wider by disguised or open criticism of their medical brethren. Medical men had long understood the difficulties and dangers of disagreement and criticism among colleagues consulting at the bedside of a patient.[42] In the mid-Victorian years these relatively private wrangles were overshadowed by the public feuds among medical men that often found coverage in the press. As long as laymen continued to have important power over medical men, and as long as medical men continued to look for lay support in their professional work, such public airing of medical men's differences continued to be the order of the day.

In the 1870's and 1880's, Sir William Withey Gull, FRCP, Dr. George Johnson, FRCP, and Frederick Pavy, FRCP, became embroiled in professional disputes in public, and the Royal College of Physicians was called upon to adjudicate. In the process of settling these physicians' complaints about one another, the College rulers strongly indicated their concern that such matters be settled in private—that matters of professional dispute and ill feeling should remain "strictly *intra muros*."[43] They encouraged medical men to consider the by-laws on bedside consultation to apply, in spirit, to all occasions when medical men appeared in public in a professional role. In 1884, when Horatio Bryan Donkin, FRCP, admitted having published an anonymous letter in the *Standard* expressing severe criticism of two Fellows of the College of Physicians, the College voted to censure him for having reflected "injuriously on the conduct of Members of the profession."[44]

Some of these public disputes grew out of honest professional disagreement and the desire to protect one's reputation. Medical entrepreneurs took such criticism one step further by denigrating the profession at large and by using such attacks as a way of selling their books and medicines and luring patients into their own surgeries. Abercrombie was relatively modest in this respect. He informed lay readers that his book would enable them to "supersede the necessity of consulting a surgeon in the majority of such diseases under ordinary circumstances, thereby avoiding useless expense."[45] While not exactly criticizing his colleagues, Abercrombie hinted that some medical consultations could be a waste of money. Harry Lobb expressed implied criticism of his colleagues by indicating that he was an enlightened medical man in writing of a subject "seldom adverted to by medical authors, and universally tabooed by the profession."[46]

While Lobb and Abercrombie may have been subtle, Abraham La'Mert was not. In his book on "secret infirmities" he described specific cases of surgical "mismanagement" of sex-related diseases. He went on to dismiss most of the profession as ineffective in such cases by reminding his readers that "it is absurd to expect rational treatment . . . from practitioners, who are either wilfully or innocently ignorant of the cause of disorder."[47] Such remarks could only lead to the credulous reader's belief in the superiority of the author and the malice or incompetence of other practitioners, and hence, to the competitive advantage of the self-promoting profiteer.

The ultimate step of the medical businessman was the adoption of a secret remedy or an exclusive mode of treatment. Long the modus operandi of quack practitioners,[48] offers of patent medicines or exclusive forms of treatment sometimes appeared in print under the aegis of licensed medical men. Abercrombie lured readers of the *Popular Treatise* to his surgery by promising them a remedy available "only from his address."[49] Some adopted flagrant forms of patent medicine vending, giving some exotic or pseudo-scientific name to their drug. John Young, MRCS, offered the "Indian Rose Pad" to sick patients. He lost his license to practice.[50] Edwin W. Alabone, MRCS, claimed to have discovered a cure for consumption in his patented "Lachnanthes." His book on consumption went into its eighth edition before the College of Surgeons called him to account, in 1885, for keeping his "discovery" secret. Alabone avoided censure by pleading ignorance of the by-laws and a promise to mend his ways. Perhaps his remedy was too lucrative; he kept the formula secret and continued to advertise, and his license was revoked.[51]

Thomas Clarkson, MRCS, tried to escape collegiate discipline for his nostrum for "bad legs" by falling back on his reputation as "a Specialist for forty years" and by informing the College Council of the nature of his remedy. But the profession's knowledge of Clarkson's recipe was not enough. When he continued to insert his patent remedy advertisements in the public press, the Council agreed that they were derogatory and disgraceful and voted his removal from Membership.[52]

Secret remedies violated professional standards of behavior; in offering a secret remedy, a medical man was acting like a quack. Medical quackery was not, it would seem, primarily a matter of the qualifications of the patent medicine vendor, the efficacy of the cure, or the intention to deceive patients.* The Royal Colleges, when investigating medical men who advertised secret cures, never inquired into a practitioner's belief in the cure, nor did they subject a patent rem-

---

*That efficacy was irrelevant is suggested by the refusal of the College of Physicians to evaluate patent medicine when asked to do so by the Foreign Office or the War Office. See: RCP, Annals, XXVIII (22 December 1864), 229–230; and XXIX (6 January 1869), 319–320. Deceit is an integral part of dictionary definitions of quackery and is central in discussions such as: James H. Young, *The Toadstool Millionaires. A Social History of Patent Medicines in America before Federal Regulation* (Princeton, N.J., 1961), e.g., pp. 167–168; Eric Jameson, *The Natural History of Quackery* (London, 1961), p. 14; Walter Rivington, *The Medical Profession* (Dublin, 1879), p. 79; and Forbes Winslow, *Physic and Physicians* (London, 1839), i, 305.

edy to chemical analysis to ascertain its curative properties. The essence of quackery was tradesmanship.* And secret remedies in the hands of licensed medical men threatened to bring the profession back to the world of trade. The dispenser of a secret cure encouraged his patients to view him as a shopkeeper rather than as a source of diagnosis and advice. The ideal of the liberally-educated medical consultant was thus undermined by the tradesman's tactics of those practitioners who offered nostrums for sale. The fathers of the profession spoke their minds when they condemned such a practice as derogatory to the status and dignity of the profession.[53]

At another level, patent medicines raised the issue of professional cohesion versus trade competition. The secret remedy gave a single practitioner presumed advantage in the eyes of the public, for he had sole monopoly over the power to cure leg ulcers, spermatorrhea, or consumption. Shared professional knowledge—and therefore corporate solidarity—was undermined by an individual practitioner's search for profit in the health care marketplace. Medical individualism in the form of patent medicines, advertising, and public criticism of colleagues all militated against the construction and maintenance of the corporate cooperation and discipline that differentiated professional men from businessmen.

Finally, the peddling of secret remedies undermined the authority of the profession over practitioners and patients alike. Secret remedies, by their very nature, were not subject to the scrutiny and evaluation of medical colleagues. Equally serious, the power to judge was placed in the hands of the buying public. Pamphlets and books addressed to lay readers appealed to them, rather than their medical man, to judge the virtue of a patent drug. Printed testimonials bore further witness to the authority of the public to judge the medical man's

---

*The derivations of the words "quack," "charlatan," and "mountebank" all point to their origins in the practice of "crying out in the market place." See, e.g., *Webster's New World Dictionary of the English Language*.

work. While hospital consultants and poor law medical men alike were seeking to establish an arena of independence and power for themselves as professional men, the licensed practitioner who offered a patent remedy was selling away professional autonomy for the sake of trade profit.

Medical men who attempted to use the avenue of trade to achieve some form of "professional" survival or success may have attained their pecuniary goals. Many paid a price, however, in their ultimate isolation from the profession to which they belonged. The Royal Colleges, in conjunction with the General Medical Council, removed their names from the *Medical Register*. These practitioners had broken rank by engaging in competition with their fellow-professionals. They had turned to the public as the primary source of judgment on their practice. The profession, working toward independence and laboring to lift its coattails out of the mud of trade, made these men outcasts from their ranks. They took a lone path, and the medical elites made their isolation from the profession a legal reality.

III

A second group of medical entrepreneurs made their appearance in large numbers in the mid-Victorian years. These men, unlike the medical profiteers, eschewed business and trade, and all the commercial activities that those involved. Unlike the profiteers, they did not operate alone. Their primary form of "medical enterprise"[54] was the hospital, and in establishing these charity institutions they affiliated themselves with other professional men and with laymen as well. Their attempts to make names for themselves involved a form of self-advertising, it is true, but by imitating the elites of the London medical establishment in associating themselves with charity medicine, they followed an accepted pattern of reputation-building. A few of these Victorian hospital entrepreneurs established new general hospitals, but the great majority sought a professional place in the sun through the vehicle of medical specialization.

Specialism was not new in the mid-Victorian era. Some forms of special practice were carried on in classical times and in England in the sixteenth century.[55] In the eighteenth century, unlicensed practitioners who engaged in bonesetting, dentistry, oculism, and the like were also considered specialists.[56] These early specialties developed outside the medical establishment in areas of little interest to qualified practitioners. In the late eighteenth and early nineteenth centuries, a few medical men began to encroach on the territories of unqualified practitioners, particularly the oculists and midwives, and began to practice as ophthalmic surgeons and accoucheurs.[57] Qualified medical men served in the new hospitals and infirmaries that appeared in this period to care for those charity patients that the voluntary hospitals of London refused to accept—maternity cases, venereal disease victims, incurables, the insane, fever cases, and the like.[58] These charity establishments managed to live amicably alongside the great general hospitals of London, perhaps because their functions complemented one another.

Unlicensed practice in such fields as oculism and bonesetting, together with the "specialist" claims of some quack practitioners, gave mid-Victorian specialism an unsavory character in the eyes of some medical observers. It smacked of self-promotion and the profit motive.[59] The new specialists, however mixed their motives might have been, could point to developments in France and Germany as a scientific justification for specializing.[60] They could also point to the private practices of eminent London consultants—many of whom built their careers on their knowledge or experience of a single disease—as "veiled specialism."[61]

The crucial difference between quack "specialists," early forms of qualified specialism, the "veiled specialism" of London consultants, and the new specialties of mid-Victorian England was that the latter involved the development and elaboration of institutions—hospitals, societies, and journals—devoted to their subject. Moreover, their stated goal went beyond caretaking to the advancement of knowledge and innovation in the treatment of specific organs. The mid-Victorian age saw an explosion of these specialist institutions at a rate unmatched in previous eras.

Of those special hospitals established in London before

1800, twelve survived to the middle of the nineteenth century. During the first half of the nineteenth century, special hospitals appeared at the rate of about five per decade. During the period 1850 to 1890, the pace more than doubled, at least twelve new specialist charities appearing in each decade. The high point of special hospital growth came in the 1860's, when twenty-two new institutions devoted to the treatment of special disorders appeared in the metropolis. (See Table 15 for details.)

Unlike most of the great general hospitals of London, these new establishments owed their existence in great measure to the initiative of medical men. For example, Charles West, a staff member at the Royal Universal Dispensary for Children, tried to convert the dispensary into an in-patient institution. When he failed, he decided to create a hospital for sick children elsewhere. He joined forces with Henry Bence Jones, FRCP, and together they began plans for the Great Ormond Street Hospital for Children.[62] John Laws Milton, MRCS, author of a work on spermatorrhea, established St. John's Hospital for Diseases of the Skin in 1863.[63]

Many of these new institutions were small and hence involved relatively minor costs in their foundation. Morrell Mackenzie, in establishing his throat hospital in the 1860's, looked for a house in a neighborhood where charity care was likely to be welcome—and competition from an established institution minimal. He rented a house in King Street, set aside two rooms for the medical charity, and sublet the remainder. A sign on the outside of the building, seating accommodations for patients inside, and a few basic instruments and drugs completed the preparations for opening the facility to out-patients.[64] While the new institutions called themselves hospitals, some had no facilities for in-patient care in their early years. St. John's Hospital had no beds and treated skin diseases only on an out-patient basis during the first three years of its existence. In 1866 three beds were installed, and in the next year the number increased to twelve.[65] St. Peter's Hospital for Stone, although primarily devoted to the surgical treatment of kidney disorders, did not have an operating theater for the first nine years of its existence.[66]

TABLE 15 The Foundation of Specialist Charity Hospitals, Dispensaries, and Infirmaries in London and Great Britain to 1890

Subject[a]	Before 1800	1800–1849	1850–1859	1860–1869	1870–1879	1880–1889	Total
Smallpox	1	—	—	—	1	—	2
V.D.	1	—	—	1	—	—	2
Insanity[b]	2	—	—	1	—	—	3
Nervous diseases	—	—	2	1	1	1	5
Fever[b]	—	1	—	—	—	—	1
Maternity, lying-in	7	—	—	2	—	2	11
Women	—	2	1	—	4	—	7
Women and children	—	2	1	3	1	2	9
Children	—	—	1	4	2	4	11
Truss	1	2	—	1	—	—	4
Urinary, rectal	—	1	—	1	—	1	3
Vaccine	—	2	—	—	—	—	2
Glandular disease	—	1	—	—	—	—	1
Chest diseases, TB	—	4	—	2	—	—	6
Eye	—	5	2	—	—	—	7
Skin	—	1	2	3	—	1	7
Ear	—	1	—	—	—	—	1
Ear and throat	—	1	—	—	3	—	4

Throat	—	—	—	2	—	1	3
Orthopedic	—	3	1	1	—	—	5
Cancer	—	1	1	—	—	—	1
Leg diseases	—	—	1	—	—	—	1
Accident	—	—	1	1	—	—	1
Dental	—	—	—	—	—	—	2
Mixed[d]	—	—	—	—	1	—	1
TOTAL LONDON	12	27	14	22	13	12	100
Provincial Special Hospitals	unknown	22	12	12	13	17	76
Scotland, Ireland, Wales	unknown	8	1	6	12	7	34
TOTAL GREAT BRITAIN	12	47	27	40	38	36	210

NOTE: Not all hospitals founded in this period survived to 1890.

SOURCES: Low's *Handbook of Charities*, 1855–1895; and R. Kershaw, *Special Hospitals*, Ch. 2. Because of the lack of information regarding early nineteenth-century foundations, all hospitals listed as founded before 1850 are those which survived until at least 1855.

[a] Subject as indicated in hospital name. It is not always clear, for example, that a women's hospital is a gynecological hospital or just a hospital for women with any illness.

[b] Not including government hospitals for lunatics and fever cases.

[c] For children only.

[d] St. Savior's Hospital (for "cancer, paralysis, . . . nervous diseases, throat, etc.").

Early publicity was an important step in setting a new charity on its feet. The hospital sign, together with handbills and newspaper notices, informed the ailing public of the availability of charity medical care for kidney stones, skin disorders, throat afflictions, or whatever other special problem the new hospital would treat.[67] The success of the hospital depended on effective patient recruitment. Growing numbers of patients provided "clinical materials" for the specialist, offered evidence of the utility of the charity, and justified its claim to public support. Initially, funds for these new enterprises might come from the medical man's own pocketbook, but, like the older hospitals, the special charities depended on philanthropy for their operating expenses.[68]

Following the example of the general hospitals, the new hospitals sought the support of charitable laymen. Charles West and Henry Bence Jones enlisted the help of the Hon. J. W. Percy, Mr. J. Hoare, Captain Holland, Rev. W. Niven, and others in the early stages of planning their hospital for children.[69] The National Hospital, Queen Square, established to treat nervous diseases, enjoyed the patronage of Lord Halsbury, Members of Parliament, and influential City businessmen.[70] The Duke of Marlborough became a patron of S. F. Statham's creation, the Great Northern Hospital, and the Princess Royal gave her patronage to the Royal London Eye Hospital.[71] The support of eminent people served as a guarantee of good management and thus a source of public confidence and continued support.[72] Lay patrons served on the hospital's board of management, made individual contributions to the charity, and sponsored fund-raising events to draw additional support from the public. By the 1870's the number of benefit events for specialist charities had proliferated to such a degree that *Punch* carried a tasteless joke about fashionable people going to the "Throat and Ear Ball" and the "Epileptic Dance."[73]

The response of the public was, in short, enthusiastic. As early as 1861, Sir William Gull observed the existence of a "popular prejudice for specialists."[74] Patients sought help from these institutions, first by the hundreds, then by the thousands. Charitable donors subscribed to the growing number of specialist hospitals, and many could claim income of several thousands of pounds each year. Even when the agricultural depression of the 1880's brought a decline in the incomes of the general hospitals, many of the new specialist establishments could boast increasing annual revenues from their supporters.[75]

Founders of special hospitals did not neglect to enlist cooperation and assistance from their medical brethren. John Milton invited Erasmus Wilson, Tilbury Fox, and J. Mill Brodsham to serve on the staff of St. John's Hospital for Skin Diseases.[76] Julius Althaus, the founder of the Maida Vale Hospital for Nervous Diseases, served as the hospital's sole physician for a brief time after establishment in 1866, but soon Dr. Benjamin Richardson joined the staff as Assistant Physician, and a dental surgeon was appointed as well. When Edward Meryon joined the Maida Vale staff, he did not bring a distinguished medical reputation, but his degrees—M.D. (London) and FRCP—his membership at the Athenaeum, and his popularity added luster to the struggling institution.[77]

In a rather acid report on activities at St. John's Hospital for Diseases of the Skin, the *BMJ* noted in 1864 that:

> The medical staff and their supporters, properly wise in their generation, show a knowledge of the means by which success is to be sought in the present day. A saint lends his name. A large room at the Westminster Palace Hotel is engaged for the opening lecture; the attractions of a conversazione are added; and a numerous company invited.[78]

The *BMJ*'s sketch suggests what a careful analysis of specialist foundations makes clear—that these new hospitals and their founders followed the path laid down before them in the development of the great general hospitals of London. By conscious or unconscious imitation, St. Bartholomew's Hospital and St. Mary's Hospital shared the task of charity medicine with the newly founded St. John's Hospital for Diseases of the Skin and St. Peter's Hospital for Stone. Like the endowed hospitals, the special hospitals recruited wide support from the upper ranks of society. Social events, laid on by the ancient hospitals and the Royal Colleges to bring medical men and laymen together, were also a vehicle for the specialists to mix with charitable donors.

The specialist hospitals did not serve their founders' and associates' pecuniary needs directly. Like consultants at the general hospitals, the senior staffs at these new institutions might receive small honoraria but otherwise earned no income for their service. The career benefits of the special hospital were the institutional connections and professional visibility they provided. Success did not always follow. J. Z. Lawrence, founder in 1857 of the London Eye Hospital and considered by some to have produced excellent work on ophthalmology, endocrinology, and genetics, never achieved fame or financial success. R. B. Carter, on the other hand, went from a "conspicuously unsuccessful" career in general practice to prosperity in his ophthalmic specialty.[79] The most dazzling success in special practice was Morrell Mackenzie. Founder of the Golden Square Hospital for Throat Diseases, he built the hospital into a successful venture and enlarged his private practice as well. He treated the well-known figures of the Victorian stage and eventually enjoyed an appointment as medical adviser to the royal family and the honor of a knighthood.[80]

One goal of specialist activities was the development of a sphere of medical repute, and in this effort the new specialists did not stop with the establishment of special hospitals. Through the media of specialist medical societies and specialist journals, the medical entrepreneurs sought to create instruments for publicizing their own work and to gather around them the support of like-minded colleagues.[81] The special hospital often provided a base and a nucleus of medical men who became the founding members of a specialist society. The Ophthalmic Society of the United Kingdom grew out of the Moorfields Club established at the eye hospital.[82] Similarly, St. John's Hospital for Skin Diseases fostered the establishment of more than one dermatological society. The first, the Willan Society, devoted to dermatology and syphilis, appeared in 1883 and lasted less than a year. Another attempt in 1911 led to the foundation of the London Dermatological Society.[83] Medical men employed in the older "special" hospitals devoted to the care of the mentally ill under the aegis of the government, organized themselves as the Association of Officers of Hospitals for the Insane in 1841. By 1857 their perspectives and goals had shifted from the fact of their employment to the specialist and scientific aspirations of their practice, and they changed the name of their society to the Medico-Psychological Association and renamed their periodical the *Journal of Mental Science*.[84] The evolution of obstetrics out of maternity and lying-in hospital practice represents a similar transformation.[85] The first specialist society appeared in the 1820's, and a handful arose in the decades after 1850. The great era of specialist society formation came in the decade of the 1880's, when six new associations devoted to specialist interests appeared. (See Table 16 for details.)

In order to succeed, a specialist society required high interest in a single locale, while a specialist periodical could draw on a national audience. Periodicals had the disadvantage, however, of requiring a strong base of professional support from subscribers and authors in order to survive. Hence, they often had a patchier history than did societies devoted to special diseases. The first periodical devoted to skin diseases appeared in the 1860's and survived for nearly a decade. A second dermatology journal appeared in 1873 but died almost immediately. Only the third attempt, the *British Journal of Dermatology*, founded in 1888, survived into the twentieth century.[86] Specialist periodicals sometimes grew out of the activities of a society—as in the case of the *Journal of Mental Science*—and at other times were produced at the initiative of one specialist. J. Z. Lawrence, the ophthalmologist, for example, founded the *Ophthalmic Review* in 1864 and published some of his own writings in its pages.[87] Specialist periodicals began to appear with some regularity in the 1840's. The 1870's and 1890's were peak periods in the appearance of new publications addressed to specialists. (For details see Table 17.)

Not all specialist enterprises led to the elaboration of modern specialties. One early establishment, St. John's Hospital for Diseases of the Eyes, Legs, and Breasts, led to nothing but a poor reputation for its founder.[88] The Dispensary for

TABLE 16 The Foundation of Medical Societies in London, 1800–1900

Types of Organizations and Societies	Before 1800	1800–1809	1810–1819	1820–1829	1830–1839	1840–1849	1850–1859	1860–1869	1870–1879	1880–1889	1890–1899
General	5	2	1	1	2	1	1	4	—	3	2
Medical school and graduates	3	—	—	2	1	—	2	3	2	1	—
Self-help	1	—	—	—	—	—	1	1	2	—	1
Regional	—	—	—	—	1	1	3	4	—	1	7
Occupational[a]	1	—	—	—	—	1	2	2	2	3	2
Specialist[b]	—	—	—	1	—	—	3	—	2	6	3
Other special interest[c]	—	—	—	—	—	1	1	—	4	3	2

SOURCES: *Medical Institutions of London* (London, 1895); Samuel D. Clippingdale, Medical Court Roll, Vol. 1, typescript (n.d.); and *London and Provincial Medical Directory*, various years.

[a] In their order of appearance, societies of Naval Surgeons, Medical Officers of Hospitals for the Insane, Medical Officers of Health, Army Medical Officers, Medical Teachers Association, Poor Law Medical Officers, Medical Officers of Schools, Infirmary Superintendents, Metropolitan Police Surgeons, Police Surgeons, Public Vaccinators.

[b] Societies of Obstetrics, Epidemiology, Odontology, Obstetrics, Medico-Psychology, Sanitary Medicine, Dental Surgery, Ophthalmology, Dermatology, Gynecology, Neurology, Laryngology-Rhinology, Laryngology, Orthopedics.

[c] These societies, in their order of appearance, were related to the following special interests, as indicated by their names: Pathology, Christian, Miscroscopy, Temperance, Physiology, Medical Women, Drunkenness, Anatomy, Medical Phonography, Roentgen Society (X-Ray), Consumption.

Diseases and Ulceration of the Legs had a short and unproductive life.[89] In the 1870's the founder of St. Saviour's Hospital devoted that charity to the "treatment of cancer, paralysis, diseases of the nervous system, throat, etc."[90] Such ventures betray more eagerness and ambition than good judgment or medical acumen on the part of their founders.

Successful specialist activities went beyond hospitals, private practice, societies, and journals into the arena of medical education. With students in the wards of a special hospital, new knowledge could be passed on to the next generation of practitioners and, in the process, specialists gained professional stature and influence. In 1876, St. John's Hospital inaugurated a series of lectures on skin diseases which was offered free of charge to medical students and qualified practitioners in the metropolis. The next step, St. John's Hospital School of Dermatology, came in 1885, and by 1888 the school offered daily clinical instruction and practical lectures twice a week.[91] Few specialties had the benefit of a champion so well connected and so wealthy as Erasmus Wilson, FRCS. A surgeon and dermatologist, he donated a portion of his large fortune to the Royal College of Surgeons for the creation of a lectureship in dermatology.[92]

While students might frequent the wards of special hospitals at will, status only came to a specialty when it became incorporated into the curriculum for a medical license, whether as a required unit of study or as an optional subject in the examinations. Formal recognition by the licensing bodies could give impetus to student interest in special areas of medicine. Specialists in obstetrics, lunacy, ophthalmology, and other new specialties urged the Royal Colleges to include their areas of interest in the curriculum from the 1870's on.*

*RCP, Annals, XXXII (22 December 1876), 6–8 (re psychological medicine); (25 October 1877), 89, and (6 March 1879), 188–189 (re obstetrics); (31 July 1879), 241–242, and XXXIII (28 April 1881), 20–21 (re ophthalmology and obstetrics); and (23 May 1882), 128–129 (re public health). As an interim step, specialist societies sometimes offered their own unofficial diplomas, such as the Medico-Psychological Association's "Certificate of Efficiency in Psychological Medicine." See: BMJ, "Advertiser," November 17, 1888, no pagination; cf. BMJ, 1876, i, 689 and 698–699.

TABLE 17 The Foundation of Specialist Medical Periodicals in the United Kingdom in the Nineteenth Century

Subject	Before 1800	1800–1809	1810–1819	1820–1829	1830–1839	1840–1849	1850–1859	1860–1869	1870–1879	1880–1889	1890–1899
Smallpox, V.D. and dermatology	2	—	—	—	—	—	—	—	—	—	—
Dermatology	—	1	—	—	—	—	—	1	1	1	2
Fever	—	—	—	—	1	—	—	—	—	—	—
Ophthalmology	—	—	—	—	1	—	1	2	1	2	1
Dentistry	—	—	—	—	—	2	3	1	1	1	5
Public health, epidemiology	—	—	—	—	—	2	2	3	13	4	5
Obstetrics, gynecology	—	—	—	—	—	1	1	1	2	1	3
Psychology, neurology	—	—	—	—	—	1	2	—	5	—	2

Military and tropical medicine	—	—	—	—	—	—	—	1	—	—	4
Chest, tuberculosis	—	—	—	—	—	—	—	—	1	—	1
Mixed special subjects	—	—	—	—	—	—	—	—	—	1	—
Laryngology, nose and throat	—	—	—	—	—	—	—	—	—	1	2
Orthopedic	—	—	—	—	—	—	—	—	—	—	1
Radiology	—	—	—	—	—	—	—	—	—	—	1
Anesthetics	—	—	—	—	—	—	—	—	—	—	1
Pediatrics	—	—	—	—	—	—	—	—	—	—	1
Otology	—	—	—	—	—	—	—	—	—	—	1
TOTAL	2	1	0	0	2	6	9	9	23	12	30

Compiled from: W. R. Lefanu, *British Periodicals of Medicine. A Chronological List* (Baltimore, 1938).

Such acceptance would have marked unqualified endorsement of the importance of these subjects and of the specialist's role in medical education and knowledge.

IV

However humane, scientific, or idealistic the specialists' motives and activities might have been, the response of the non-specialist majority-of the profession reflected a sense of terrible threat from their activities. As unhappy as general practitioners had been over the loss of paying patients to the charity wards of the general hospitals, their grumbling grew noisier when they saw their patients lost to these parvenus in the specialist hospitals. General practitioners were vehement, outspoken, and bitter. Special hospitals were "a monstrous evil—an evil which springs from within the profession."[93] W. O. Markham, later editor of the *BMJ*, spoke angrily of the new specialists at a BMA meeting: "[T]he gentlemen engaged in those special hospitals got their names spread all over England, but in the meantime the profession was being ruined."[94] The term "guinea pig" labelled the specialist as a greedy profiteer, seeking only to line his pockets.[95]

Laryngologist Morrell Mackenzie, not without some bitterness of his own, described the conflict between the general practitioner and the specialist:

> Not so very long ago the general practitioner looked upon his patient as his private property. . . . He now feels that his position has lost something of its security, for he knows that if his patient does not rapidly mend, inquiry will be made for the name and address of the greatest authority on the disease in question, to whose care his patient will straightaway commit himself. The family doctor thus comes to look on the specialist as a receiver of stolen goods, if not as the actual thief.[96]

The poor received free care at the special hospital, and paying patients sought the advice of the medical specialist whose reputation was bolstered—if not created—by his affiliation with the hospital.

General practitioners who appeared before the House of Lords Select Committee on Metropolitan Hospitals in the early 1890's expressed their conviction that the existence of special hospitals had robbed them of income in their private practices. The Rev. S. D. Bhakha, clergyman and general practitioner, told the committee that the general and special hospitals "starve" the general practitioner.[97] Cottenham Farmer, MRCS, who practiced in the neighborhood of Gray's Inn Road, testified that the special hospitals drove general practitioners to peddle bottles of medicine in their desperate search for income.[98]

General practitioners' objections to specialism did not rest wholly on their sense of personal injury. They also criticized specialists on scientific and medical grounds. One periodical, *The General Practitioner*, insisted on the importance of the "family doctor[s] . . . , all-round men, who understand that the body is a unit, the parts of which are related, and must work together harmoniously to produce health."[99] Specialists, by contrast, often served "no preliminary apprenticeship to general medicine," and, as a consequence, "Their minds are narrowed, judgment biased and unbalanced by disproportionate knowledge of one subject. The specialist is too apt to trace all symptoms to the eye, the nerves, the reproductive organs, as the case may be."[100] In the end, the patient suffers, for unlike the patient's family doctor, the specialist "knows nothing of the constitutional idiosyncracies of the individual, which are essential to correct diagnosis and treatment."[101]

While general practitioners and hospital consultants found themselves at odds on many issues, they agreed on the matter of specialism. The consultants, too, attacked specialism on scientific grounds. Sir William Gull, FRCP, asked his fellow-physicians, "Who can treat as a specialty the derangements and diseases of the stomach, whilst its relations and sympathies are so universal? . . . How can there be a special 'brain doctor,' whilst the functions of the brain are so dependent upon parts the most distant, and influences the most various?"[102] Sir Benjamin Brodie, Bart., FRCS, argued forcefully that:

Diseases generally are so connected with each other, and a knowledge of one is so necessary to the right understanding of another, that no one who limits his attention to any given disease, can be so competent to investigate its nature, and to improve the methods of treating it, as those are who have a wider field of observation, and who are better acquainted with general pathology.[103]

Such statements as these reflect the continuing adherence of many leaders of the profession to the idea of disease as the manifestation of a widespread underlying state, in the face of growing localism which provided the theoretical justification for specialism.[104] Theoretical disagreement with the specialists was not enough, in itself, to provoke the hospital consultants' great outpouring of protest against the special hospitals. Indeed, the corporate elites studiously avoided dictating to the profession on matters of medical theory and modes of treatment.[105] The hospital and medical school elites objected to specialism, not primarily on theoretical grounds, but because specialism took organizational forms which threatened their institutions and their authority.

Nowhere is this clearer than in the nationwide campaign launched in June, 1860, in response to news of the imminent establishment of St. Peter's Hospital for Stone. A committee of "Representatives of Medical Staffs of General Hospitals" composed a statement of protest against the proliferation of special hospitals. Nineteen of England's most eminent consultants, including Thomas Mayo, President of the Royal College of Physicians, John Flint South, President of the Royal College of Surgeons, and Sir James Clark, Bart., and Sir Henry Holland, Bart., Physicians in Ordinary to the Queen, signed the statement. Copies were printed and sent to hospital consultants throughout England. By mid-October, 1860, at least 415 hospital doctors in London and the country had added their names to the document, and funds were contributed in order to publicize the profession's disapproval of special hospitals in the *Times* and the medical press.[106]

The objections voiced in this campaign letter revealed the hospital consultants' concern for the impact of special hospitals on the funding, reputations, and teaching functions of their own institutions. The circular claimed that special hospitals were "injurious" to the public and the profession, first, "because in the maintenance of numerous small establishments the funds designed for the direct relief of the sick poor, are wasted in the useless multiplication of expensive Buildings, Salaries, and Hospital Appliances, and in the custom of constantly advertising to attract Public attention."[107] In fact, the consultants argued, everything needed for the treatment of disease "is already supplied in the existing General Hospitals."[108] The message was clear: philanthropic individuals must choose between contributing to the special hospitals—and thereby paying for wasteful duplication of expensive buildings and equipment—or supporting the established general hospitals, where they could be sure that their gifts brought direct relief to the sick poor. In their private correspondence, medical men expressed more bluntly their belief that special hospitals diverted needed funds away from the general hospitals. "I hear," wrote one angry medical man, "of subscriptions and contributions withheld from an old established Hospital and given to the Cancer, the Orthopaedic, and lately the recently 'got-up' specialty for Bladder disorders!"[109]

The consultants also feared for the reputations of the general hospitals: "[T]he Public," their circular asserted, "is led to believe that particular classes of disease can be more successfully treated in the small special Institutions than in the General Hospitals, an assumption directly contrary to evidence."[110] The consultants insisted on the point, "the fact being that the resources of the General Hospitals are in every respect superior to those of the special Institutions."[111] Public conversion to the idea of special hospitals would mean the loss of patients, who were the lifeblood of philanthropy, the source of clinical materials, and the foundation of clinical medical education in the general hospitals. It was "essential for the interests of the Public, with a view to the efficient education of Students preparing themselves for the practice of the Medical profession, that all forms of disease should, as far as possible, be collected in the General Hospitals to which Medical Schools are attached."[112] For the good of patients, the benefit of students, and the superior reputation of the medical schools, the special hospitals could not be permitted to draw away valuable clinical illustrations of kidney, throat, or skin disease.

The strength of the general hospitals lay in the quantity and diversity of medical and surgical cases. A successful special hospital would, by offering unparalleled opportunities to observe a particular disease, command the attention of medical students and draw them away from the general hospitals. In the long run, such decentralization would undermine the consultants' claims to supremacy in medical education. Privately, medical men admitted that specialism was equally dangerous in the short run. As E. H. Sieveking wrote in a letter to John Erichsen, "I have long held that the Special Hospitals are the source of much injury to the student . . . by engendering distrust in his teachers. . . ."[113] The special hospitals, in short, posed the possibility of an alternative authority in knowledge of disease, treatment, and medical science, and in so doing threatened the supreme authority of the hospital consultants.

Public condemnation was the first weapon in the armory of the consultants in their battle to dissuade medical men from adopting specialism and to influence donors to withhold their support. Privately, consultants could boycott specialists by refusing to send patients to them and by denying consultations with them.[114] Specialists could be excluded from the social and professional benefits of medical associations. Morrell Mackenzie warned his young protégé Felix Semon to "get yourself elected to the Royal Medical and Chirurgical Society before it becomes known that you are attached to our [throat] hospital."[115]

Consultants took direct action to isolate the special hospitals from any connections, through their personnel, with the teaching hospitals of London. Social pressure on medical men with dual appointments forced them to choose between their general hospital ties and specialism. Thomas William Nunn, FRCS, had held the post of Assistant Surgeon at the Middlesex Hospital for eight years when he was invited to join the staff of St. Peter's Hospital for Stone in 1866. He accepted, but resigned within the year in order, he said, to avoid an "open rupture" with his colleagues at the Middlesex.[116] Dr. J. L. W. Thudichum withstood such professional pressure for only two months. He resigned his post at St. Peter's because "I am threatened with serious injury in my profession and to my prospects in life."[117] His obeisance to professional opinion seems to have served him well. Five years after he left St. Peter's, he gained an appointment at St. Thomas's Hospital Medical School. His London practice grew large, and eventually he enjoyed the honor of a Fellowship in the Royal College of Physicians.[118]

Through public censure, social pressure, and ostracism, the old guard of the profession tried to contain the growth of specialism, to undermine its chances for public support and success, and to prevent those pursuing specialties within the framework of the special hospitals from achieving positions of prestige and power in the teaching hospitals and the Royal Colleges.* While attempting to forestall the rise to eminence of the renegade founders of special hospitals, the consultants of London took the apparently contradictory measure of supporting the introduction of special wards in the teaching hospitals. Early on, hospitals had appointed men to serve as dentists, ophthalmologists, lithotomists, and the like, but excluded them from places in the hierarchy of general medicine or surgery and from medical teaching. Teaching activities in ophthalmology, laryngology, and other special subjects were placed in the hands of the assistant physicians and surgeons, who achieved those positions "by accident" and without regard to their fitness for these roles. The concessions to specialism came grudgingly: the instructors "taught in inconvenient places" and the subjects were given lower priority than their other duties.[119] By placing specialties in the hands of assistant physicians and surgeons, they remained under the control of the senior staff. The consultants thus maintained the supremacy of general medicine and surgery over specialties, while at the same time incorporating them into their institutions.[120]

* Of the specialists who held the FRCP or FRCS, few held offices or examinerships in the Royal Colleges up to 1890.

By the 1870's, special departments with beds devoted to specific disorders began to form a part of the general hospitals' in-patient service and teaching resources, and young medical men interested in special medicine could find at least a limited place for their work within the establishment. Needless to say, the posts in the new special wards did not go to men like Morrell Mackenzie, who had been leaders in creating the problem of specialism in the first place. In 1882, when the treasurer and senior staff of St. Thomas's Hospital agreed to entrust the throat department to a specialist in laryngology, they did not offer the post to Mackenzie. Instead, the appointment went to Felix Semon, a man trained in laryngology by Mackenzie, but one who had impeccable credentials and connections in Germany and who had established family and professional connections with St. Thomas's from his earliest days in London.[121]

Typically, general hospitals established ophthalmic departments first among the specialties. St. Thomas's organized such a department in 1871. After a slow beginning, the 1880's and 1890's saw special departments multiply. St. Thomas's created the throat department in 1882, the skin and ear department in 1884, a gynecology department in 1888, and, in the 1890's, departments for dentistry, electrotherapy, x-ray, vaccination, and mental diseases.[122] Guy's Hospital, after an early start in offering gynecological and ophthalmological care, followed a similar chronology in the creation of other departments. Guy's established an ear department in 1863, and skin and throat departments came in the 1880's. Although teaching in psychological medicine had been carried on at Guy's since 1871, no psychiatrist served the medical staff until 1896—and even then he had no separate ward. A special department for genito-urinary diseases did not appear until 1908, and neurology did not have a separate ward until the 1930's.[123]

Not surprisingly, the medical establishment was not eager to incorporate the new specialties into the examining system. Obstetrics, a standard part of the general practitioner's work, became a required unit of the licensing examinations only in 1886.[124] Attempts on the part of specialists to gain a place in the system of medical education and licensing through the issuance of special diplomas met with thoroughgoing resistance from the Royal Colleges. The Royal College of Surgeons' dental license, created in 1859, represents the first—and for decades sole—step in the direction of special qualification. In the 1870's, Trinity College, Dublin, and Cambridge University established diplomas in state medicine and public health, and the Royal Colleges followed suit in 1886 with a registrable Certificate in Hygiene (later changed to Public Health).* These qualifications, together with the Diploma in Tropical Medicine created in 1910, suggest that government employment spurred the integration of some specialties into the curriculum.

Specialties in psychological medicine, ophthalmology, gynecology, and obstetrics had less success in gaining collegiate recognition. In 1879, ophthalmologists and members of the Obstetrical Society called on the Royal College of Physicians to establish diplomas in their specialties. Their requests were refused, and only after long negotiations did the College establish the Diploma in Ophthalmic Medicine and Surgery in 1920, and in Obstetrics and Gynecology in 1930. A diploma in psychiatry was also created in 1920.[125]

The professional elite was relatively helpless to contain the growth of special hospitals as long as medical men dared to found them and as long as patrons would supply the funds. They held, of course, the ultimate weapon of control over the special hospitals' role in medical education, and they moved astutely to bring the specialties—if not the specialists—under the aegis of the general hospitals. In so doing they preserved their own institutions and in the end brought the specialties under their control.

The specialists had challenged the consultants on their own ground, for they had embraced the ideals of charity, science, and the public good. The specialists' scientific claims helped shake the English medical establishment loose from its

---

*Alexander M. Cooke, *A History of the Royal College of Physicians of London* (Oxford, 1972), III, 885–889. Many of the examiners did not hold the diploma for which they served as judges.

devotion to "the practical aspects of diagnosis and treatment" and prompted English medicine to engage more actively in the search for "scientific explanations."[126]

Advertising was the medium through which tradesmen made their goods visible to the public, and self-publicizing was common both to medical profiteering and to specialism. The profession in the nineteenth century had, through its corporate regulations and through "consciousness-raising" discussions in the medical press, sought to divorce itself from trade and to emphasize its professional character. Medical men knew that tradesmen were not gentlemen, and most eschewed the tactics of the marketplace in their efforts to conform to the standards of that social rank to which they aspired.*

The leadership responded to the advertising activities of medical men by prohibiting not only tradesmanlike selling but the self-promotion that formed an integral part of entrepreneurial medical behavior. In the attempt, information about medical books, debates, and medical self-criticism began to disappear from the public press, the public view, and from the sphere of public judgment. The motive for such action may have been to protect the status and dignity of the profession by avoiding ungentlemanly behavior. Indeed, medical men understood that medical "ethics" promoted "the cultivation of that courtesy between professional brethren which rules the conduct of one gentleman towards another, and which knows no laws between those of good breeding and honour."[127]

While the ideal of gentlemanly honor may have motivated the rules against publicity, the justification lay in the realm of expertise. Commenting on advertising, one medical writer in 1907 explained: "In the case of most trade articles purchasers are competent judges of the quality of goods," but

---

*Robert Saundby, *Medical Ethics: A Guide to Professional Conduct*, 2nd ed. (London, 1907), pp. 5–6, said that advertising lowers "the standard of the profession" by attracting to its ranks the "sharp business men" who elbow out "the true scientific worker."

"the public cannot judge" the value of patent remedies, nor can they judge the qualities of a medical man.[128] That power belonged to medical men alone. As R. B. Carter put it in 1903 in his book, *Doctors and Their Work*:

> Professional eminence in medicine . . . in its true sense, should denote a combination of the greatest attainable knowledge of truth, in relation to the problems presented by disease, with the most carefully trained powers of observation and of recollection. It can only be obtained by a small number of persons, and can only be fully appreciated by knowledge and powers possibly far inferior in degree, but nevertheless of kindred character. In other words, it can only be certainly predicated by the medical profession itself.[129]

Out of the challenges of medical entrepreneurship, the profession began to articulate the foundations of professional authority in its knowledge of the human body and disease. While specialists and patent medicine vendors alike relied on popular appeal and lay testimonials, the profession, by elaborating its regulations regarding medical men's relations with the public, began to isolate professional life from the judgment of the public. And by the elaboration and enforcement of special rules of behavior for all medical men, the profession reasserted the unity of all medical practitioners which differences of income and rank had tended to undermine.

Serious question can be raised as to whether the profession's arrogation to itself of all power to judge the character and quality of medical work served the public interest, but there is no question that the profession gained by it. During the mid-Victorian years the leaders of the profession in London had begun to gain control over the hospital as the agency of health care delivery, medical education, and professional mobility. Through the instrumentality of professional censure and boycott, the elites also began to gain a measure of control over the behavior and mentality of the rank and file. In the process, the leaders of the profession had to abandon to a large degree the lay standards that had ruled their lives in their pursuit of lay patronage and prestige in the eyes of the public. Instead, they came to rely on the one instrument of judgment that set them apart from the rest of society—their knowledge of medicine. Only their medical knowledge justified their claims to exclusive authority over the patient, the pharmacopoeia, the hospitals, and their colleagues in the profession.

With the end of publicity, with the withdrawal of medical debate from the public sphere, and with the increasing identity of medical men as men of science, medicine became a "SACRED" profession, set apart, its membership a "priesthood,"* and its knowledge a mystery. For the public this meant dependence on the expert—the medical man. For the medical profession it was the apotheosis of authority and liberty from lay control.

*Thomas Underhill, *On Hospitals and Medical Education* (Birmingham, [1870]), p. 27. Cf. Ouida [Marie Louise de la Ramée], *The New Priesthood* (London, 1893), pp. 4 and 27–28. Ouida compares science to religion in its "fanaticism." She attacks physicians and physiologists for, among other things, their "clannish, cliquish, irrational, blind partisanship": "A gang never confesses that one of its members is in the wrong," and the doctor/scientists "constitute one of the largest, strongest, most widely spread, and most formidably armed gangs that the world has ever seen." She contrasts the ideal of the tender, merciful doctor with the "reality of the scientific experimentalist, whether surgeon or doctor, . . . who regards all suffering with curiosity, inquisitiveness, and . . . indifference."

Conclusion

In Thomas Hardy's novel, *The Woodlanders* (1887), the young doctor Fitzpiers holds a fascination for Grace Melbury because of his profession. That fascination is redoubled when she finds that old Grammer Oliver has sold her brain to the young doctor for his scientific research after her death. He comes to have the aspect of "a remorseless Jehovah of the sciences, who would not have mercy, and would have sacrifice."[1] In fact as well as fiction, medical men had come a long way from the bumbling Mr. Candy, Wilkie Collins's surgeon of the 1840's, to the sinister figure of Fitzpiers with his scalpel and his science.

In the early Victorian years, the old estate order of the medical profession appeared to be crumbling under the weight of practitioners' discontents and the new demands of medical practice in industrial society. The centrifugal force of rank and file aspirations and needs threatened to bring about a new order in the medical world in which the old corporations would be wiped away and a new, more homogeneous structure for medical practice would be instituted with greater power for the ordinary general practitioners. Legislation to that end was never passed, because of the corporate influence of the Royal College elites. Meanwhile, outside the realm of legislation, the elites of London had begun to build a new foundation for their leadership in the medical schools of London. Their authority there gave them a stronghold over the new generations of medical men who took their training in London. The medical schools thus laid the groundwork for their lifelong authority in the eyes of students who later filled the ranks of practitioners.

The medical schools provided an independent base for physicians and surgeons who began to expand their powers of patronage and influence, not only within the schools, but within the hospitals as well. During the mid-Victorian years, the medical elites began to establish a separate source of authority for themselves—an authority based on their medical knowledge—that served as the foundation for their growing claims to a role in the governance of medical institutions and, thereby, over their professional lives and those of their colleagues and successors. Medical knowledge was not intrinsically valued, either by medical men or by lay society, and the achievement of professional power involved the evolution of independent power within the sphere of the medical school and the assertion of influence within the hospital. Perhaps the governors' very philanthropy itself made them amenable to medical men's claims to superior knowledge of what the sick needed and, therefore, the right to consult and decide.

The problem of power in medical institutions was only one of several faced by medical men in the mid-Victorian years. Craft and trade traditions in medicine left a legacy of low incomes and lack of patient respect that men combatted in a variety of ways. Efforts to improve the liberal education and self-image of medical men fostered a sense of pride. Professional organizations brought medical men together, increased their sense of corporate unity, and focussed their attention on their medical and scientific roles. Such measures could only accomplish part of the goal as long as medical men continued, under the pressures of professional overcrowding, to compete with one another, to sell drugs, and to bow to the authority of their lay employers in the infirmaries and sick clubs. The problem of medical income and medical independence was not solved in the Victorian years. Only the passage of National Health Insurance in 1911 liberated many general practitioners from the drug trade and from dependence based on poverty.[2]

Low incomes and differential status created serious tensions within the medical profession. Some abandoned their profession for the sake of profit through trade. Other ambitious men sought to solve the problem by building independent medical institutions outside the establishment. The new specialist establishments appealed to the Victorian public's growing interest in science and benefited from popular belief in technical expertise. At the same time, however, they threatened to undermine the position of the consulting elite by drawing money and influence away from the established hospitals. By sanction, boycott, and cooptation, the elites managed to maintain their hegemony over the profession, but in the process received additional impetus toward the development of specialist studies within the general hospitals and the exclusion of laymen from the shrine of medical knowledge.

Perhaps the growth of specialism, together with the profession's increasingly acknowledged claims to authority based on knowledge, provided the stimulus for medical research. Certainly the late Victorian years saw the blossoming of research institutions and scientific aggressiveness among English medical men not seen in earlier decades.[3] Government support reflected public commitment to the utility of science in probing questions of life, disease, and death. Medical men had, for much of the century, remained wedded to the ideal of the gentleman, but they could only fulfill their aspirations to the independence and authority of the gentleman by committing themselves to the ungentlemanly virtues of practical skills and technical knowledge.

Medical independence was purchased at the expense of laymen, in institutions and in private life as well. Medical men became the new priesthood, ministering to the physical and psychic needs of patients.[4] Some of their patients found solace in being able to lean on their medical consultant. Others raged against the helplessness of patients in the hands of the profession. G. B. Shaw damned a society in which medical men defined their own work:

It may . . . be necessary to hang a man or pull down a house. But we take care not to make the hangman and the housebreaker the judges of that. If we did no man's neck would be safe and no man's house stable. But we do make the doctor the judge, and fine him . . . if he decides in our favor.[5]

The decision to amputate and the fees for doing so both came to the medical man, and Shaw saw in that the unmitigated power of medical men over the public.

The medical profession's story sheds light not only on the changing status and self-image of medical men, but also on the larger issue of the rise of the expert in Victorian society. Rank and file medical men, like other aspiring occupational groups, long made claims to merit as the sole legitimization of professional prestige and power. The claims came early, but the realities came late. Ideals of gentility, character, and the power of connection were a long time dying. Members of the elite clung to the status afforded them by their public school and university ties and by their acceptance in the upper echelons of society. The efforts of ordinary medical men to gain recognition based upon their science bore little fruit until their own leadership discovered the social value of their knowledge. Additionally, the rise of the expert required social acceptance, not of the *fact* of expertise—medical men had always been knowledgeable about disease and treatment—but of the equation of expertise and authority. Authority came to the experts as the public was increasingly closed off from knowledge of their work. The power of the experts was not the power to do, but the power to know, and therefore to judge. Finally, the experts reaped the benefits of the decline of religion and the growing secularization of society. Knowledge, expertise, and science all offered an alternative system for understanding and explaining the "real" world, no longer defined in transcendental terms but in terms of the body and the material universe. The experts gained stature not because they could always act effectively, but because only they could name, describe, and explain.

The fabled birth of class society and modernization in nineteenth-century England also has a relationship to the medical profession's story. The Victorian era is said to have been a time when "the old vertical connections of dependency or patronage" were replaced by the "horizontal solidarities of class."[6] Through struggles for power, law, codes of ethics, and the restructuring of their professional community, medical men created a new corporate structure. The modern professions—whose archetype is medicine—fostered group solidarity, loyalty, and exclusiveness, regardless of differences in general education, ascribed social rank, or economic standing. In the face of laissez-faire ideals and the competition of the modern marketplace, the professions created a special place for themselves in which "modern" science justified a "traditional" structure of authority and social relations. Universalism born of professional ambition and esoteric skill gave exclusive power to the possessors of knowledge, who perpetuated the old vertical connections of dependency and patronage in the name of expertise.

Appendix A

Medical Licensing Bodies and Licenses and Degrees in the United Kingdom in the Nineteenth Century*

MEDICAL CORPORATIONS	LICENSES
England	
The Royal College of Physicians of London	FRCP, MRCP, LRCP, Extra-Lic., RCP
The Royal College of Surgeons of England	FRCS, MRCS, Lic., Midwifery
The Society of Apothecaries [London]	LSA
Archbishop of Canterbury	MD Lambeth—granted prior to August 1, 1858
Scotland	
Royal College of Physicians of Edinburgh	FRCP Edin., MRCP Edin.
Royal College of Surgeons of Edinburgh	FRCS Edin., LRCS Edin.
Faculty of Physicians and Surgeons of Glasgow	FFPSG, LFPSG
Ireland	
King's and Queen's College of Physicians of Ireland	FKQCP Ire., LKQCP Ire.
Royal College of Surgeons of Ireland	FRCS Ire., LRCS Ire.
Apothecaries' Hall [Dublin]	LAH

Universities		Degrees
England	Oxford Cambridge London Victoria Durham	MB, MD, and BCh, MCh, and Lic. Med.
Scotland	Edinburgh Aberdeen Glasgow St. Andrew's	
Ireland	Dublin	

Key: F = Fellow; M = Member; L or Lic. = Licentiate

*Source: W. E. Steavenson, *The Medical Act (1858) Amendment Bill and Reform; a paper read before the Abernethian Society* ... (London, 1880), pp. 30–31.

Appendix B

Social Origins of Physicians (FRCP), Surgeons (FRCS), and Registered Apothecaries' Apprentices in the Nineteenth Century*

Father's Occupation	Physicians	Surgeons	Apothecaries
Medical profession			
MD, physician, FRCS	89	103	32
"Surgeon," medic, general practitioner, apothecary	80	184	405
Clergy			
Upper clergy	—	4	1
Vicar, curate	66	77	77
Cleric and schoolmaster	1	3	—
Dissenting minister	2	8	1
Schoolmaster	1	7	7
Legal profession			
Barrister	11	6	2
Solicitor, attorney	9	20	32
Services	19	36	51
Scholar, university professor	7	5	—
Miscellaneous new professions and para-professionals			
Author	2	—	—
Architect	5	2	4
Accountant	—	1	3
Actuary, underwriter	1	3	—
Engineer	3	2	4
Journalist	3	—	—
Surveyor	1	1	2

Father's Occupation	Physicians	Surgeons	Apothecaries
Hospital manager, steward	—	—	2
Scientist, anatomy teacher	—	2	—
Mineralogist	—	1	—
Veterinary surgeon	—	—	3
Agricultural chemist	1	—	—
Dentist	—	6	3
Actor	—	1	—
Artist, musician	—	4	10
Civil service and local government			
Miscellaneous	14	—	16
Writer to Signet	—	2	—
County clerk, town recorder	—	2	—
Irish Exchequer	—	1	—
Justice of the Peace	4	—	1
Secretary, customs	—	1	—
Secretary, customs commission	—	1	—
Indian civil service	—	2	—
Private Messenger to King	—	1	—
Assistant Secretary, Navy Board	—	1	—
Colonial government	—	3	—
Customs collector	—	1	—
Police magistrate	1	—	1
Admiralty (no detail)	—	1	—
Foreign Office	—	1	—
Mint employee	—	1	—
Arsenal employee	—	1	—
GPO Chief Clerk	—	1	—
Business and manufacturers			
Merchant, banker, broker	35	46	53
Bank manager	1	1	—
Stockbroker	1	—	9
"Business"	—	11	—
Manufacturer	15	7	17
Brewer	—	4	—
Shipowner	1	2	1

Father's Occupation	Physicians	Surgeons	Apothecaries
Builder	—	2	—
Shipbuilder	1	3	—
Contractor	—	—	2
Publisher	—	4	—
Ship agent	—	—	1
Estate or land agent	—	6	1
Trade, craft, and labor			
Craftsman, artisan	8	13	39
Tradesman	13	9	37
Wharfinger & barge owner	1	—	1
Master mariner	—	—	2
Mariner	2	—	—
Currier, grazier	—	—	4
Coal viewer	—	—	1
Private soldier	—	2	—
Herbalist	—	2	—
Gentleman, esquire	17	26	213
Landowner	8	3	—
Kt., Bart., MP (and no other occupation known)	5	2	1
Planter	—	2	5
Farmer, yeoman	6	20	22
Miscellaneous occupations			
Auctioneer	—	—	3
Bank cashier	—	1	1
Chiropodist	—	—	1
Clerk	—	1	2
Cupper	—	—	1
Dock officer	—	1	—
Ordnance officer, Tower	—	1	—
Piano teacher	—	—	1
Political agent	1	—	—
Proctor	—	—	1
Unknown	321	1786	165
TOTALS	756	2452	1241

*SOURCES: *Munk's Roll*; *Plarr's Lives*; and Society of Apothecaries, Minutes.

A note on the scope of these statistics:

Physicians—All Fellows of the Royal College of Physicians elected from 1800 through 1889.

Surgeons—All Fellows of the Royal College of Surgeons, from the institution of the Fellowship (1843) through 1889 (but excluding those Fellows who died after 1930).

Apothecaries—All apothecaries whose apprenticeships were registered at the London Society of Apothecaries from 1817 through 1889.

Appendix C

Basic Organizational Structure of a Hospital and Medical School*

PATRONS

BOARD OF GOVERNORS

TREASURER

HOSPITAL	MEDICAL SCHOOL

ADMINISTRATION

Hospital superintendent
Secretary

MEDICAL STAFF

Consulting physicians and
  surgeons (retired honorary staff)
Physicians and surgeons
  (in-patient care)
Physicians and surgeons in
  charge of special wards
Assistant physicians and assistant
  surgeons (out-patient care)

JUNIOR MEDICAL STAFF

Registrar
House physician, house surgeon
Obstetric assistant, other house
  posts in special wards

STUDENTS

Clinical clerk, dresser

TEACHING STAFF

Professors (various subjects)
Lecturers
Demonstrators (anatomy,
  physiology, surgery)

ADMINISTRATION

Dean of the medical school
Curator of the museum
Librarian

NOTE: The hospital posts related to special subjects (ophthalmology, obstetrics, laryngology, etc.) were introduced in the latter half of the nineteenth century and varied from hospital to hospital.

*This chart does *not* show lines of authority in the hospital or the medical school.

Appendix D

The Growth of Staffs in the London Teaching Hospitals, 1855–1889*

	Numbers on the staff					
Positions	1855	1875	Percent of increase	1889	Percent of increase	1855–89 Percent of increase
A. Consultants						
Physicians	33	42		51		
Assistants	26	36		34		
Surgeons	33	40		43		
Assistants	24	28		36		
Total physicians, surgeons, and assistants	116	146	25.9	164	12.3	41.4
B. Special Departments						
Surgeon-accoucheurs, physician-accoucheurs, or obstetric physicians	12	12		12		
Assistants	0	7		6		
Dental surgeons	6	6		13		
Assistants	0	2		2		
Ophthalmic surgeons	4	11		12		
Assistants	0	1		4		

Aural surgeons	1	4		8		
Assistants	0	0		1		
Skin surgeons, physicians	0	3		6		
Assistants	0	1		0		
Anesthetists or chloroformists	0	1		4		
Orthopedic	0	0		1		
Throat	0	0		3		
Mental	0	1		0		
Electro-therapists	0	0		1		
Casualty physicians	0	3		3		
Total physicians and surgeons in charge of special departments	23	52	126.1	76	46.2	230.4
C. *"Consulting"* (i.e., retired) physicians and surgeons	5	43	760.0	64	204.8	1180.0
Total: General and special staff	144	241	67.4	304	26.1	111.1

*SOURCE: *London and Provincial Medical Directory*, 1855, 1875, 1889.

Appendix E

The Foundation of General and Specialist Periodicals in the United Kingdom in the Nineteenth Century*

Subject	Before 1800	1800– 1809	1810– 1819	1820– 1829	1830– 1839	1840– 1849	1850– 1859	1860– 1869	1870– 1879	1880– 1889	1890– 1899
						Date of Foundation					
General medicine and surgery	31	7	12	19	28	18	15	16	19	24	46
Auxiliary medical sciences						10	7	4	5	2	6
Specialist journals†	2	1			2	6	9	9	23	12	30
Miscellaneous: alcoholism, hygiene, water cure, spas, phrenology, vegetarian, mesmerist, and other "fringe" journals			1	2		15	14	9	8	13	15
TOTALS	33	8	13	21	30	49	45	38	55	51	97

*SOURCE: W. R. Lefanu, *British Periodicals of Medicine. A chronological list* (Baltimore, 1938).
† See Table 17 for details.

Notes

(NB: To avoid unnecessary duplication, authors' first names and the titles of their works have been abbreviated here. For complete citations, consult the Bibliography.)

Introduction

1. D. Sayers, *Whose Body?* (New York, 1923), p. 133.

2. K. Thomas, *Religion and the Decline of Magic* (London, 1971), p. 49. But see: E. Freidson, *Profession of Medicine* (New York, 1970), pp. 16 and 21–22.

Chapter I

1. The most recent studies of the history of the English medical profession are: J. Berlant, *Profession and Monopoly* (Berkeley and Los Angeles, 1975); and N. Parry and J. Parry, *The Rise of the Medical Profession* (London, 1976). Berlant's is the superior work. See also: W. J. Reader, *Professional Men* (London, 1966); A. M. Carr-Saunders and P. A. Wilson, *The Professions* (Oxford, 1933); R. H. Shryock, *The Development of Modern Medicine* (London, 1948); and G. Clark, "The History of the Medical Profession," *Medical History*, 10:3 (1966), 213–220.

2. I. Waddington, "The Struggle to Reform the Royal College of Physicians, 1767–1771," *Medical History*, 17:2 (1973), 108; and S. W. F. Holloway, "Medical Education in England, 1830–1858," *History*, 49 (1964), 299–324.

3. R. Dahrendorf, *Class and Class Conflict in Industrial Society* (Stanford, 1959), pp. 6–7; T. H. Marshall, *Class, Citizenship, and Social Development. Essays by T. H. Marshall*, ed. S. M. Lipset (Garden

City, N.Y., 1964), p. 193; and Max Weber, *From Max Weber: Essays in Sociology*, ed. and trans. H. H. Gerth and C. Wright Mills (New York, 1958), pp. 190 ff. As Dahrendorf points out, Weber's term *stände*, rendered "status" by his translators, can also be read "estate." For rigid legal stratification as an aspect of traditional pre-industrial societies, see, e.g., C. E. Black, *The Dynamics of Modernization* (New York, 1966); and R. Mousnier, *Les Hierarchies Sociales de 1450 à nos jours* (Paris, 1969), pp. 19–23 and Chapter X.

4. Marshall, *Essays*, p. 193; Dahrendorf, *Class Conflict*, p. 7; and Weber, *Essays in Sociology*, pp. 190–191 and 193. S. W. F. Holloway, while recognizing the estate order of the profession, considers the period before 1858 to be a time of unification ("Medical Education," p. 299).

5. For a history of the College from its foundation to 1858, see: G. Clark, *A History of the Royal College of Physicians of London* (Oxford, 1966), 2 vols. The third volume, by A. M. Cooke (Oxford, 1972), covers the period from 1858 to 1948.

6. Clark, *A History*, I, 60, 81, 138, 190, and 281; and II, 519, 533, and 738–739. See also: J. Chapman, *Medical Institutions of the United Kingdom* (London, 1870), pp. 32–33; and W. Rivington, *The Medical Profession* (Dublin, 1879), pp. 16–17.

7. Marshall, *Essays*, p. 194: in an estate system, "change of status must be by a legal or official act."

8. 14 & 15 Henry VIII, c. 5, quoted in Carr-Saunders and Wilson, *The Professions*, p. 68.

9. This idea is clear in the *Report of the Select Committee on Medical Education*, 1834 (602.I), xiii, Part I, pp. 9 ff. (Sir Henry Halford). See also: Clark, *A History*, II, 685–688; C. Newman, *The Evolution of Medical Education in the Nineteenth Century* (London, 1957), pp. 8–9; and Reader, *Professional Men*, p. 17. The College emphasized classical learning over practical knowledge in its examinations. At some periods, Oxbridge taught no medicine at all. Regarding Edinburgh medical education, see: D. Guthrie, "Scottish Influence on the Evolution of British Medicine," in *The Evolution of Medical Practice in Britain*, ed. F. N. L. Poynter (London, 1961), pp. 150 ff.

10. Z. Cope, *The Royal College of Surgeons of England* (London, 1959), pp. 1–26 passim, is the source of my material on the Royal College of Surgeons. For information on the practice of surgeons, see: C. B. Keetley, *The Student's and Junior Practitioner's Guide to the Medical Profession*, 2nd ed. (London, 1885), p. 39.

11. B. Abel-Smith, *The Hospitals, 1800–1948* (London, 1964), p. 2. Cf. *Report of the Select Committee on Medical Education*, 1834 (602.II), xii, Part II, Appendices 2 and 44.

12. Cope, *The Royal College*, pp. 42 ff. See also: Sir D'Arcy Power, *The Evolution of the Surgeon in London* (London, 1912), p. 30.

13. For histories of the Society of Apothecaries, see: C. Wall, *A History of the Worshipful Society of Apothecaries of London*, Vol. 1: 1617–1815 (no other volume published), abstracted, arranged, and edited by H. C. Cameron and E. A. Underwood (London, 1963); C. Wall, *The London Apothecaries* (London, 1932); C. R. B. Barrett, *History of the Society of Apothecaries* (London, 1905), W. S. C. Copeman, *The Worshipful Society of Apothecaries of London* (Oxford, 1967); and L. G. Matthews, *The Royal Apothecaries* (London, 1967).

14. *Select Committee on Medical Education*, 1834 (602.III), xiii, Part III, Appendix 6. The proportion who held both the LSA and the MRCS is an approximation by RCS officials. See: ibid., Part II, Appendix 44. See also: A. H. T. Robb-Smith, "Medical Education at Oxford and Cambridge Prior to 1850," in *The Evolution of Medical Education in Britain*, ed. F. N. L. Poynter (London, 1966), p. 51; and Abel-Smith, *The Hospitals*, p. 2.

15. Wall, *A History*, pp. 81–82. Cf. Weber, *Essays in Sociology*, pp. 190 ff.

16. See, e.g., H. Eckstein, *Pressure Group Politics* (Stanford, 1960), p. 50n.; and Newman, *Medical Education*, p. 75. Cf. S. W. F. Holloway, "The Apothecaries' Act of 1815," Parts I and II, *Medical History*, 10:2 (1966), 107–129; and 10:3 (1966), 221–236.

17. Holloway, "Apothecaries' Act of 1815," Part I, shows this clearly. See also: Royal College of Physicians of Edinburgh, *Historical Sketch and Laws of the Royal College of Physicians from Its Institution to December 1865* (Edinburgh, 1867), p. 46; Chapman, *Medical Institutions*, p. 22; and N. G. Horner, *The Growth of the General Practitioner of Medicine in England* (London, 1922), pp. 35 ff.

18. Abel-Smith, *The Hospitals*, is the most complete. Others are: J. Woodward, *To Do the Sick No Harm* (London and Boston, 1974); A. G. L. Ives, *British Hospitals* (London, 1948); and C. Dainton, *The Story of England's Hospitals* (London, 1961).

19. Newman, *Medical Education*, pp. 84 and 96.

20. For a sophisticated discussion of this development, see: K. Figlio, "The Historiography of Scientific Medicine," *Comp. Stud. Soc. and Hist.*, 19:3 (July, 1977). See also: I. Waddington, "The Role of

the Hospital in the Development of Modern Medicine," *Sociology*, 7:2 (1973), 211–225.

21. For the growth of medical schools, see: Newman, *Medical Education*, pp. 112–122. Also see the histories of individual hospitals, for example: H. C. Cameron, *Mr. Guy's Hospital, 1726–1948* (London, 1954); E. M. McInnes, *St. Thomas' Hospital* (London, 1963); and J. Langdon-Davies, *Westminster Hospital* (London, 1952). For first-hand accounts, see: St. Thomas's Hospital, Minutes of the Grand Committee (H.1/ST/A6/11), 10 May 1842, p. 7, passim; and St. Bartholomew's Hospital Manuscripts. Medical School. Copies of entries in the Journals concerning the Medical School, 1842–1851 (M.S.3/1).

22. Society of Apothecaries, Minute Books, show apprenticeships recorded into the 1880's.

23. See: [RCS], *A Few Words on the Fellowship, with a Suggestion Concerning the Present Crisis . . .* (London, 1845), pp. 8–9. See also: T. McKeown, "A Sociological Approach to the History of Medicine," *Medical History*, 14:4 (1970), 346–347; and Abel-Smith, *The Hospitals*, pp. 17 ff.

24. McKeown, "History of Medicine," p. 347, considers these distinctions "well established" by 1886. He attributes increased unity, in part, to the Medical Act Amendment Act of 1886. On the continued competition among the corporations, see: R. Quain, *Observations on Medical Education* (London, 1865), p. 44, note A.

25. R. B. Carter, *Doctors and Their Work* (London, 1903), pp. 11–12, thought that the social distance between the "higher" and "lower" grades of medical man increased during the course of the nineteenth century.

26. Cope, *The Royal College*, p. 41. Cf. Waddington, "Struggle to Reform," p. 123. After the establishment of the new LRCP in 1861, similar relations existed within the College of Physicians.

27. Holloway, "Apothecaries' Act of 1815," pp. 224 ff. and 235.

28. The Royal College of Physicians had its "College Club"; see: J. F. Payne, *History of the College Club of the Royal College of Physicians of London* (London, 1909); and Clark, *A History*, II, 559–560. The Society of Apothecaries had its "Friendly Medical Society"; see: Society of Apothecaries, Friendly Medical Society: Minute Books, 1775–1917, 5 vols., Guildhall Ms. 8278.

29. W. H. McMenemey, *The Life and Times of Sir Charles Hastings* (Edinburgh and London, 1959), gives the most detail regarding

these groups. Other information regarding medical societies may be found in *The London and Provincial Medical Directory* [also known as *Churchill's Medical Directory*] and in *Medical Institutions of London* (London, 1895), pp. 31–46. These two sources are of limited value for the early nineteenth-century societies, however, because *Churchill's* first appeared in 1846, and because the BMA list includes only those societies that survived until 1895. Table 16, below, showing the foundation of medical societies in the nineteenth century, does not include the many ephemeral early associations.

30. Holloway, "Apothecaries' Act of 1815," p. 109.

31. Ibid., p. 111; Clark, *A History*, II, 559 and 615 ff.; and McMenemey, *Sir Charles Hastings*, p. 146. See also: Cope, *The Royal College*, p. 87.

32. Holloway, "Apothecaries' Act of 1815," p. 116; and McMenemy, *Sir Charles Hastings*, pp. 152 and 178–179.

33. E. Harrison, *An Address Delivered to the Lincolnshire Benevolent Medical Society . . . in 1809* (1810), p. 88, quoted in Holloway, "Apothecaries' Act of 1815," p. 117.

34. Royal College of Physicians of London. Treasurer's Documents, Box 4, Envelope 41, quoted in Holloway, "Apothecaries' Act of 1815," p. 118.

35. Holloway, "Apothecaries' Act of 1815," pp. 119–125. I have drawn heavily on Holloway's excellent account of the 1815 Act in this section.

36. Newman, *Medical Education*, pp. 75–77 and 134. See also: F. N. L. Poynter, "The Centenary of the General Medical Council," *BMJ*, 1958, ii, 1245; and others cited by Holloway in "Apothecaries' Act of 1815," pp. 231 ff.

37. Holloway, "Apothecaries' Act of 1815," p. 128. See also: Carr-Saunders and Wilson, *The Professions*, pp. 77 ff. The Act did nothing to limit the activities of chemists and druggists who competed with the apothecaries.

38. [RCS], *A Few Words on the Fellowship . . .* , pp. 17 and 19.

39. McMenemey, *Sir Charles Hastings*, pp. 68–69 and 145. See also pp. 72–73 and 96.

40. On the poor law medical men, see: R. Hodgkinson, *The Origins of the National Health Service* (London, 1967); and J. Rogers, *Reminiscences of a Workhouse Medical Officer* (London, 1889). See also: McMenemey, *Sir Charles Hastings*, p. 474.

41. McMenemey, *Sir Charles Hastings*, pp. 40, 87, 142, and 143.

See also: *Memoirs of the Life of a Country Surgeon* (London, 1845), especially the dedication and pp. 19–20.

42. Rivington, *The Medical Profession*, pp. 248 and 255. Histories of the British Medical Association are: E. M. Little, comp., *History of the British Medical Association, 1832–1932* (London, [1932]); P. Vaughan, *Doctors' Commons* (London, 1959); and Eckstein, *Pressure Group Politics*. For earlier accounts, see: G. N. Stephen, *The British Medical Association and the Medical Profession* (London, 1914); and R. Coombe, *Medico-Political History of the British Medical Association* (London, 1921). W. H. McMenemey's *Sir Charles Hastings*, a biography of the BMA's founder, is very complete for the early years.

43. Quoted in McMenemey, *Sir Charles Hastings*, p. 99.

44. Idem. See also pp. 149 and 300.

45. Quoted in McMenemey, *Sir Charles Hastings*, p. 149. See also: [RCS], *A Few Words on the Fellowship*, pp. 8 and 33.

46. Biographies of Wakley include: S. S. Sprigge, *The Life and Times of Thomas Wakley* (London, 1899); C. Brook, *Battling Surgeon* (Glasgow, 1945); and E. C. Sherrington, "Thomas Wakley and Reform, 1832 to 1862" (Oxford D.Phil. thesis, 1973). Sherrington has the clearest recognition of Wakley's counterproductive inflammatory style, while Sprigge tends to gloss a bit, and Brook has an even more favorable view. Newman, *Medical Education*, pp. 140–142, views Wakley with obvious disapproval, while McMenemey, *Sir Charles Hastings*, allows Wakley's writings to serve as a foil to show the moderation of Hastings and the PMSA.

47. *Lancet*, 1831–32, i, 2, quoted in I. Waddington, "The Development of Medical Ethics," *Medical History*, 19:1 (1975), 44.

48. McMenemey, *Sir Charles Hastings*, p. 217.

49. Holloway summarizes these developments in "Medical Education," pp. 299–306.

50. Newman, *Medical Education*, pp. 134–140.

51. The material in this section is drawn from: Newman, *Medical Education*, pp. 154–193; and W. L. Burn, *The Age of Equipoise* (New York, 1965), pp. 202 ff.

52. *Edinburgh Medical and Surgical Journal*, lxiv, 255, quoted in Burn, *Age of Equipoise*, p. 209.

53. Newman, *Medical Education*, p. 136.

54. Ibid., pp. 136–137; and Burn, *Age of Equipoise*, p. 208.

55. Burn, *Age of Equipoise*, p. 208; and Newman, *Medical Education*, pp. 175–176 and 183–184.

56. Newman, *Medical Education*, p. 188; see also pp. 174, 177, and 182–184.

57. Holloway, "Medical Education," p. 299.

58. E. Freidson, *Profession of Medicine* (New York, 1970), p. 72.

59. Ibid., p. 21. Freidson says that efficacy of practice is fundamental to social acceptance.

60. Ibid., p. 84, passim.

61. R. K. Merton discusses the matter of universalism in science, and by extension in medicine, in "The Institutional Imperatives of Science," in *Sociology of Science: Selected Readings*, ed. Barry Barnes (Harmondsworth, 1972), pp. 65–80, especially pp. 68–72. See also: T. Parsons, *The Social System* (Glencoe, Ill., 1958), pp. 198 ff.; and Freidson, *Profession of Medicine*, p. 21.

Chapter II

1. "The Physiology of the London Medical Student," *Punch*, I (1841), 184.

2. B. Abel-Smith, *The Hospitals, 1800–1948* (London, 1964), illustration facing p. 130.

3. See S. Rothblatt, *The Revolution of the Dons* (New York, 1968), pp. 89–90, note 3. See also: N. G. Annan, "The Intellectual Aristocracy," in *Studies in Social History*, ed. J. H. Plumb (London, 1955), pp. 243–265; *Plarr's Lives*, s.v. William Rose, Jr.; and S. M. Lipset and R. Bendix, *Social Mobility in Industrial Society* (Berkeley and Los Angeles, 1967), p. 40.

4. *Plarr's Lives*, s.v. Henry Cline. See also s.v. William Webb.

5. Ibid., s.v. Bransby Cooper and C. A. Key. See also s.v. George Y. Heath.

6. See J. A. Banks, *Prosperity and Parenthood* (London, 1954), Chapter XI, for costs of education for various professions. Cf. A. Marder, *From the Dreadnought to Scapa Flow* (London, 1961), I, 30–31.

7. S. Paget, *Sir Victor Horsley* (London, 1919), p. 16. Cf. F. J. Gant, *Autobiography* (London, 1905), pp. 17–18.

8. J. Bland-Sutton, *The Story of a Surgeon* (London, 1930), pp. 24–25.

9. *Plarr's Lives*, s.v. Thomas Heckstall Smith, and s.v. David Goodsall. See also: J. D. Carr, *The Life of Sir Arthur Conan Doyle* (New York, 1949), p. 20; and G. Haight, *George Eliot and John Chapman* (New Haven, 1940), p. 95.

10. C. B. Keetley, *The Student's and Junior Practitioner's Guide to the Medical Profession*, 2nd ed. (London, 1885), pp. 13–14.

11. Sir John Cockburn, quoted in *Plarr's Lives*, s.v. William Rose, Jr.

12. Ibid. See also the remarks regarding Walsham in A. Doran, *Life Memories* (Typescript, RCS Library, 1923), p. 5.

13. A. C. Doyle, *The Stark Munro Letters* (New York, 1895), p. 160. See also: *Confessions of an English Doctor* (London, 1904), p. 26; and Bland-Sutton, *Surgeon*, p. 59, regarding E. H. Greenhow.

14. H. E. Counsell, *37 The Broad* (London, 1943), pp. 9–10. See also: R. Farquharson, *In and Out of Parliament* (London, 1911), p. 44.

15. Bland-Sutton, *Surgeon*, pp. 1, 4–5, and 24.

16. *Plarr's Lives*, s.v. William Henry Stone. For a similar case, see: C. J. B. Williams, *Memoirs of Life and Work* (London, 1884), pp. 3–5.

17. J. Beddoe, *Memories of Eighty Years* (Bristol, 1910), p. 26. See also: Bland-Sutton, *Surgeon*, p. 12; and G. Makins, *Autobiography* (RCS Library, n.d.), p. 12.

18. J. Simon, *Personal Recollections of Sir John Simon, KCB* (London, privately printed, 1894), pp. 9–12. Cf. Sir Benjamin Brodie's remarks in T. Holmes, *Sir Benjamin Collins Brodie* (London, 1897), Appendix A, p. 226.

19. B. Brodie, *Autobiography of the Late Sir Benjamin Brodie, Bart.* (London, 1865), pp. 20–22.

20. G. K. Rainow [pseud.], *"G.P."* (London and Glasgow, 1939), p. 1.

21. Keetley, *Guide*, p. 95.

22. H. B. Thomson, *The Choice of a Profession* (London, 1857), p. 145.

23. Ibid., p. 142. Cf. Rainow, *"G.P.,"* p. 75.

24. *Dr. Watson's Address, March 26th, 1866* (Privately printed for the RCP, n.d.), p. 3. *Note*: All proceedings of the Royal College of Physicians, including presidential addresses, are *secreta collegii*, and they are cited here by the kind permission of the Royal College of Physicians, London.

25. W. Jenner, Presidential Addresses (RCP Mss. 1928/181), Vol. 1, 1885, pp. 3–4. For similar remarks about other physicians, see: ibid., Vol. 1, 1882, irreg. pag., regarding Dr. Archibald Billing and Dr. R. W. Falconer; and 1885, irreg. pag., regarding Dr. Daniel

Noble, Dr. Thomas Bishop, and Dr. Thomas Watson. See also: *Munk's Roll*, III, s.v. Sir Henry Holland; and *Plarr's Lives*, s.v. Charles Brooke, Frederick H. Marsh, Thomas Rivington Wheeler, Alfred Winkfield, John Briscoe, and E. L. Hussey, for further examples.

26. Brodie, *Autobiography*, p. 20. See also: Holmes, *Sir Benjamin*, Appendix I, p. 236; and Haight, *Eliot and Chapman*, p. 114. Sir William Jenner, in his eulogy to Dr. Hall Davis, spoke of a medical career as "the race for fame or fortune" (Presidential Addresses, Vol. 1, 1885, irreg. pag.).

27. Beddoe, *Memories*, p. 27.

28. J. De Styrap, *The Young Practitioner* (London, 1890), pp. vii–viii.

29. For studies of Victorian secondary education, see: T. W. Bamford, *The Rise of the Public Schools* (London, 1967); S. J. Curtis, *The History of Education in Great Britain*, 7th ed. (London, 1967); R. Wilkinson, *Gentlemanly Power* (London and New York, 1964); and I. Weinberg, *The English Public Schools* (New York, 1967).

30. P. Eade, *The Autobiography of Sir Peter Eade* (London, 1916), pp. 21–22. It is not clear from Eade's account whether he boarded at school or lived at home.

31. Makins, *Autobiography*, pp. 5, 8, and 9.

32. Beddoe, *Memories*, p. 173.

33. *Plarr's Lives*, s.v. John Postgate.

34. F. Musgrove, "Middle Class Education and Employment in the Nineteenth Century," *Econ. Hist. Rev.*, 2nd ser., 12 (1959), 99. See also: W. J. Reader, *Professional Men* (London, 1966), p. 157; and Banks, *Prosperity and Parenthood*, pp. 191 ff.

35. Williams, *Memoirs*, p. 3.

36. Idem.

37. Thomson, *Choice of a Profession*, p. 140. See also: W. Dale, *The State of the Medical Profession in Great Britain* (Dublin, 1875), p. 38. For earlier expressions of similar views on the virtues of a good preliminary education, see: *Select Committee on Medical Education*, 1834, (602–I), xiii, Part 1, p. 8, Q. 109, p. 30, Q. 466–469 (Macmichael). Conversely, the author of *A Few Words on the Fellowship*, p. 19, refers to "the degrading habits of a low education."

38. Thomson, *Choice of a Profession*, p. 140. See also: *Select Committee on Medical Education*, 1834, Part 1, p. 27, Q. 356 (Halford).

39. B. Brodie, *Introductory Discourse on Duties and Conduct of Medical Students and Practitioners* (London, 1843), p. 19.

40. Dale, *The Medical Profession*, pp. 38–39. See also: *BMJ*, 1876, i, 736; and *BMJ*, 1884, ii, 546.

41. [J. Vaughan-Hughes], *Seventy Years of Life in the Victorian Era* (London, 1893), p. 2. See also: *Munk's Roll*, III, s.v. Peter Mere Latham; and *Select Committee on Medical Education*, 1834, Part 1, pp. 73 and 76, Q. 1111–1116 and 1198–1200 (Seymour) regarding classical education and gentlemanliness.

42. British Medical Association, *Medicine in Modern Times* (London, 1869), pp. 5–6.

43. Keetley, *Guide*, p. 16. In 1860, articled students registered with the Royal College of Surgeons were required to demonstrate "proficiency" in Latin: RCS, *Bye-Laws of the Royal College of Surgeons of England* (London, [1860]), p. 13. Cf. S. T. Taylor, *The Diary of a Medical Student during the Mid-Victorian Period, 1860–64* (Norwich, 1927), p. 2.

44. G. Turner, *Unorthodox Reminiscences* (London, 1931), p. 71.

45. Holmes, *Sir Benjamin*, pp. 129–130.

46. Keetley, *Guide*, pp. 16, 49, and 60.

47. Ibid., p. 60. See also: R. Quain, *Observations on Medical Education* (London, 1865), p. 47, note B.

48. *BMJ*, 1884, ii, 546. See also: *Select Committee on Medical Education*, 1834, Part 1, p. 27, Q. 356 (Halford).

49. In BMA, *Medicine in Modern Times*, p. 43. See also: T. C. Allbutt, "Medicine in the 19th Century," *J. Med. Educ.*, 31 (1956), 466 ff.

50. J. B. Atlay, *Sir Henry Wentworth Acland* (London, 1903), p. 76.

51. Z. Cope, *The Royal College of Surgeons of England* (London, 1959), p. 134.

52. Keetley, *Guide*, p. 52. For the history of medical education, C. Newman's *The Evolution of Medical Education in the Nineteenth Century* (London, 1957) is the standard work. See also: S. W. F. Holloway, "Medical Education in England, 1830–1858," *History*, 49 (1964), 299–324. H. H. Bellot, *University College London, 1826–1926* (London, 1929), gives a detailed account of medical education there. For further information, see: F. N. L. Poynter, ed., *The Evolution of Medical Education in Britain* (London, 1966); H. D. Rolleston, *The Cambridge Medical School* (Cambridge, 1932); A. H. T. Robb-Smith, *A Short History of the Radcliffe Infirmary* (Oxford, 1970); A. Rook, ed., *Cambridge and Its Contribution to Medicine* (London, 1971); and T.

Puschmann, *A History of Medical Education from the Most Remote to the Most Recent Times* (London, 1891). Histories of hospitals also include some information on medical education.

53. Newman, *Medical Education*, pp. 8–12, 74, 107, and 122–133; Cope, *The Royal College*, pp. 134–135.

54. Newman, *Medical Education*, pp. 74, 107–108, 211 ff., and 296; *BMJ*, 1884, ii, 504; and Bellot, *University College London*, Chart 6.

55. Newman, *Medical Education*, pp. 107–108.

56. St. Thomas's Hospital, Minute Books of the Grand Committee (H.1/ST/A6/11), 13 July 1842, p. 17; (H.1/ST/A6/13), 12 February 1856, p. 60, and 14 February 1860, pp. 204–205; (H.1/ST/A6/15), 28 July 1870, p. 195; and (H.1/ST/A6/16), 13 March 1877, p. 227.

57. E. M. McInnes, *St. Thomas' Hospital* (London, 1963), pp. 74–82 and 92–95; J. Langdon-Davies, *Westminster Hospital* (London, 1952), pp. 105–117; Z. Cope, *The History of St. Mary's Hospital Medical School* (London, 1954), pp. 4–8 and 20 ff.; H. C. Cameron, *Mr. Guy's Hospital, 1726–1948* (London, 1954), pp. 88 ff.; N. Moore, *History of St. Bartholomew's Hospital* (London, 1918), II, 803; and Abel-Smith, *The Hospitals*, pp. 16–18.

58. For a brief discussion of apprenticeship, see: Cope, *The Royal College*, pp. 11 and 135.

59. Cameron, *Mr. Guy's Hospital*, pp. 87–88 and 158–159.

60. Keetley, *Guide*, p. 12; and Taylor, *Diary, 1860–64*, pp. 6–7.

61. E. M. Brockbank, *The Foundation of Provincial Medical Education in England, and of the Manchester School in Particular* (Manchester, 1936).

62. Makins, *Autobiography*, p. 19.

63. Keetley, *Guide*, pp. 18 and 51. See also: Newman, *Medical Education*, pp. 102, 124–130, and 276 ff.

64. Keetley, *Guide*, p. 56; also see pp. 49–51. Cf. T. C. Allbutt, *On Professional Education* (London, 1906), pp. 10 ff.

65. Keetley, *Guide*, p. 18.

66. See: Keetley, *Guide*, p. 15; and authors cited by Banks, *Prosperity and Parenthood*, pp. 177–178; and by Reader, *Professional Men*, p. 120.

67. Cope, *St. Mary's*, pp. 4 ff. and Chapter IV; McInnes, *St. Thomas' Hospital*, pp. 81, 92, and 95; Langdon-Davies, *Westminster Hospital*, p. 122; and Moore, *St. Bartholomew's*, II, 812 and 814–815.

68. Apprenticeship contract of Richard Hughes, bound to Henry Reynolds, November 4, 1851, Society of Apothecaries, in: Guildhall Mss.

69. *London and Provincial Medical Directory*, 1855, p. 562; and 1860, p. 300.

70. Ibid., 1860, p. 300; and Keetley, *Guide*, p. 14.

71. Keetley, *Guide*, p. 14. Also see James Paget's survey of living costs of medical students in 1843 in: St. Bartholomew's Hospital Mss., Copies of Entries . . . (M.S. 3/1), pp. 12–13 and 35.

72. Banks, *Prosperity and Parenthood*, pp. 59 and 74.

73. Ibid., p. 59; and Keetley, *Guide*, p. 15. See also: E. H. Hunt, *Regional Wage Variation in Britain, 1840–1914* (Oxford, 1973), passim.

74. See, e.g., *Plarr's Lives*, s.v. Edward Stephens. Also see: H. R. Haweis, *Sir Morrell Mackenzie, Physician and Operator*, 2nd ed. (London, 1894), p. 46. Sir Felix Semon tells of how his relatives made loans to him for his London studies and early years of practice (*The Autobiography of Sir Felix Semon* [London, 1926], pp. 99–101). See also: *Munk's Roll*, IV, s.v. S. Ringer.

75. *London and Provincial Medical Directory*, 1860, p. 302.

76. Ibid., p. 326.

77. Ibid., 1875, p. 238.

78. *Plarr's Lives*, s.v. William Warwick Wagstaffe, Sr. See also: *Munk's Roll*, IV, s.v. J. L. H. Langdon-Down.

79. See, e.g., St. Thomas's Hospital, Minute Books of the Grand Committee (H.1/ST/A6/11), 13 July 1842, pp. 17–18.

80. *Plarr's Lives*, s.v. E. Cock. Cf. s.v. J. H. Green, Thomas Bellot, and T. B. Curling.

81. Ibid. See also: s.v. Robert C. Brown and Richard Quain. Thomas Bryant, Oliver Pemberton, Charles Frederick Maunder, and Matthew Berkeley Hill are examples of the many medical students who were apprenticed locally in what seem to be indentures with previous family connections. Cf. Charles Dickens, *Bleak House*, Chapter 13.

82. *Plarr's Lives*, s.v. Samuel Solly and John Birkett.

83. Ibid., s.v. W. Rivington.

84. Ibid. Also see: entries in *Plarr's Lives* regarding Marcus Beck and Rickman Godlee, who studied at Glasgow where their cousin Joseph Lister was professor of Surgery; and s.v. Caesar H. Hawkins,

Louis S. Little, Sir Charles Sissmore Tomes, Thomas Rivington Wheeler, Benjamin Travers, Jr., Sir William Thorburn, and Arthur F. McGill. Edward Cock, apprenticed to his uncle Sir Astley Cooper, also went to lectures at St. Thomas's, where another relative, Henry Cline, was Surgeon and teacher.

85. Ibid. Cf. s.v. Thomas Eastes, and *Munk's Roll*, IV, s.v. Herbert Davies.

86. Ibid., s.v. Dennis Hovell, John Hammond Morgan, and Adams.

87. Makins, *Autobiography*, p. 19. See also: *Plarr's Lives*, s.v. Honoratus Leigh Thomas. Also: Counsell, *Memoirs*, pp. 9–10; A. H. G. Doran, *Life Memories* (RCS Library, 1923), p. 3; and Carr, *Arthur Conan Coyle*, p. 18.

88. Bland-Sutton, *Surgeon*, pp. 26 and 28.

89. Keetley, *Guide*, pp. 21–22. The numbering and order are Keetley's.

90. Ibid., p. 24.

91. Ibid., p. 23.   93. Ibid., p. 23.

92. Ibid., pp. 22–23.   94. Idem.

95. See Newman, *Medical Education*, pp. 39 ff., for a brief sketch. See also: *Select Committee on Medical Education, Schools of Anatomy*, 1828, vii (568), for a description of pre-reform conditions.

96. Taylor, *Diary, 1860–64*, p. 9. For other accounts of medical student life, see: S. T. Taylor, *Diary of a Norwich Hospital Medical Student, 1858–1860* (London, 1930); and S. H. Snell, *A Doctor at Work and Play* (London, 1937), pp. 13 ff.

97. See: St. Bartholomew's Hospital Mss., Copies of Entries . . . (M.S. 3/1), pp. 12 ff.

98. St. Bartholomew's Hospital Mss., Regulations, Medical College Hall (M.S. 2).

99. Keetley, *Guide*, p. 37. See also: J. Paget, "The Advantages of Medical Societies" [an address] (RCS ms., n.d.), f. 5.

100. Keetley, *Guide*, p. 37.

101. *Plarr's Lives*, s.v., e.g., E. B. Owen, J. C. Forster, and J. R. Lane; and *Munk's Roll*, IV, s.v. William Wadham. By 1898, St. Thomas's Hospital students had twelve clubs, ranging from the Lawn Tennis Club and the Rifle Club to the Medical and Physical Society. See: St. Thomas's Hospital Medical School, *Prospectus for the Year Commencing October 1st, 1898* (London, [1898]), p. 4 [RCS Library, St. Thomas's Hospital, Reports and Papers, 1863–1898].

102. *Plarr's Lives*, s.v. Sir Alfred Cooper (regarding the Masonic Lodge at St. Bartholomew's Hospital) and s.v. E. B. Owen (regarding the lodge at St. Mary's). For other references to Masonic activities, see: *Plarr's Lives*, s.v. Edmund J. Furner, George Woods, H. W. Dodd, W. A. Duncan, R. H. Whitelock, H. B. Robinson, F. C. Vinrace, W. H. H. Jessop, E. G. Whittle, C. E. L. B. Hudson, William Rawes, J. E. Lane, Sir C. P. Lukes, James Turton, and T. F. Pearse.

103. Taylor, *Diary, 1860–64*, pp. 2, 6, and 36.

104. E.g., Snell, *Doctor at Work*, pp. 16 and 18.

105. S. S. Sprigge, *Physic and Fiction* (London, 1921), p. 150.

106. Idem. Peter Eade was optimistic about his London career because he was a prizeman (*Autobiography*, p. 47).

107. Keetley, *Guide*, p. 28.

108. Sprigge, *Physic and Fiction*, p. 153. Cf. Sir Benjamin Brodie's views in: Holmes, *Sir Benjamin*, Appendix D, p. 230.

109. Cope, *St. Mary's*, p. 50; Quain, *Observations*, p. 24; and S. Paget, *Sir Victor Horsley*, p. 17.

110. Sprigge, *Physic and Fiction*, p. 152.

111. Makins, *Autobiography*, p. 23.

112. *Plarr's Lives*, s.v. William B. Page.

113. General Medical Council, *Minutes of the General Medical Council . . . for the Year 1885*, Vol. XXII (London, 1886), p. 139. [Hereafter: GMC, *Minutes*.]

114. Keetley, *Guide*, p. 87. See also: A. M. Cooke, "The College and Europe," *J. Royal Coll. Phys. London*, 4:2 (1970), 105–113 passim.

115. Abel-Smith, *The Hospitals*, Chapter 2.

116. Makins, *Autobiography*, p. 29.

117. Examples include: Edgar Barker; John Barnes; Edward R. Bickersteth and his son; John Lawrence and his son; and George F. Bodington—q.v. in *Plarr's Lives*.

118. Examples (from *Plarr's Lives*): Alfred Baker; Frank Barendt; Samuel Barnes; Alexander H. Bartlet; William Bates; Alexander Best; and George Mallett.

119. The phrase is from Snell, *Doctor at Work*, p. 28.

120. Counsell, *Memoirs*, pp. 21–22.

121. Ibid., p. 22.

122. Idem.

123. Keetley, *Guide*, p. 52. Also see p. 56.

Chapter III

1. A report of the Royal College of Physicians indicates that there were 10,000 to 15,000 midwives practicing in England and Wales, most of them untrained and unlicensed. See: A. M. Cooke, *A History of the Royal College of Physicians of London* (Oxford, 1972), III, 896. For further information on unlicensed practice, see: Great Britain, Privy Council, *Report as to the Practice of Medicine and Surgery by Unqualified Persons in the United Kingdom* (London, 1910). See also: S. W. F. Holloway, "The Apothecaries' Act of 1815," *Medical History*, 10:3 (1966), 230.

2. In Wilkie Collins, *The Moonstone* (London, n.d.), pp. 70–71. Cf. Salisbury's comment to Lord Lytton in 1877: "[Y]ou never should trust experts. If you believe the doctors, nothing is wholesome" (in: Lady Gwendolyn Cecil, *Life of Robert, Marquis of Salisbury* [London, 1921–23], II, 153). See also: F. Turner, "Rainfall, Plagues, and the Prince of Wales," *Journal of British Studies*, 13:2 (May, 1974), 46–65.

3. E. Freidson, *Profession of Medicine* (New York, 1970), p. 72.

4. *Select Committee on Medical Education*, 1834, Part I, pp. 13–14, Q. 111–113 (Halford); and p. 87, Q. 1450 (Warren).

5. C. B. Keetley, *The Student's and Junior Practitioner's Guide to the Medical Profession*, 2nd ed. (London, 1885), p. 45. Cf. H. B. Thomson, *The Choice of a Profession* (London, 1857), pp. 161–162.

6. Thomson, *Choice of a Profession*, p. 162.

7. Keetley, *Guide*, p. 45.

8. Idem.

9. A. C. Doyle, *The Stark Munro Letters* (New York, 1895). For similar but less detailed accounts, see: *Memoirs of the Life of a Country Surgeon* (London, 1845); G. K. Rainow [pseud.], "*G.P.*" (London and Glasgow, 1939), pp. 77 ff.; and F. Winslow, *Physic and Physicians* (London, 1839), I, 137–140.

10. A. C. Doyle, *Memories and Adventures* (Boston, 1924), pp. 56–65; and J. D. Carr, *The Life of Sir Arthur Conan Doyle* (New York, 1949), pp. 34 ff.

11. Doyle, *Stark Munro*, pp. 228–232.

12. Ibid., p. 249. Cf. Keetley, *Guide*, pp. 45–46.

13. Doyle, *Stark Munro*, pp. 256–258 and 263–265.

14. Ibid., pp. 262, 265–266, and 275.

15. Ibid., pp. 291 and 305–306.

16. Ibid., p. 316.

17. Ibid., p. 324.

18. Ibid., pp. 297–298.

19. Ibid., pp. 302–303.

20. Ibid., p. 318.

21. Ibid., p. 321.

22. Ibid., pp. 321–322.

23. Ibid., p. 322.

24. Ibid., pp. 322–323.

25. Ibid., p. 324.

26. Ibid., p. 317.

27. Ibid., pp. 336, 342, and 348.

28. Ibid., p. 343.

29. Ibid., p. 344.

30. Idem.

31. Ibid., pp. 344–346.

32. Ibid., p. 369.

33. Cf. J. A. Banks, *Prosperity and Parenthood* (London, 1954), pp. 177–178. See also: F. Davenant, *What Shall My Son Be?* (London, 1870), p. 55.

34. L. B. Namier, *The Structure of Politics at the Accession of George III*, 2nd ed. (London, 1965), pp. 16–17.

35. See, e.g., G. Makins, *Autobiography* (RCS ms., n.d.), pp. 26–27; H. E. Counsell, *37 The Broad. The Memoirs of an Oxford Doctor* (London, 1943), p. 24; and the advertisements sections of the *Lancet* and the *BMJ*.

36. Keetley, *Guide*, p. 43. Thomson, *Choice of a Profession*, p. 165, indicates that, in the 1850's, practices were sold for two to three years' purchase. Earlier in the century, Wakley bought a practice for less than one year's purchase; see S. S. Sprigge, *The Life and Times of Thomas Wakley* (London, 1899), p. 35.

37. *BMJ*, "Advertiser" section, February 12, 1876, no pagination.

38. Idem. Cf. S. H. Snell, *A Doctor at Work and Play* (London, 1937), pp. 43 and 199. For further discussion of income, see Chapter V, below.

39. Keetley, *Guide*, pp. 44–45. F. Ashurst, *Memoirs of a Young Surgeon* (London, 1898), p. 51, writes of "the weary grind of a middle class city practice." Cf. W. Rivington, *The Medical Profession* (Dublin, 1879), p. 84.

40. *BMJ*, "Advertiser" section, February 12, 1876, no pagination. Snell, *Doctor at Work*, pp. 43–44, mentions a practice with an obstetric load of 300 cases. Advertisements suggest that thirty was a moderate number.

41. *BMJ*, "Advertiser" section, February 12, 1876, no pagination.

42. Idem.

43. P. Eade, *The Autobiography of Sir Peter Eade* (London, 1916), p. 56.

44. *BMJ*, "Advertiser" section, February 12, 1876, no pagination. Cf. Snell, *Doctor at Work*, pp. 43 and 199.

45. Keetley, *Guide*, p. 44. Cf. Thomson, *Choice of a Profession*, pp. 166–167.

46. Snell, *Doctor at Work*, pp. 43–44. See also: Keetley, *Guide*, p. 44; and Ashurst, *Memoirs*, p. 35.

47. *BMJ*, "Advertiser" section, February 12, 1876, no pagination.

48. Buxton Shillitoe, for example, spent only one weekend a year in Brighton for many years of his medical life. See his Visiting Lists and Diaries, Wellcome Historical Medical Library, Mod. Mss. 4526, 4529 et seq. Cf. Keetley, *Guide*, p. 44.

49. Thomson, *Choice of a Profession*, pp. 166–167; and Keetley, *Guide*, pp. 43–45.

50. Keetley, *Guide*, p. 43; and Thomson, *Choice of a Profession*, pp. 166–167.

51. *BMJ*, "Advertiser" section, February 12, 1876, no pagination.

52. *Lancet*, 1881, i, 195.

53. *Plarr's Lives*, s.v. Also see s.v.: the Burds (Salop); the Coates (Salisbury); the Colbys (Malton, Yorkshire); the Chevasses (Birmingham); the Bickersteths (Liverpool); the Bullars (Southampton); the Bulleys (Reading); and the Barneses (Bath) for other illustrative cases. For other multi-generation medical families, not necessarily in a single town, see *Plarr's Lives*, s.v.: C. H. Marriott; T. R. Teale; H. M. Greenhow; W. H. Power; J. B. Maurice; Thomas Sympson; and S. B. Gwynn. In *Munk's Roll*, IV, see s.v.: J. A. Symonds; Henry Munro; and E. H. Greenhow (three generations in North Shields).

54. *Plarr's Lives*, s.v. Other surgeons include: E. W. and A. B. Duffin (London) and the Thomas Wheelers (London). For physicians, see: *Munk's Roll*, III, s.v. Thomas Mayo; and *Munk's Roll*, IV, s.v. Sir James Alderson and William Ord.

55. Computed from information in *Plarr's Lives*.

56. *Plarr's Lives*, s.v. See also s.v.: Edgar Barker; John Barnes; George Bodington; Archibald Dalrymple; William Percival; and William Pettigrew—a few of the many cases. For physicians, see: *Munk's Roll*, IV, s.v. James Johnstone and C. J. B. Williams.

57. J. Beddoe, *Memories of Eighty Years* (Bristol, 1910), pp.

50–51, 125–126, 139, and 161–162; and *Munk's Roll*, IV, s.v. E. L. Fox. Beddoe later gained a post at the Infirmary.

58. Keetley, *Guide*, p. 46 (emphasis added). Cf. Wilkie Collins's struggling young doctor who had "not a friend in the place" (*Moonstone*, p. 305).

59. *Plarr's Lives*, s.v. See also s.v.: John B. Eastlin; W. H. Bellot; James E. Moreton; and James Stephens. For cases of brothers in practice, see s.v.: Archibald Dalrymple; F. C. Julius; J. H. Ceeley; William Willis; and Alexander Thom Thomson (in partnership with a brother-in-law). Samuel Hey, FRCS, shared a practice with his cousin.

60. *Report of the Committee Appointed by the Secretary of State to Enquire into the Causes which Tend to Prevent Sufficient Eligible Candidates from Coming Forward for the Army Medical Department* [C. 2200], 1878–79, xliv, 28.

61. *Plarr's Lives*, s.v. For further examples, see s.v. James Turton and Francis M. B. Sims. For another sort of father-in-law assistance, see: Sprigge, *Thomas Wakley*, pp. 35, 43, and 64–66.

62. Compiled from *Plarr's Lives*. For physicians who practiced in towns where they had relatives or other ties, see *Munk's Roll*, IV, s.v.: J. R. Reynolds; Samuel Wilks; Samuel Fenwick; George Shaw; Marshall Hall; D. J. Leach; and T. R. Glynn.

63. *Plarr's Lives*, interleaved copy, RCS Library, with additional ms. notes regarding the Shillitoe family, s.v. Buxton Shillitoe and his brother Richard Rickman Shillitoe. For the Quaker connection in London, see: Buxton Shillitoe Mss., Wellcome Historical Medical Library, Mod. Ms. 4517, Visiting List, 1865, which contains a letter from a Quaker patient. Also the names in his Visiting Lists include those of several families known to be Quakers: WHML Mod. Ms. 4520, Visiting List, 1867 (Hoare and Rickman) and WHML Mod. Ms. 4533, Pocket Diary, 1881 (Gurney and Hoare) (no pagination).

64. *Plarr's Lives* and *Munk's Roll*, IV, s.v. See also: *Plarr's Lives*, s.v. J. S. N. Boyd and Marcus Beck.

65. *Plarr's Lives*, s.v.

66. F. Semon, *The Autobiography of Sir Felix Semon* (London, 1926), p. 97.

67. Keetley, *Guide*, p. 40. See also: R. G. Hodgkinson, *The Origins of the National Health Service* (Berkeley and Los Angeles, 1967), p. 85.

68. E. Freidson, "The Organization of Medical Practice," in

Handbook of Medical Sociology, ed. H. E. Freeman et al. (Englewood Cliffs, N.J., 1963), pp. 307–309.

69. See examples in *Plarr's Lives*, s.v.: A. Buchanan; Charles H. Buncombe; Alfred Crabb; C. S. Barter; George Beaman; John Bishop; and Francis Beard.

70. G. Ayers, *England's First State Hospitals and the Metropolitan Asylums Board, 1867–1930* (London, 1971), pp. 139–154.

71. S. S. Sprigge, *Medicine and the Public* (London, 1906), p. 146, quoted in J. L. Brand, *Doctors and the State* (Baltimore, 1965), p. 88. Cf. Keetley, *Guide*, p. 42; and *Plarr's Lives*, s.v. J. W. Barnes. For further information on the growth of state medicine in England, see: Hodgkinson, *National Health Service*; D. Roberts, *Victorian Origins of the British Welfare State* (New Haven, 1960); R. Lambert, *Sir John Simon and English Social Administration, 1816–1904* (London, 1963); S. E. Finer, *Life and Times of Edwin Chadwick* (London, 1952); A. S. MacNalty, *The History of State Medicine in England* (London, 1948); R. M. McLeod, "The Anatomy of State Medicine," in *Medicine and Science in the 1860's*, ed. F. N. L. Poynter (London, 1968), pp. 199–228; and R. M. McLeod, "The Frustration of State Medicine, 1880–1899," *Medical History*, 11 (1967), 15–40.

72. Brand, *Doctors and the State*, pp. 88 and 109; Keetley, *Guide*, pp. 40 and 42; and Hodgkinson, *National Health Service*, pp. 73 and 105–106.

73. Brand, *Doctors and the State*, p. 88; Hodgkinson, *National Health Service*, pp. 102–116 passim; B. Abel-Smith, *The Hospitals, 1800–1948* (London, 1964), pp. 58 ff.; and Keetley, *Guide*, p. 40. The system of "tender" (bidding for posts) was the norm until the 1840's and may have continued, irregularly, after that time. See the 1848 cartoon in *Mr. Punch among the Doctors* (London, 1933), p. 3.

74. Keetley, *Guide*, p. 42; and Brand, *Doctors and the State*, p. 110. Cf. Lambert, *Sir John Simon*, p. 538.

75. Hodgkinson, *National Health Service*, pp. 59 and 344–351 passim; Brand, *Doctors and the State*, p. 85; and Ayers, *First State Hospitals*, p. 3.

76. J. Rogers, *Reminiscences of a Workhouse Medical Officer* (London, 1889), pp. 8, 29, 77, and 105. Rogers' reforming interests brought him into constant conflict with his board. For other sources regarding poor law practice, see: A. Sheen, *The Workhouse and Its Medical Officer* (Cardiff, 1875); and L. Twining, *Recollections of Workhouse Visiting and Management during Twenty-five Years* (London, 1880).

77. S. Novak, "Professionalism and Bureaucracy," *Journal of Social History*, 6:4 (1973), 445. See also: W. J. Reader, *Professional Men* (London, 1966), p. 23.

78. Hodgkinson, *National Health Service*, pp. 8–9, 118, 649, passim.

79. Freidson, "Medical Practice," p. 316.

80. Hodgkinson, *National Health Service*, pp. 73–78, 82, and 340 ff.; and Abel-Smith, *The Hospitals*, p. 58.

81. Hodgkinson, *National Health Service*, pp. 73 and 340 ff.; and Abel-Smith, *The Hospitals*, p. 63.

82. Hodgkinson, *National Health Service*, pp. 363–370; and Abel-Smith, *The Hospitals*, p. 228. This was still an issue in 1911; see: A. M. Cooke, *A History of the Royal College of Physicians of London* (Oxford, 1972), III, 1007.

83. Novak, "Professionalism," p. 452; Lambert, *Sir John Simon*, pp. 62–63 and 534–540; and Ayers, *First State Hospitals*, pp. 5 and 9.

84. Hodgkinson, *National Health Service*, pp. 20 ff.; and Ayers, *First State Hospitals*, p. 120.

85. Lambert, *Sir John Simon*, pp. 63n and 573–577. John Simon's administration was, of course, an exception.

86. Novak, "Professionalism," p. 453; Abel-Smith, *The Hospitals*, pp. 60, 62, 90–91, and 225; Hodgkinson, *National Health Service*, pp. 19–28 and 276–279; and Ayers, *First State Hospitals*, pp. 140 ff.

87. *BMJ*, 1873, ii, 192, quoted in Novak, "Professionalism," p. 452.

88. Hodgkinson, *National Health Service*, p. 649; and Brand, *Doctors and the State*, pp. 112–116.

89. Regarding asylums for inebriates, see: B. Harrison, *Drink and the Victorians* (London, 1971), p. 22. See also: W. Parry-Jones, *The Trade in Lunacy* (London, 1972); and K. Jones, *A History of the Mental Health Services* (London and Boston, 1972).

90. *Plarr's Lives* is filled with illustrations.

91. A. J. Cronin describes such practice, in *Adventures in Two Worlds* (Boston, 1952), pp. 135 ff. Cf. the prosperous colliery surgeon in A. Conan Doyle's *Stark Munro*, pp. 100 ff. See also: Hodgkinson, *National Health Service*, pp. 223–224 and 236–239; and Freidson, "Medical Practice," pp. 308–309.

92. The following is taken from Hodgkinson's extended discussion in *National Health Service*, pp. 215–239 and 602–610. See also: Abel-Smith, *The Hospitals*, pp. 93 and 153.

93. [W. Martin], Untitled book of accounts, 1888–1914, RCP Ms., especially pp. 569–574 and 575. Biographical information is from *The London and Provincial Medical Directory*, 1888.

94. Hodgkinson, *National Health Service*, p. 606.

95. Abel-Smith, *The Hospitals*, pp. 93 and 107. See also: Freidson, "Medical Practice," p. 303.

96. *Report of the Special Commission Set Up by the "Lancet" to Inquire into Medical Association and the Profession*, 1895. Reprinted as "The Battle of the Clubs," *Lancet*, 1895, ii, passim. Quoted in Hodgkinson, *National Health Service*, pp. 615–616.

97. *BMJ*, 10 April 1875, p. 484. Quoted in Abel-Smith, *The Hospitals*, p. 107.

98. Hodgkinson, *National Health Service*, p. 683; Abel-Smith, *The Hospitals*, p. 107; and Cooke, *A History*, III, 840–841 and 1079.

99. Abel-Smith, *The Hospitals*, pp. 107–108; and Hodgkinson, *National Health Service*, pp. 13–14, 220–221, 607–610, and 683.

100. Lambert, *Sir John Simon*, pp. 246, 299, 315–327 passim, and 386.

101. Hodgkinson, *National Health Service*, p. 444.

102. *Lancet*, 1869, i, 25–26. Quoted in Hodgkinson, *National Health Service*, p. 445.

103. Hodgkinson, *National Health Service*, pp. 445–446.

104. Keetley, *Guide*, pp. 43 ff. Cf. Doyle, *Stark Munro*, p. 100; and Cronin, *Adventures*, pp. 40 ff., for a description of assistancy work in a Scots country practice. See also: *Memoirs of the Life of a Country Surgeon*, pp. 16–17.

105. *Plarr's Lives*, s.v.

106. Ibid., s.v.

107. Ibid., s.v. Middlemore. H. E. Counsell had the assistance of his teachers at Guy's Hospital in building his country practice (*Memoirs*, p. 28). See also: Beddoe, *Memories*, p. 125; and *Plarr's Lives*, s.v. Sir Edwin Saunders, Theodore Duka, W. H. Crowfoot, Simon Nicholson, and Peter Redfern. Sir William Turner, FRCS, and Sir William Withey Gull, FRCP, are excellent examples of the combined value of patronage and a brilliant student career in the life of "poor and friendless" students.

108. *Munk's Roll*, III, s.v.

109. Keetley, *Guide*, p. 41. See *Plarr's Lives*, s.v. Charles H. Rogers-Harrison, William Newman, Eustace Smith, and E. C. Johnson. See also: *Munk's Roll*, III, s.v. Robert Bree, William Mac-

Michael, Thomas C. Morgan, G. D. Yeats, Charles Badham, J. A. Wilson, Henry Holland, and Peter M. Roget; and *Munk's Roll*, IV, s.v. H. A. Pitman and W. B. Cheadle. Also see a fictional example of aristocratic patronage in W. M. Thackeray's *The History of Pendennis* (New York, 1917), Chapter II; and Stark Munro's dream of treating "a fair countess;" in A. Conan Doyle's *Stark Munro*, p. 324. Private attendance on high-ranking Army and Navy officers could also lead to help in practice. See: *Plarr's Lives*, s.v. J. R. Rogers-Harrison, Thomas Spencer Wells, and E. M. Wrench.

110. *Plarr's Lives*, s.v.

111. Makins, *Autobiography*, p. 29. See also: Z. Cope, *The Versatile Victorian* (London, 1951), p. 28. Sir Henry Thompson (Cope's "versatile Victorian") by chance met the Chairman of the Board of Guardians of the Marylebone Workhouse Infirmary just before a vacancy occurred there; his connection got him the appointment.

112. St. Thomas's Hospital Ms. (H1/ST/Y36), Miscellanea associated with St. Thomas's Hospital. Certificates . . . including a letter of reference signed by Astley Cooper, 1838. The quotations come from letters by Francis Ramage, 4 August 1835; Astley Cooper, 17 June 1838; E. D. Dermott, 28 July 1835; and one, signature illegible (J. Rayner?), 10 May 1836.

113. Ibid., letters from F. Ramage, 4 August 1835; and (Rayner?), 10 May 1836.

114. Ibid., letter from James J. Power to the Infirmary, 18 June 1838.

115. St. Bartholomew's Hospital Manuscripts (M.C. 5/9/2), Correspondence. Paget testimonials. See also: Lambert, *Sir John Simon*, pp. 103–104 and 108 (quotations from Sir John Simon's dossier).

116. *Plarr's Lives*, s.v. Plarr records over sixty cases of Fellows who established themselves in provincial practice this way.

117. Keetley, *Guide*, pp. 97–98.

118. Ibid., pp. 46 and 100. See also: R. G. Glenn, *A Manual of the Laws Affecting Medical Men* (London, 1871), pp. x–xiii. For a detailed study of Army medical careers, see: N. D. Lankford, "Status, Bureaucracy, and Professionalism" (Ph.D. dissertation, Indiana University, 1976). For other histories of the medical services, see: D. G. Crawford, *History of the Indian Medical Service, 1600–1913* (London, 1914), 2 vols.; C. Lloyd and J. L. S. Coulter, *Medicine and the Navy, 1200–1900* (Edinburgh, 1963), 4 vols.; and J. Laffin, *Surgeons in the Field* (London, 1969).

119. *Plarr's Lives*, s.v. Nottidge Charles Macnamara, Thomas Spencer Wells, and the young surgeon in Dickens' *Bleak House*, Mr. Allan Woodcourt.

120. Compiled from *Plarr's Lives*.

121. Keetley, *Guide*, pp. 95–99. See also: Thomson, *Choice of a Profession*, pp. 139 and 169 ff.

122. Keetley, *Guide*, p. 97.

123. Ibid., pp. 97–98; and *BMJ*, 1857, i, 3.

124. Keetley, *Guide*, p. 100; and Glenn, *Manual*, pp. x–xiii. See, e.g., *Plarr's Lives*, s.v. R. H. Castellote.

125. *Plarr's Lives*, e.g., s.v. Charles Clark. A. Conan Doyle and A. J. Cronin began this way; see: Carr, *Arthur Conan Doyle*, pp. 28–29; and Cronin, *Adventures*, pp. 29 ff.

126. Examples from *Plarr's Lives* include: Edward J. Waring; James T. Ruddall; John Davies; Thomas Wigg, Jr.; John S. Wilkinson; Richard Rendle; Henry W. Saunders; Frederick Wadham; John Johnson; Herbert Fox; James Robertson; D. J. Williams; Charles Knight; Horatio Clarke; and Henry Challinor. In A. Conan Doyle's *Stark Munro*, p. 379, the unscrupulous Cullingworth finally takes up ophthalmology and emigrates. See also: Thomson, *Choice of a Profession*, p. 9; and *My Doctors*, "By a Patient" (London, 1891), p. 6.

127. Keetley, *Guide*, p. 46. Cf. J. H. Salter, *Dr. Salter of Tolleshunt D'Arcy* (London, 1933), p. 35.

128. [Martin], Book of accounts, var. pag.

129. *Plarr's Lives*, s.v.

130. Idem.

131. Counsell, *Memoirs*, pp. 26–27.

132. A. Conan Doyle describes a case of devious publicity-seeking, in *Stark Munro*, p. 165.

133. Counsell, *Memoirs*, p. 50; and Eade, *Autobiography*, pp. 54–55, 82–83, and 85–86. See also: A. Thackray, "Natural Knowledge in Cultural Context," *American Historical Review*, 79:3 (1974), 672–709.

134. Eade, *Autobiography*, p. 35.

135. Quoted in G. Haight, *George Eliot and John Chapman* (New Haven, 1940), p. 113. See also: Doyle, *Stark Munro*, pp. 93 and 97; and Thomson, *Choice of a Profession*, p. 163.

136. Written in 1878, the letter is quoted in Carr, *Arthur Conan Doyle*, p. 24. See also: Ashurst, *Memoirs*, pp. 35–36; Snell, *Doctor at*

Work, p. 43; and the ugly doctor in Collins, *Moonstone*, pp. 305–306. For examples of how social grace, or the lack of it, influenced practice, see: *Munk's Roll*, III, s.v. Charles Locock; and *Munk's Roll*, IV, s.v. John Curnow, Frederic Weber, and I. B. Yeo.

137. Quoted in *Historical Review of British Obstetrics and Gynaecology, 1800–1950*, ed. J. M. M. Kerr et al. (Edinburgh and London, 1954), p. 317. See also: Ashurst, *Memoirs*, p. 35.

138. Thomson, *Choice of a Profession*, pp. 144–145 and 162. See also: *Plarr's Lives*, s.v. B. T. Lowne.

139. C. Darwin, *The Life and Letters of Charles Darwin* (New York, 1959), I, 12, 17, and 19. See also: *Dictionary of National Biography*, s.v. Charles Darwin.

140. Quoted in T. Holmes, *Sir Benjamin Collins Brodie* (London, 1897), p. 164.

141. Keetley, *Guide*, pp. 60–61. See also: Rivington, *The Medical Profession*, pp. 48–50.

142. Keetley, *Guide*, p. 19.

143. Quoted in L. V. Fildes, *Luke Fildes, R.A.* (London, 1968), p. 118. The painting is reproduced facing p. 115. The teacher is not identified.

144. Idem.

145. I. Ashe, *Medical Education and Medical Interests* (Dublin, 1868), p. 1.

146. Ibid., pp. 1–2.

147. Ibid., p. 2.

148. Drawn from William Martin, Book of accounts, var. pag. His income in 1888 was £200; in 1889, over £500.

149. *BMJ*, 1857, ii, 25. See also: *Confessions of an English Doctor* (London, 1904), p. 27.

150. A. Doran, *Life Memories* (RCS Library, 1923), p. 2; and Ashurst, *Memoirs*, p. 23.

151. S. S. Sprigge, *Physic and Fiction* (London, 1921), p. 167. Cf. R. B. Carter, *Doctors and Their Work* (London, 1903), p. 153.

152. Abel-Smith, *The Hospitals*, pp. 96–97. See also: Ayers, *First State Hospitals*, pp. 55 and 142 ff.; but also see pp. 42, 43, and 60.

Chapter IV

1. E. Longford, *Victoria R.I.* (London, 1964), pp. 294–299.

2. Ibid., p. 389; and *Munk's Roll*, IV, s.v. William W. Gull. See

also: F. M. Turner, "Rainfall, Plagues, and the Prince of Wales," *J. Brit. Stud.*, 13:2 (1974), 46–65.

3. For examples, see: *Munk's Roll*, IV, s.v. Sir Hermann Weber, Isaac B. Yeo, and Sir Andrew Clark, Bt.; and *Plarr's Lives*, s.v. Sir Alfred Cooper, John S. Wells, and Edward Cutler. For a list of royal medical men, see: S. D. Clippingdale, "Medical Court Roll" (Typescript, RCS Library ms., n.d.), II, 51 ff.

4. For examples, see: *Munk's Roll*, IV, s.v. Thomas H. Green and Robert Liveing; and *Plarr's Lives*, s.v. Sir Henry Thompson, Bt., Sir James Paget, Bt., Isaac B. Brown, Sir Anthony Bowlby, Bt., William Rose, Jr., Benjamin Wainewright, and John Goldwyer Andrews. For a fictional account, see: G. Allen, *The Woman Who Did* (London, 1895), pp. 15, 92–93, 161, and 228.

5. Computed from data for the sample year 1878 in: W. Rivington, *The Medical Profession* (Dublin, 1879), p. 1; RCS, *Calendar of the Royal College of Surgeons of England* (London, 1878); and A. M. Cooke, *A History of the Royal College of Physicians of London* (Oxford, 1972), III, 1132–33.

6. B. Abel-Smith, *The Hospitals, 1800–1948* (London, 1964), p. 5. For more detail see individual hospital histories, e.g.: H. C. Cameron, *Mr. Guy's Hospital, 1726–1948* (London, 1954), Chapter I; and J. Langdon-Davies, *Westminster Hospital* (London, 1952), Chapter I.

7. At Guy's there were a minimum of forty and a maximum of sixty governors (Cameron, *Mr. Guy's Hospital*, p. 50). At Bart's there were 281 governors (*32nd Report of the Charity Commissioners*, Pt. VI, 1840 [219.], xix, Part I, p. 48). St. Mary's Hospital had one of the largest boards, with upwards of 1,500 members (Z. Cope, *History of St. Mary's Hospital Medical School* [London, 1964], p. 17). See also: Langdon-Davies, *Westminster Hospital*, pp. 142–143; E. W. Morris, *A History of the London Hospital*, 2nd ed. (London, 1910), pp. 71 and 119–121; and E. M. McInnes, *St. Thomas' Hospital* (London, 1963), pp. 25 and 141–142. The Report of the Charity Commissioners cited above gives extended details on the endowed hospitals in 1840.

8. *32nd Report of the Charity Commissioners*, 1840, pp. 48–49 (Bart's); pp. 668–669 (St. Thomas's); and pp. 731–734 (Guy's). See also: McInnes, *St. Thomas' Hospital*, pp. 141–142; Langdon-Davies, *Westminster Hospital*, pp. 150–151; and Morris, *London Hospital*, p. 96. N. Moore, *History of St. Bartholomew's Hospital* (London, 1918), II, 397–400, illustrates relations of the Court and House Committee.

9. *32nd Report of the Charity Commissioners*, 1840, p. 50; and

Moore, *St. Bartholomew's*, II, 168 and 802. The almoners often served *ex officio* on the House Committee.

10. *32nd Report of the Charity Commissioners*, 1840, p. 738; and Cameron, *Mr. Guy's Hospital*, pp. 43 and 59.

11. Abel-Smith, *The Hospitals*, pp. 10, 14–15, and 36–37; and *32nd Report of the Charity Commissioners*, 1840, pp. 671 and 738.

12. *32nd Report of the Charity Commissioners*, 1840, p. 30 (*re* maternity) and p. 678 (*re* other diseases); Langdon-Davies, *Westminster Hospital*, pp. 58–60 (*re* venereal disease) and pp. 49–51 (*re* religion); and Abel-Smith, *The Hospitals*, pp. 12–15.

13. Langdon-Davies, *Westminster Hospital*, pp. 58–60; also see p. 3.

14. See, e.g., St. Bartholomew's Hospital Mss., Minutes of the Board of Governors (Ha 1/25), 10 March 1881, p. 188. For an example of charges to hospital officers, see: St. Thomas's Hospital Records (H.1/ST/A28/1), "Rules and Orders for the Government of St. Thomas's Hospital, 1844," pp. 17–21.

15. St. Thomas's Hospital Records, Minutes of the General Court (H1/ST/A1). 28 August 1834, p. 314; St. Thomas's Hospital Records, "Rules and Orders . . . 1844" (H1/ST/A28/1), p. 18; St. Thomas's Hospital Records, "Rules and Orders . . . 1853" (H1/ST/A28/2), p. 17; and *32nd Report of the Charity Commissioners*, 1840, pp. 734–735.

16. St. Thomas's Hospital Records, Minutes of the Grand Committee (H1/ST/A6/17), 1 November 1882, p. 158. Cf. H. H. Bellot, *University College London, 1826–1926* (London, 1929), p. 158; and McInnes, *St. Thomas' Hospital*, p. 133.

17. Abel-Smith, *The Hospitals*, p. 33, expresses a different view.

18. Bellot, *University College London*, p. 163. *Munk's Roll*, III, s.v. J. Elliotson, says his colleagues also objected.

19. See, e.g., Langdon-Davies, *Westminster Hospital*, pp. 171–172 and 181–182; St. Thomas's Hospital Records, Minutes of the General Court (H1/ST/A1/9), 25 May 1858, pp. 143–151; and *32nd Report of the Charity Commissioners*, 1840, p. 684.

20. *32nd Report of the Charity Commissioners*, 1840, p. 53; St. Bartholomew's Hospital Mss., Minutes of the Board of Governors (Ha 1/17), 13 December 1816, p. 91; and St. Bartholomew's Hospital Mss., Minutes of the Medical Council (M.C. 1/1), 2 July 1870, p. 219.

21. *32nd Report of the Charity Commissioners*, 1840, pp. 667–669; and W. Hunter, *Historical Account of Charing Cross Hospital and Medi-*

cal School (London, 1914), p. 15. There were exceptions: at Guy's, five retired members of the staff became hospital governors between 1800 and 1900 (Cameron, *Mr. Guy's Hospital*, p. 98*n*). At St. George's Hospital, all who donated £5 a year could become governors, and a number of medical men used this avenue to the board; see the *Times*, July 27, 1880, p. 4. See also: R. J. Minney, *The Two Pillars of Charing Cross* (London, 1967), p. 10. Bart's also elevated retired staff to the board on occasion; see note 29, below.

22. Compiled from Moore, *St. Bartholomew's*, II, Chapter XXV, and from *Plarr's Lives*.

23. Compiled from *Plarr's Lives* and hospital histories. See also: F. Semon, *The Autobiography of Sir Felix Semon* (London, 1926), p. 81; and Abel-Smith, *The Hospitals*, p. 19. At Charing Cross, governors could also nominate students; see: Hunter, *Charing Cross Hospital*, pp. 54–55.

24. *32nd Report of the Charity Commissioners*, 1840, p. 52.

25. Abel-Smith, *The Hospitals*, p. 20. See also: Morris, *London Hospital*, pp. 116–117; Minney, *Two Pillars*, p. 10; and Langdon-Davies, *Westminster Hospital*, pp. 2 and 10. Cf. the *Times*, July 27, 1880, p. 4.

26. Langdon-Davies, *Westminster Hospital*, p. 157. Cf. Morris, *London Hospital*, p. 119.

27. *32nd Report of the Charity Commissioners*, 1840, p. 48 (*re* Bart's); p. 667 (*re* St. Thomas's); and p. 731 (*re* Guy's).

28. Ibid., p. 684.

29. St. Bartholomew's Hospital Mss., Minutes of the Board of Governors (Ha 1/17), 17 July 1815, pp. 27–29, 31 and 32 (*re* Earle); 30 November 1824, pp. 529–530 (*re* Latham); cf. pp. 501 and 504.

30. Ibid. (Ha 1/16), 14 August 1801, p. 14; and (Ha 1/17), 16 April 1819, p. 217 (*re* R. Powell). See also the case of James Risdon Bennett in: St. Thomas's Hospital Records, Minutes of the General Court (H1/ST/A1/8), 13 May 1844, pp. 429–431. For an illustration of the extensive family connections among governors, see: St. Thomas's Hospital Records, *List of Governors of St. Thomas's Hospital in Southwark* (London, 1853), (H1/ST/A65/12), especially the Pott family.

31. St. Thomas's Hospital Records, Minutes of the General Court (H1/ST/A1/8), 24 January 1884, p. 420; cf. p. 416.

32. E.g., Cameron, *Mr. Guy's Hospital*, pp. 98*n* and 134, regarding the Babingtons.

33. Langdon-Davies, *Westminster Hospital*, pp. 185–189, passim.

34. Cameron, *Mr. Guy's Hospital*, pp. 132–133 and 137.

35. *32nd Report of the Charity Commissioners*, 1840, p. 684.

36. Ibid., pp. 49, 668–669, 734–735, and 750. See also: Langdon-Davies, *Westminster Hospital*, p. 149.

37. Cameron, *Mr. Guy's Hospital*, pp. 105–107.

38. *Select Committee (H.L.) on Metropolitan Hospitals*, 1890 (392), xvi, p. 345, Q. 5976 (Roberts); and Langdon-Davies, *Westminster Hospital*, pp. 148–150.

39. Cameron, *Mr. Guy's Hospital*, pp. 105 and 166.

40. Ibid., p. 110; and *Dictionary of National Biography*, s.v. T. Addison.

41. Cameron, *Mr. Guy's Hospital*, p. 110.

42. *Munk's Roll*, IV, s.v.

43. Compiled from Cameron, *Mr. Guy's Hospital*, p. 498; and from *Plarr's Lives*, s.v.

44. Compiled from data in *Plarr's Lives*. Brodie's students later appointed were: P. G. Hewett; Caesar Hawkins; Thomas Tatum; Edward Cutler; G. D. Pollock; and Timothy Holmes. Abernethy's were: W. Lawrence; Edward Stanley; F. C. Skey; E. A. Lloyd; and Thomas Wormald. Cf. at St. Thomas's: Henry Cline, Sr., whose students (Henry Cline, Jr. and J. H. Green) gained posts on the senior staff.

45. *Plarr's Lives*, s.v. Charles Aston Key. Cf. C. Newman, *The Evolution of Medical Education in the Nineteenth Century* (London, 1957), p. 143.

46. In addition to Astley Cooper's group at Guy's, the following appointees were relatives of hospital staff: Edward Stanley and Henry Earle (Bart's); Robert Keate, Thomas Tatum, and Caesar H. Hawkins (St. George's); Henry Cline, Jr., J. H. Green, and John Flint South (St. Thomas's); Thomas Blizard Curling (London); S. A. Lane (St. Mary's); Thomas Morton (University College Hospital); and Alexander Shaw (Middlesex). For the above, see: *Plarr's Lives*, s.v.; and G. Gordon-Taylor, *Sir Charles Bell* (Edinburgh, 1958), p. 108 (*re* Shaw). See also: B. Brodie, *Autobiography of the Late Sir Benjamin Brodie, Bart.* (London, 1865), pp. 78–79 (*re* Robert Keate). Thomas Callaway, Sr., assistant surgeon at Guy's, was the grandson of Guy's steward (Cameron, *Mr. Guy's Hospital*, p. 140), and his son, Thomas Callaway, Jr., became assistant surgeon to Guy's in 1853 (ibid., pp. 246–247).

47. *Plarr's Lives*, s.v.

48. Langdon-Davies, *Westminster Hospital*, p. 185.

49. Moore, *St. Bartholomew's*, II, 547–549; and *Munk's Roll*, III, s.v. P. M. Latham. Peter Latham's grandson also became a member of Bart's staff.

50. Cameron, *Mr. Guy's Hospital*, p. 134; and *Munk's Roll*, III, s.v.

51. *Munk's Roll*, IV, s.v. Family succession also occurred outside the teaching hospitals; see, e.g.: *Munk's Roll*, III, s.v. Alexander J. Sutherland; and *Munk's Roll*, IV, s.v. Adam Neale.

52. N. G. Annan, "The Intellectual Aristocracy," in *Studies in Social History*, ed. J. H. Plumb (London, 1955), p. 243.

53. *32nd Report of the Charity Commissioners*, 1840, pp. 684 and 750.

54. Evaluations are drawn from *Munk's Roll*, *Plarr's Lives*, and Cameron, *Mr. Guy's Hospital*, pp. 128 ff., 137, and 139.

55. Cameron, *Mr. Guy's Hospital*, p. 140 (*re* Cooper); and *Munk's Roll*, IV (*re* Babington).

56. *Munk's Roll*, III, s.v. John Scott.

57. Quoted in Cameron, *Mr. Guy's Hospital*, p. 104.

58. Ibid., p. 136.

59. Langdon-Davies, *Westminster Hospital*, pp. 185–188. For other examples, see: T. G. Wilson, *Victorian Doctor* (New York, 1946), p. 89, which describes F. Tyrrell as "such a clumsy and unlucky operator that he was debarred from performing major operations for a year." See also: Bellot, *University College London*, p. 161 (*re* R. Quain); and F. Winslow, *Physic and Physicians* (London, 1839), I, 131–133, 154, and 345. For others of limited ability, see: *Plarr's Lives*, s.v. Charles Brooke, Alfred Winkfield, E. L. Hussey, and John Briscoe.

60. Cameron, *Mr. Guy's Hospital*, pp. 132–133 and 157–158. George MacIlwain stated: "[T]here is not one single surgeoncy that is fairly and *bona fide* open to scientific competition" (*Memoirs of John Abernethy, F.R.S.* [New York, 1853], p. 335). See also: MacIlwain, *Memoirs*, pp. 337 and 341–343; and *Plarr's Lives*, s.v. Francis Kiernan and A. M. McWhinnie.

61. Langdon-Davies, *Westminster Hospital*, p. 185. See also: *32nd Report of the Charity Commissioners*, 1840, p. 52.

62. *32nd Report of the Charity Commissioners*, 1840, p. 684.

63. Idem.

64. S. S. Sprigge, *The Life and Times of Thomas Wakley* (London, 1899), p. 109; and Newman, *Medical Education*, pp. 140–154.

65. RCS, *List of Officers, &c. of the Royal College of Surgeons of England, 1800–1895* (London, 1896), pp. 4 ff., 11, and 15. Lucas's father had also served.

66. For those never elected FRCP who had hospital posts, see: *Munk's Roll*, III, s.v. Benjamin Robinson, Richard Dennison, Hugh Ley, John Ashburner, John Conquest, William Back, and David Davis. Charles D. Badham (q.v. *Munk's Roll*, IV) never practiced medicine but was elected FRCP. See also: *Munk's Roll*, II, s.v. Charles Gower; and *Munk's Roll*, III, s.v. Richard Simmons and Thomas Young.

67. Quoted in *Select Committee on Medical Education*, 1834 (602–I), xiii, Part I, p. 288, Q. 4281.

68. Ibid. For an example, see: *Munk's Roll*, III, s.v. William Maton.

69. *Select Committee on Medical Education*, 1834, Part I, p. 288, Q. 4281.

70. E.g., *Munk's Roll*, III, s.v. Peter M. Latham, Charles Price, Archibald Billing, and Richard Bright; and *Munk's Roll*, IV, s.v. Sir George E. Paget.

71. *Munk's Roll*, II, s.v. Charles Gower; and *Munk's Roll*, III, s.v. Thomas Young, John Scott, James Tattersall, Robert Williams, and Joseph Hurlock.

72. *Munk's Roll*, III, s.v. William Shearman, John Macullock, and Robert M. Kerrison.

73. *Select Committee on Medical Education*, 1834, Part I, p. 40, Q. 568 (Macmichael). For an assessment of the relationship of patronage and science in the eighteenth century, see: J. D. Newson, "Medical Knowledge and the Patronage System in 18th-Century England," *Sociology*, 8:3 (1974), 369–385.

74. For example, see *Munk's Roll*, IV, s.v. Henry Jeaffreson, Algernon Frampton, Robert Nairne, and William E. Page.

75. *Select Committee on Medical Education*, 1834, Part I, p. 42, Q. 589; p. 54, Q. 748–772 (Macmichael); and p. 97, Q. 1483 (Warren).

76. Ibid., p. 9, Q. 109 (Halford).

77. Ibid., p. 9, Q. 110 (Halford); and p. 35, Q. 506 ff. (Macmichael).

78. Ibid., p. 25, Q. 348 (Halford).

79. Ibid., p. 35, Q. 511.

80. For example, see: *Munk's Roll*, III, s.v. Henry H. Southey, William Macmichael, John A. Paris, and Sir Charles Locock, Bart.

81. *Munk's Roll*, III, s.v. For illustrations of how royal influence could lead to the Fellowship, see *Munk's Roll*, III, s.v. Andrew Bain, who was M.D. Edin., but elected FRCP because he was a royal physician. See also: *Select Committee on Medical Education*, 1834, Part I, p. 15, Q. 201 (Halford). However, a number of physicians to the crown were never elected FRCP. See: *Select Committee on Medical Education*, Part I, Appendix 5, p. 13.

82. *Munk's Roll*, III, s.v. W. M. Maton, W. F. Chambers, and J. A. Paris. Sir Benjamin Brodie seems also to have befriended Chambers. For other examples, see: *Munk's Roll*, III, s.v. Joseph Ager and Charles Gower.

83. Newman, *Medical Education*, p. 137. See also: *Munk's Roll*, III, s.v. Charles Gower, Richard Simmons, and Thomas Young.

84. *Munk's Roll*, III, s.v. For other examples of aristocratic patronage, see: *Munk's Roll*, III, s.v. Robert Bree, Thomas Hume, and James H. Wilson.

85. [T. Watson], *Dr. Watson's Address, March 26th, 1866* (Privately printed, n.d.), p. 3. *Munk's Roll*, III, s.v. Henry Herbert Southey, indicates that Lord Brougham was one of his patrons. Cf. Brodie, *Autobiography*, pp. 78–79, for an example of a surgeon enjoying aristocratic patronage.

86. [Watson], *Address*, p. 3. For other examples of early aristocratic service, see: *Munk's Roll*, III, s.v. Grant David Yeats, William Macmichael, Charles Badham, Edward J. Seymour, J. A. Wilson, Peter Mark Roget, Charles D. Nevison, and Thomas Young (a Quaker physician, who may have benefited from his early service to the Barclay and Gurney families). See also: Moore, *St. Bartholomew's*, II, 551–552.

87. *Select Committee on Medical Education*, 1834, Part I, p. 25, Q. 356 (Halford); also see p. 70, Q. 1114 and 1116 (Seymour).

88. Ibid., p. 91, Q. 1450 (Warren); also see Q. 1449–1453.

89. One Dr. Wells was described as an "extremely irritable man" and therefore not elected FRCP. See: *Select Committee on Medical Education*, 1834, Part I, p. 39, Q. 558 (Macmichael). See also: p. 40, Q. 570; and p. 87, Q. 1387 and 1450 (Warren).

90. B. Brodie, *Introductory Discourse* (London, 1843), quoted in

T. Holmes, *Sir Benjamin Collins Brodie* (London, 1897), Appendix L, p. 239. Cf. I. Ashe, *Medical Education and Medical Interests* (Dublin, 1868), p. 2. See also: L. Namier, *The Structure of Politics at the Accession of George III*, 2nd ed. (London, 1965), p. 18. Anthropologists have studied the social implications of patronage and friendship in premodern societies. See, e.g., J. A. Pitt-Rivers, *The People of the Sierra* (London, 1954), pp. 107 ff.; and J. K. Campbell, *Honour, Family, and Patronage* (Oxford, 1964), pp. 257 ff. Note also the definitions of "friend" (usage 3 and 5) and "friendship" (usage 3) in the *Oxford English Dictionary*.

91. *Select Committee on Medical Education*, 1834, p. 289, Q. 4283.

92. Langdon-Davies, *Westminster Hospital*, pp. 172–176, 181, and 188, and G. Clark, *A History of the Royal College of Physicians of London* (Oxford, 1966), II, 617–620 and 664–665, offer illustrations.

93. See, e.g., Langdon-Davies, *Westminster Hospital*, pp. 106–109; Cope, *St. Mary's*, pp. 20–22; Morris, *London Hospital*, p. 145; Hunter, *Charing Cross Hospital*, pp. 1, 4, 8–10, and 22; McInnes, *St. Thomas' Hospital*, pp. 74 ff.; Moore, *St. Bartholomew's*, II, 648–649 and 803 ff.; and Cameron, *Mr. Guy's Hospital*, pp. 88 ff. See also: *32nd Report of the Charity Commissioners*, 1840, pp. 70 and 748; and Newman, *Medical Education*, pp. 33 ff.

94. *32nd Report of the Charity Commissioners*, 1840, pp. 70, 683, and 750. But see: Langdon-Davies, *Westminster Hospital*, pp. 161–162.

95. Langdon-Davies, *Westminster Hospital*, pp. 117–122; Hunter, *Charing Cross Hospital*, pp. 10 and 22; Cameron, *Mr. Guy's Hospital*, pp. 124 and 222–223; and McInnes, *St. Thomas' Hospital*, p. 92. Harrison, the treasurer at Guy's, controlled teaching appointments until his retirement in 1846, when, by default, the medical faculty took over management. See: *32nd Report of the Charity Commissioners*, 1840, pp. 734–735, 748, and 750; and Cameron, *Mr. Guy's Hospital*, pp. 177–180 and 186. At University College, laymen controlled the school, but medical men had a free hand over hospital staff appointments; see: Bellot, *University College London*, pp. 37 and 152.

96. Over 1,000 students passed through St. Bartholomew's Hospital Medical School between 1839 and 1859. See: J. Paget, "What Becomes of Medical Students," *St. Bartholomew's Hospital Reports*, 5 (1869), 238. The essay is reprinted in: J. Paget, *Selected Essays and Addresses* (London, 1902), p. 27. For data on medical students later in the century, see: S. S. Sprigge, *Physic and Fiction* (London, 1921), pp. 166 ff. From 1870 on, the General Medical Council, *Medi-*

cal Register, includes data on medical students. For individual medical schools, see: Moore, *St. Bartholomew's*, II, 814; St. Bartholomew's Hospital Mss., Number of Students, 1851–1904 (M.S. 4/1); Cope, *St. Mary's*, p. 22 and passim; and Hunter, *Charing Cross Hospital*, p. 160 and Chart I facing.

97. S. T. Taylor, *The Diary of a Medical Student during the Mid-Victorian Period, 1860–64* (Norwich, 1927), pp. 10–11.

98. *Plarr's Lives*, s.v. Butlin became Surgeon to St. Bartholomew's Hospital, President of the RCS, Baronet, and left an estate valued at over £90,000. The stimulus of medical school sometimes complemented family ambitions; Butlin had an ambitious mother. See also: Z. Cope, *The Versatile Victorian* (London, 1951), p. 24; Semon, *Autobiography*, pp. 17–18, 84, and 89; J. Paget, *Memoirs* (RCS Library ms., n.d.), irreg. pag.; and *Munk's Roll*, IV, s.v. Sir William Withey Gull and Sir Dyce Duckworth.

99. P. Eade, *The Autobiography of Sir Peter Eade* (London, 1916), pp. 46–48; F. J. Gant, *Auto-Biography* (London, 1905), p. 19; and G. Makins, *Autobiography* (RCS ms., n.d.), pp. 19–20.

100. *32nd Report of the Charity Commissioners*, 1840, pp. 51, 684, and 736; Cameron, *Mr. Guy's Hospital*, p. 185; Hunter, *Charing Cross Hospital*, p. 154; and McInnes, *St. Thomas' Hospital*, p. 96.

101. Cameron, *Mr. Guy's Hospital*, p. 229.

102. *32nd Report of the Charity Commissioners*, 1840, pp. 51 and 53. House surgeons' posts were created earlier than house physicians'. At Bart's each surgeon had his own houseman in 1836, at Guy's in 1856, but the apothecary was often the only adjunct to the physicians' staff in the first half of the nineteenth century. See also: Cameron, *Mr. Guy's Hospital*, p. 207.

103. Medical school entries in *The London and Provincial Medical Directory* for various years provide at least partial information on hospitals' junior staff posts. Guy's established the post of registrar in 1853; see: Cameron, *Mr. Guy's Hospital*, p. 179. Full reports on all cases were first required at Bart's in 1867; see: Moore, *St. Bartholomew's*, II, 751; and Cope, *St. Mary's*, p. 50.

104. See, e.g., *The London and Provincial Medical Directory*, 1855, pp. 559–566, for lists of hospital and teaching staffs. Cf. Langdon-Davies, *Westminster Hospital*, pp. 115–119; *32nd Report of the Charity Commissioners*, 1840, p. 750; and McInnes, *St. Thomas' Hospital*, pp. 81 and 91–92.

105. Moore, *St. Bartholomew's*, II, 813; and J. Simon, *Personal Recollections of Sir John Simon, KCB* (London, 1894), pp. 9–10. *The*

London and Provincial Medical Directory for various years is a good index of the growth and variety of these posts.

106. The pattern of junior status with subjects taught emerges in the biographies of surgeons and physicians in *Plarr's Lives* and *Munk's Roll*. The relative pay for these subjects is also an index to the seniority of the teacher; see: *Select Committee on Metropolitan Hospitals (H. L.)*, 2nd Report, 1890–91 (457), xiii, p. 21, Q. 10195–98 (Perry), and p. 142, Q. 13100–01 (Gould); and Cope, *St. Mary's*, p. 26.

107. See, e.g., *Plarr's Lives*, s.v. Sir James Paget; and *Select Committee on Metropolitan Hospitals*, 1890–91, pp. 17 (Perry) and 37 (Moore) for illustrations. Junior staffing of these posts is a consistent pattern emerging in *Plarr's Lives* and *Munk's Roll*.

108. C. B. Keetley, *The Student's and Junior Practitioner's Guide to the Medical Profession*, 2nd ed. (London, 1885), p. 40. See also: G. MacDonald, *Reminiscences of a Specialist* (London, 1936), p. 127; Gant, *Auto-Biography*, p. 107; Cope, *Versatile Victorian*, p. 24; J. Bland-Sutton, *The Story of a Surgeon* (London, 1930), p. 30; and A. C. Doyle, *The Hound of the Baskervilles*, in *The Complete Sherlock Holmes* (New York, n.d.), II, 671.

109. *Select Committee on Metropolitan Hospitals*, 1890 (392), xvi, p. 20, Q. 181–182 (Montefiore); p. 163, Q. 2506 (Waterlow); 1890–91, p. 22, Q. 10225 (Perry); and Semon, *Autobiography*, p. 81. See also: St. Thomas's Hospital Records, Minute Books of the Grand Committee (H1/ST/A6/12), 10 August 1847, p. 3.

110. Computed from *Plarr's Lives* (N = 17) and *Munk's Roll* (N = 21) for the 1840's; Physicians N = 27, Surgeons N = 20 for the 1870's. These delays came despite the institution of mandatory retirement of senior men at age sixty or sixty-five, and sometimes could cause trouble. See: Langdon-Davies, *Westminster Hospital*, p. 165; and Makins, *Autobiography*, p. 55.

111. The phrase is common; see: Simon, *Recollections*, p. 11; J. Paget, *Memoirs*, irreg. pag.; and MacDonald, *Reminiscences*, p. 127.

112. Bland-Sutton, *Surgeon*, pp. 27, 30, and 52; Eade, *Autobiography*, pp. 47–48; and MacDonald, *Reminiscences*, p. 127. For a discussion of income of junior staff, see: *Select Committee on Metropolitan Hospitals*, 1890, p. 31, Q. 275 (Steele); and p. 567, Q. 9751 (Clark).

113. Makins, *Autobiography*, p. 55; and Simon, *Recollections*, p. 14. Bland-Sutton, *Surgeon*, pp. 65 ff., describes his hospital work and studies for advanced qualification. For regulations regarding advanced RCS and RCP requirements, see: Royal College of Surgeons of England, *Bye-Laws* (London, [1860]), pp. 7 ff.; and Royal College

of Physicians of London, *The Charter, Bye-Laws, and Regulations* (London, 1892), pp. 44 and 66 ff.

114. Simon, *Recollections*, p. 14. Cf. Makins, *Autobiography*, pp. 48–50 and 54. See also: J. A. Banks, *Prosperity and Parenthood* (London, 1954), pp. 41 ff., 119, and 124.

115. Based on scattered data in *Plarr's Lives* and *Munk's Roll*.

116. These figures are based on material from *Plarr's Lives*.

117. S. Paget, *Sir Victor Horsley* (London, 1919), p. 36. Paget was a surgeon as well as a biographer. Cf. Langdon-Davies, *Westminster Hospital*, p. 151.

118. Moore, *St. Bartholomew's*, II, 813–814.

119. St. Bartholomew's Hospital Mss., Minutes of the Medical Council (M.C. 1/1), July 2, 1870, pp. 218–219; October 5, 1874, p. 277; and *Select Committee on Metropolitan Hospitals*, 1890–91, p. 38, Q. 10597 (Moore); p. 146, Q. 13191 (Gould).

120. Sprigge, *Thomas Wakley*, p. 172, quoted in R. Stevens, *Medical Practice in Modern England* (New Haven and London, 1966), p. 19*n*.

121. *Plarr's Lives*, s.v.; and Moore, *St. Bartholomew's*, II, 683 and 685–686. Other instances include: Walter Hamilton Acland Jacobson (godson of Henry Wentworth Acland) and T. D. Acland (son of H. W. Acland and son-in-law of W. W. Gull); see *Plarr's Lives* and *Munk's Roll*, IV, respectively. For further instances of family-related appointments among surgeons, see: *Plarr's Lives*, s.v. H. Haynes Walton, Walter Rivington, J. E. Adams, Marcus Beck, Edward Clapton, Thomas Morton, Rickman Godlee, Sydney Jones, L. S. Little, Prescott G. Hewett, and J. E. Lane. Also see: Cameron, *Mr. Guy's Hospital*, p. 253, regarding Cuthbert Golding-Bird. Physicians appointed with relatives in hospitals include: Edmund A. Parkes, John William Ogle, Cyril Ogle, Reginald Southey, and A. B. Duffin, for whom see *Munk's Roll*, IV. See also Charles Newman's fascinating remarks on the value of nepotism (*Medical Education*, pp. 143–145).

122. *Plarr's Lives*, s.v.; and Cameron, *Mr. Guy's Hospital*, p. 251. Davies-Colley's son later held a post at Guy's.

123. *Plarr's Lives*, s.v. Alfred Willett. See also: *Plarr's Lives*, s.v. Walter Rivington; and *Munk's Roll*, IV, s.v. W. H. Dickinson (son-in-law of J. A. Wilson). Cf. *Munk's Roll*, IV, s.v. Cyril Ogle, A. B. Duffin, and J. A. Ormerod.

124. E.g., T. D. Acland in *Munk's Roll*, IV.

125. D'Arcy Power and W. R. Lefanu, *Lives of the Fellows of the*

Royal College of Surgeons of England, 1930–1951 (London, 1953), s.v. Sir James Berry. (Hereafter cited as *Plarr's Lives*, III.)

126. Idem. Bart's medical staff did not select senior staff but were "informally" consulted on the decision by the treasurer and governors; see: *Select Committee on Metropolitan Hospitals*, 1890, p. 134, Q. 2068 (Clarke), and p. 162, Q. 2503 (Waterlow).

127. For examples, see: Bland-Sutton, *Surgeon*, pp. 27, 29, and 64–65; J. Paget, *Memoirs and Letters* (London, 1901), pp. 39 ff.; S. Paget, *Sir Victor Horsley*, pp. 36–37 and 43; *Plarr's Lives*, III, s.v. Watson Cheyne; and A. Doran, *Life Memories* (RCS Library, 1923), pp. 3 and 67. See also: remark on "favoritism" in *Select Committee on Metropolitan Hospitals*, 1890, p. 135, Q. 2089 (Clarke); and p. 508, Q. 8791–97 (Buxton).

128. MacDonald, *Reminiscences*, p. 215. Cf. *Plarr's Lives*, s.v. Edmund Roughton; and *Plarr's Lives*, III, s.v. Charles J. Heath.

129. See, e.g., *Plarr's Lives*, s.v. Frederick LeGros Clark, W. S. Savory, John Cooper Forster, Thomas Pickering Pick, and C. T. Dent; and *Munk's Roll*, IV, s.v. Sir Dyce Duckworth, Sir William Selby Church, Sir William Overend Priestley, and Sir Richard Douglas Powell. Keetley, *Guide*, pp. 9–10, said that the important prerequisites for success in medicine were judgment, decisiveness, memory for fact, "tenderness of heart," personal gifts such as kindliness, cheerfulness, "the manly figure," common sense, and, last of all, "interest in the healing art." Keetley thought this last would grow with experience. RCP presidential addresses also include reflections of this sort; see: W. Jenner, Presidential Addresses to the Royal College of Physicians (RCP Ms., 1883), irreg. pag., regarding Sir James Alderson and Sir Thomas Watson; ibid., 1885, irreg. pag., for general remarks; and ibid., 1886, irreg. pag., regarding A. B. Shepherd.

130. For early expressions of this view, see: *Select Committee on Medical Education*, 1834, Part I, p. 9, Q. 109–110 (Halford). Cf. Royal College of Physicians of London, *Charter*, p. 55; and Jenner, Presidential Addresses.

131. *Plarr's Lives*, s.v. He was rich, the son of a prosperous Lambeth general practitioner, and a student of Aston Key.

132. *Plarr's Lives*, s.v.; and Moore, *St. Bartholomew's*, II, 677–678. Coote's patron was the powerful Sir William Lawrence. Cf. *Munk's Roll*, IV, s.v. John Harley, whose medical ideas were considered outrageous.

133. For instances of sons and nephews who failed, despite influential relatives, to get hospital posts, see: *Plarr's Lives*, s.v.

Stephen Paget; and *Plarr's Lives*, III, s.v. John Poland, Edwin Holt-house, and Harry Page.

134. Bland-Sutton, *Surgeon*, pp. 27, 29, and 64–65.

135. *Munk's Roll*, IV, s.v.

136. Ibid. Also see: Cameron, *Mr. Guy's Hospital*, pp. 211 and 243–244. Mahomed was of Indian descent. He died at the age of thirty-five. For other examples, see: *Plarr's Lives*, s.v. Sir Frederick Treves, Sydney Jones, Sir William Turner, and William H. Stone; and *Munk's Roll*, IV, s.v. Samuel Gee and Sir William R. Gowers. For modern discussions of sponsorship, see: R. Turner, "Modes of Social Ascent through Education," in *Education, Economics, and Society*, ed. N. Smelser and S. M. Lipset (New York, 1961), pp. 121–139; R. Turner, "Acceptance of Irregular Mobility in Britain and the United States," *Sociometry*, 29:4 (1966), 334–352; and O. Hall, "The Stages of a Medical Career," *Am. J. Soc.*, 53:5 (1948), 336.

137. Langdon-Davies, *Westminster Hospital*, p. 179; and Cameron, *Mr. Guy's Hospital*, p. 136.

138. For examples, see: St. Bartholomew's Hospital Mss., Minutes of the House Committee (Ha 1/25), 12 January 1882, pp. 248 ff.; and 12 March 1885, pp. 515–518. These concerns are clear in the testimony before the *Select Committee on Metropolitan Hospitals*; see, e.g., 1890, p. 207, Q. 3065 (Currie); p. 508, Q. 8791–97 (Buxton); and 1890–91, p. 65, Q. 11195 (Ord).

139. St. Thomas's Hospital Records, Minutes of the General Court (H.1/ST/A1/9), 16 November 1852, p. 45. Cf. *Select Committee on Metropolitan Hospitals*, 1890, p. 448, Q. 7561 (Fenwick).

140. St. Thomas's Hospital Records, Minutes of the General Court (H.1/ST/A1/9), 16 November 1852, p. 45. Cf. *Select Committee on Metropolitan Hospitals*, 1890, p. 207, Q. 3064 (Currie).

141. St. Bartholomew's Hospital Mss., Minutes of the House Committee (Ha 1/25), 11 December 1879, p. 81; and 13 January 1881, p. 170 (*re* study of medical staff duties). Ibid., 18 March 1880, pp. 102–103 (*re* control over outside lecturing). Ibid., 13 November 1879, pp. 77, 118, 125–126, and 247–258 (*re* the conduct of the medical school). Also see: McInnes, *St. Thomas' Hospital*, p. 133; Langdon-Davies, *Westminster Hospital*, pp. 181–182; and Cameron, *Mr. Guy's Hospital*, pp. 185–186, 222, and 227.

142. Newman, *Medical Education*, pp. 140 ff.

143. G. Millerson, *The Qualifying Associations* (London, 1964), especially Chapter 5 and Appendix II. See also: A. M. Carr-Saunders and P. A. Wilson, *The Professions* (Oxford, 1933), *passim*.

144. W. Dale, *The State of the Medical Profession in Great Britain and Ireland* (Dublin, 1875), p. 57.

145. Keetley, *Guide*, p. 31; also see p. 47. Keetley never had a hospital post until he founded his own hospital. See *Plarr's Lives*, s.v.

146. See John Bland-Sutton's remarks on the Jacksonian Prize, in *Surgeon*, pp. 67–68.

147. E.g., Simon, *Recollections*, pp. 9–12. For an illustration of the general practitioner's sense of disadvantage in medical research, see: J. Jeaffreson's remarks in *BMJ*, 1857, ii, 22.

148. S. Paget, *Sir Victor Horsley*, p. 144.

149. *Select Committee on Medical Education*, 1834, p. 221, Q. 3429 (Farre).

150. *Munk's Roll*, IV, s.v.

151. *Munk's Roll*, IV, s.v. Charles Locock, W. B. Cheadle, T. D. Acland, H. G. Sutton, and Sir Andrew Clark are examples.

152. *Munk's Roll*, IV, s.v.

153. Ibid. The eminent colleagues who consulted him included Lister, Paget, Gull, Henry Thompson, and Spencer Wells.

154. RCP, *Charter*, p. 55.

155. Keetley, *Guide*, p. 65.

156. St. Bartholomew's Hospital Mss., Minutes of the House Committee (Ha 1/25), 12 January 1882, pp. 248 ff.; *Select Committee on Metropolitan Hospitals*, 1890, p. 58, Q. 810 (Hardy); p. 87, Q. 1316–17 (Bousfield); p. 521, Q. 8979–89 (Nixon); p. 533, Q. 9184–86 (Mackenzie); and 1892, p. xci, para. 517.

157. *Select Committee on Metropolitan Hospitals*, 1890, p. 121, Q. 1814 (Currie); and p. 535, Q. 9215 (Nixon).

158. St. Bartholomew's Hospital Mss., Minutes of the House Committee (Ha 1/25), 12 March 1885, pp. 515–518. See also: *Select Committee on Metropolitan Hospitals*, 1890, p. 52, Q. 720 (Holmes).

159. *Select Committee on Metropolitan Hospitals*, 1890, p. 54, Q. 763 (Holmes); pp. 164–165, Q. 2529–31 (Waterlow); p. 511, Q. 8843, 8850, and p. 513, Q. 8816 (Nixon).

160. Ibid., 1890, p. 83, Q. 1256 (Bousfield).

161. Ibid., 1890, p. 33, Q. 315, 326 (Steele); p. 49, Q. 671–672 (Holmes); p. 82, Q. 1240, 1246, and p. 88, Q. 1326 (Bousfield); and p. 129, Q. 1945–53 (Clarke).

162. Ibid., 1890, p. 8, Q. 57 ff. (Montefiore); p. 33, Q. 315–316,

and p. 40, Q. 427 (Steele); p. 50, Q. 681 (Holmes); p. 87, Q. 1311–21 (Bousfield); p. 116, Q. 1731, and p. 120, Q. 1788–93 (Currie); p. 131, Q. 2004 (Clarke); and 1892, p. xxxii, para. 178–179.

163. Ibid., 1890, pp. 41–42, Q. 450–451, and p. 46, Q. 580, 586 (Steele); p. 83, Q. 1252 (Bousfield); and p. 114, Q. 1702 (Currie). See also: St. Bartholomew's Hospital Mss., Minutes of the House Committee (Ha 1/25), 12 January 1882, p. 252; and McInnes, *St. Thomas' Hospital*, p. 108. The evolution of the almoners is described in: E. M. Bell, *The Story of Hospital Almoners* (London, 1961).

164. Bellot, *University College London*, p. 50.

165. Abel-Smith, *The Hospitals*, p. 34; *Select Committee on Metropolitan Hospitals*, 1892, p. xxviii; and Langdon-Davies, *Westminster Hospital*, pp. 147–149.

166. Moore, *St. Bartholomew's*, II, 807.

167. Ibid., II, 809–812.

168. *Select Committee on Metropolitan Hospitals*, 1890, p. 345, Q. 5975 (Roberts).

169. Langdon-Davies, *Westminster Hospital*, p. 119. Regarding the evolution of Guy's Medical Council, see: Cameron, *Mr. Guy's Hospital*, pp. 185–186, 226, and 228–229. The Middlesex, the London, and St. George's medical schools had Committees of Management made up of governors and medical men. See: Langdon-Davies, *Westminster Hospital*, p. 122; and *Select Committee on Metropolitan Hospitals*, 1890, p. 345, Q. 5976 (Roberts), and p. 426, Q. 7221–22 (Carr-Gomm).

170. Moore, *St. Bartholomew's*, II, 811–812; and *Select Committee on Metropolitan Hospitals*, 1890, p. 345, Q. 5976 (Roberts).

171. St. Thomas's Hospital, Minute Books of the Grand Committee (H1/ST/A6/12), 10 August 1847, pp. 2–3.

172. Ibid., p. 3.

173. St. Bartholomew's Hospital Mss., Minutes of the Medical Council (M.C. 1/1), 29 June 1848, p. 30; 5 January 1878, p. 330; Minutes of the House Committee (Ha 1/25), 12 January 1882, pp. 254 and 255; 25 March 1883, pp. 515–518; and St. Thomas's Hospital Records, Minutes of the Grand Committee (H1/ST/A6/14), 13 February 1866, p. 283; and (H1/ST/A6/15), 28 July 1870, p. 33.

174. Abel-Smith, *The Hospitals*, p. 35, dates the change in the 1860's.

175. C. Woodham-Smith, *Florence Nightingale, 1820–1910* (Lon-

don, 1950), pp. 256–257 and 536–538. On the history of nursing in Britain, see: B. Abel-Smith, *A History of the Nursing Profession in Great Britain* (New York, 1960).

176. McInnes, *St. Thomas' Hospital*, pp. 116–117, 120–121, 124, and 130.

177. Ibid., pp. 139–140.

178. Cameron, *Mr. Guy's Hospital*, pp. 203–204, gives the text of the letter.

179. S. O. Habershon, "On the Nursing Crisis at Guy's Hospital" (No. II), *Nineteenth Century*, 7 (May, 1880), 897–898. See also: W. Moxon's letter in the *Times*, July 29, 1880, p. 10; and Abel-Smith, *Nursing*, p. 19n.

180. O. Sturges, "Doctors and Nurses" (No. I), *Nineteenth Century*, 7 (June, 1880), 1092; Habershon, "Nursing Crisis," p. 897; and Abel-Smith, *Nursing*, p. 19.

181. W. W. Gull, "On the Nursing Crisis at Guy's Hospital" (No. I), *Nineteenth Century*, 7 (May, 1880), 889.

182. Cameron, *Mr. Guy's Hospital*, p. 203. Cf. M. Lonsdale, "The Present Crisis at Guy's Hospital," *Nineteenth Century*, 7 (April, 1880), 679.

183. W. Moxon, "Miss Lonsdale on Guy's Hospital," *Contemporary Review*, 37 (May, 1880), 889; and Cameron, *Mr. Guy's Hospital*, p. 209.

184. Lonsdale, "Present Crisis," p. 679; and Gull, "Nursing Crisis," p. 886.

185. Moxon, "Miss Lonsdale," p. 878.

186. Lonsdale, "Present Crisis," pp. 677 and 682. There was considerable debate over the social origins of the "old" sisters. See: Habershon, "Nursing Crisis," p. 899.

187. Lonsdale, "Present Crisis," p. 683.

188. Gull, "Nursing Crisis," p. 888.

189. Ibid., p. 886; and Habershon, "Nursing Crisis," pp. 898 and 900. There was some hint that some lady nurses were related to governors.

190. Lonsdale, "Present Crisis," p. 684.

191. Ibid., p. 682. Cf. Langdon-Davies, *Westminster Hospital*, p. 138.

192. Gull, "Nursing Crisis," pp. 887–888.

193. Sturges, "Doctors and Nurses," p. 1089. A. G. Henriques,

"On the Nursing Crisis at Guy's Hospital" (No. III, concl.), *Nineteenth Century*, 7 (May, 1880), 904, discusses the London Hospital; and Moxon, "Miss Lonsdale," p. 888, discusses Bart's. See also: *Select Committee on Metropolitan Hospitals*, 1892, p. xxii, para. 92; p. xxvii, para. 129; p. lxxxii, para. 462; and Abel-Smith, *Nursing*, pp. 27 and 36.

194. Moxon, "Miss Lonsdale," pp. 885–886 and 892; Habershon, "Nursing Crisis," pp. 898 and 900; and Gull, "Nursing Crisis," p. 888.

195. Habershon, "Nursing Crisis," p. 898; and Moxon, "Miss Lonsdale," pp. 891–892.

196. Habershon, "Nursing Crisis," p. 901.

197. Idem.

198. Gull, "Nursing Crisis," pp. 887–888.

199. Habershon, "Nursing Crisis," p. 901 (emphasis his).

200. Letter from S. O. Habershon in the *Times*, July 24, 1880, p. 10; and letter from G. H. Russell, the *Times*, August 11, 1880, p. 10. See also: "Guy's Hospital," the *Times*, July 22, 1880, p. 13.

201. Quoted in Cameron, *Mr. Guy's Hospital*, pp. 205–206.

202. Moxon, "Miss Lonsdale," p. 888.

203. Habershon, "Nursing Crisis," p. 893 (emphasis his).

204. Moxon, "Miss Lonsdale," p. 883 (quoting Dr. Steele, the Medical Superintendent of Guy's). Cf. Lonsdale, "Present Crisis," p. 677.

205. Cameron, *Mr. Guy's Hospital*, pp. 205–206.

206. "The Government of Hospitals," the *Times*, July 24, 1880, p. 4.

207. Idem.

208. Cameron, *Mr. Guy's Hospital*, pp. 206–208.

209. "Guy's Hospital," the *Times*, July 22, 1880, p. 13.

210. Idem.

211. Idem.

212. Letter from S. O. Habershon, the *Times*, July 24, 1880, p. 10. See also: letter from S. Wilkes, the *Times*, July 23, 1880, p. 7. For additional correspondence in the *Times* regarding this issue, see: July 27, 1880, p. 12 (Pavy); July 28, 1880, p. 7 (Lonsdale); July 29, 1880, p. 10 (Wilks and Moxon); July 31, 1880, p. 8 (Steele and Fagge); August 2, 1880, p. 10 (Lonsdale); and August 5, 1880, p. 6 (Moxon). The issue of August 6, 1880, p. 11, carried the story of the trial of

one of Guy's nurses for manslaughter, which provoked a *Times* commentary on the general problem of medical authority on August 7, 1880, p. 9. For further correspondence, see: August 7, 1880, p. 9 (Pavy); August 9, 1880, p. 12 (Lushington and Horsey); August 11, 1880, p. 10 (Russell); August 12, 1880, p. 11 (Gull, Hayes, and Pye-Smith); and August 16, 1880, p. 11 (Moxon). See also: Cameron, *Mr. Guy's Hospital*, pp. 210–214.

213. *Select Committee on Metropolitan Hospitals*, 1890, p. 30, Q. 254 (Steele); and Cameron, *Mr. Guy's Hospital*, pp. 212–213.

214. See, e.g., Langdon-Davies, *Westminster Hospital*, pp. 127–138; McInnes, *St. Thomas' Hospital*, pp. 116–117; Abel-Smith, *Nursing*, pp. 24–29 and 36; and Cope, *St. Mary's*, p. 17. *Select Committee on Metropolitan Hospitals*, 1890, p. 255, Q. 3985–86 (Brodhurst), expresses the view that the hospital had become a "mere adjunct" to the medical school. See also: ibid., 1892, p. xci, para. 517.

215. St. Bartholomew's Hospital Mss., Minutes of the House Committee (Ha 1/25), 8 January 1880, pp. 87–88; and Minutes of the Medical Council (M.C. 1/2), 13 June 1892, p. 227. See also: *Select Committee on Metropolitan Hospitals*, 1890, p. 134, Q. 2068 (Clarke); p. 162, Q. 2503 (Waterlow); and p. 255, Q. 3990 (Brodhurst).

216. Moore, *St. Bartholomew's*, II, 807.

217. Langdon-Davies, *Westminster Hospital*, p. 195. Cf. Moore, *St. Bartholomew's*, II, 807.

218. *Select Committee on Metropolitan Hospitals*, 1890, p. 30, Q. 254, and p. 45, Q. 522 (Steele); p. 207, Q. 3062–63 (Currie); p. 348, Q. 6052–54 (Roberts); p. 505, Q. 8720 (Buxton); 1890–91, p. 4, Q. 9781–82 (Lushington); p. 21, Q. 10203 (Perry); p. 74, Q. 11361–62 (Wainwright); p. 107, Q. 12196–97 (Todd); and 1892, pp. ix–xxviii passim.

219. The *Times*, August 7, 1880, p. 9.

220. *Select Committee on Metropolitan Hospitals*, 1890, p. 162, Q. 2503. See also: p. 164, Q. 2521 (Waterlow); and p. 519, Q. 8935 (Buxton).

221. Ibid., p. 47, Q. 628 (Steele).

222. Ibid., p. 207, Q. 3065–66.

223. *BMJ*, 1857, i, 673–674.

224. For illustrations, see: Royal College of Physicians, Annals, XXXIII (January 31, 1884), 336–337 and 339; Langdon-Davies, *Westminster Hospital*, pp. 110 and 181; Bellot, *University College London*, pp. 195 ff.; and A. M. Cooke, *A History of the Royal College of Physicians of London* (Oxford, 1972), III, 902–905.

225. Cooke, *A History*, III, 902–905, and Appendix VI, p. 1184.

226. Jenner, Presidential Addresses, 1883, p. 3.

227. *Select Committee on Metropolitan Hospitals*, 1890, p. 134, Q. 2079 (Clarke).

228. Ibid., 1890, pp. 109–110, Q. 1630–31 (Woods); p. 135, Q. 2081–82 (Clarke); pp. 162–163, Q. 2505–09 (Waterlow); p. 207, Q. 3068 (Currie); and 1890–91, pp. 114–115, Q. 12371–12401 (Whipham).

229. St. Thomas's Hospital Records, Minutes of the Grand Committee (H1/ST/A6/11), 13 July 1842, pp. 16–17. See also: St. Bartholomew's Hospital Mss., Minutes of the Medical Council (M.C. 1/2), February 8, 1873, pp. 23–24.

230. *Select Committee on Metropolitan Hospitals*, 1890, p. 39, Q. 412 (Steele); 1890–91, p. 21, Q. 10195 and 10198 (Perry); p. 41, Q. 10659 (Moore); and p. 64, Q. 11175 (Ord). See also: Cope, *St. Mary's*, p. 43; and Cameron, *Mr. Guy's Hospital*, pp. 175–180. Faculty income was based on a systematic division of receipts from students' fees, by "shares." For a comment on teachers' neglect and the problems therefrom, see: St. Thomas's Hospital Records, Minutes of the General Court (H1/ST/A1/8), 28 August 1834, pp. 314–315; and *Select Committee on Metropolitan Hospitals*, 1890–91, p. 42, Q. 10672 (Moore).

231. Bellot, *University College London*, pp. 159–160; and Sprigge, *Thomas Wakley*, p. 172, quoted in Stevens, *Medical Practice*, p. 19n.

232. Sir George Burrows gives a brief sketch of developments to 1875 (*Address of the President of the Royal College of Physicians . . . 1875* [London, 1875], pp. 6–11). See also: RCS, *Annual Report . . . 1875–76* (London, 1876), p. 8 and subsequent minutes; and Cooke, *A History*, III, 845–863 passim.

233. Cooke, *A History*, III, 861. See also: J. Simon, *On the Claim, Asserted by the Royal College of Physicians, that the College of Itself . . . Can Grant Such Letters-Testimonial . . .* (London, 1892), pp. 17 and 19–20; N. G. Horner, *The Growth of the General Practitioner of Medicine in England* (London, 1922), pp. 24 ff., and C. R. B. Barrett, *The History of the Society of Apothecaries of London* (London, 1905), pp. 251 ff.

234. Burrows, *Address*, p. 12.

235. Ibid., pp. 12–13. Cf. Simon, *Recollections*, p. 17. At the same time, the College maintained the distinction between the upper orders (MRCP, FRCP) and the Licentiates, who were general practitioners. See: RCP, Annals, XXVII (March 28, 1860), 3; and Cooke, *A History*, III, 814.

Chapter V

1. J. A. Banks, *Prosperity and Parenthood* (London, 1954), pp. 86 ff.

2. Quoted in A. M. Carr-Saunders and P. A. Wilson, *The Professions* (Oxford, 1933), p. 295. See also: R. Wilkinson, *Gentlemanly Power* (London and New York, 1964), pp. 19–20 and works cited there. Matthew Arnold likened Keats's love letters to those a "surgeon's apprentice" might have written because they lacked "tone"; they were "underbred and ignoble, as of a youth ill brought up." See his "John Keats," in *Essays in Criticism* (2nd series), in *Works of Matthew Arnold* (London, 1903), IV, 75–76. Thanks are due to Professor Catherine Cox Runcie for this reference. See also: H. B. Thomson, *The Choice of a Profession* (London, 1857), p. 1; and F. Davenant, *What Shall My Son Be?* (London, 1870), pp. 48 and 54, and note the order of professions in the Table of Contents. Cf. C. Newman, *The Evolution of Medical Education in the Nineteenth Century* (London, 1957), pp. 78 and 112. W. J. Reader, *Professional Men* (London, 1966), pp. 32 and 43, accepts Thomson's idea that high status came from connection with the State; it was surely a more complex matter.

3. W. Stokes, "Valedictory Address, 1868," in BMA, *Medicine in Modern Times* (London, 1869), p. 5. See also: *BMJ*, 1857, i, 237; ii, 575; and G. R. Turner, *Unorthodox Reminiscences* (London, 1931), p. xiii.

4. Turner, *Unorthodox Reminiscences*, p. 3; also see pp. 1, 2, and 4. Cf. *BMJ*, 1872, ii, 703.

5. Turner, *Unorthodox Reminiscences*, p. 24; cf. p. 71. For other allusions to medical men's ideas of their low status, see: E. Harrison's remarks quoted in S. W. F. Holloway, "The Apothecaries' Act of 1815," *Medical History*, 10:2 (1966), 116; and the *London Medical Gazette*, 1837, quoted in W. H. McMenemy, *The Life and Times of Sir Charles Hastings* (Edinburgh and London, 1959), p. 179.

6. J. B. Atlay, *Sir Henry Wentworth Acland* (London, 1903), p. 335; and J. De Styrap, *The Young Practitioner* (London, 1890), p. viii.

7. Turner, *Unorthodox Reminiscences*, p. xiii.

8. *Memoirs of the Life of a Country Surgeon* (London, 1845), p. 18.

9. *Medical Press and Circular*, November 24, 1875, p. 432, quoted in J. L. Brand, *Doctors and the State* (Baltimore, 1965), p. 20. See also: BMA, *Medicine in Modern Times*, p. 4; *BMJ*, 1884, ii, 546–547; and I. Ashe, *Medical Education and Medical Interests* (Dublin, 1868), p. 136.

10. Ouida [Marie Louise de la Ramée], *The New Priesthood* (London, 1893), pp. 21–23.

11. [F. P. Cobbe], *The Medical Profession and Its Morality* (London, 1886), p. 12 (emphasis hers). Regarding authorship, see: R. D. French, *Antivivisection and Medical Science in Victorian Society* (Princeton, N.J., 1975), p. 247. See also: P. Vaughan, *Doctors' Commons* (London, 1959), p. 59.

12. Wilkinson, *Gentlemanly Power*, pp. 19 ff.; G. Kitson-Clark, *The Making of Victorian England* (London, 1962), pp. 258–265; G. Best, *Mid-Victorian Britain, 1851–75* (New York, 1972), pp. 245 ff.; and P. Cominos, "Late Victorian Sexual Respectability and the Social System" (Parts I and II), *Int. Rev. Social History*, 8 (1963), 18–48 and 216–250.

13. *Select Committee on Metropolitan Hospitals*, 1890, p. 508, Q. 8791–97 (Buxton); and 1890–91, p. 115, Q. 12399 and 12401 (Whipham).

14. R. B. Carter, *Doctors and Their Work* (London, 1903), p. 153.

15. De Styrap, *The Young Practitioner*, p. xi. Cf. Thomson, *Choice of a Profession*, pp. 34 ff.; Reader, *Professional Men*, pp. 10 and 206; and E. Berdoe [pseud. Scalpel Aesculapius], *St. Bernard's* (London, 1887), pp. 177 and 194–195.

16. See "profession," "liberal," and "gentleman," in the *Oxford English Dictionary*.

17. [Cobbe], *The Medical Profession*, p. 11. See also: Ouida [M. L. de la Ramée], *The New Priesthood*, pp. 21–22; and Ashe, *Medical Education*, pp. 3–4.

18. [Cobbe], *The Medical Profession*, p. 11.

19. Cf. Newman, *Medical Education*, pp. 4, 16, and 21; B. Abel-Smith, *The Hospitals, 1800–1948* (London, 1964), p. 5; and Reader, *Professional Men*, pp. 33–34, who all give impressionistic accounts of the origins of medical men.

20. S. Rothblatt, *The Revolution of the Dons* (New York, 1968), Appendix II:A, p. 280.

21. C. B. Otley, "Social Origins of British Army Officers," *Sociological Review*, 18:2 (1970), 224.

22. Ibid., p. 224n.

23. D. H. J. Morgan, "The Social and Educational Background of Anglican Bishops—Continuities and Changes," *Brit. J. Sociol.*, 20:3 (1969), 297. Morgan gives no data on manufacturing, business, trades, or laboring origins of bishops.

24. Sir Joseph Laffan and William Somerville, in *Munk's Roll*.

25. Ibid., s.v.

26. Morgan, "Anglican Bishops," p. 297, computes the landed and peerage connections (birth and marriage) as a percent of the total number of bishops. His findings: 1860–79, 112.5%; 1880–99, 96.3%.

27. Compiled from *Munk's Roll* and *Plarr's Lives*.

28. *Plarr's Lives*, s.v.; and F. M. L. Thompson, *English Landed Society in the Nineteenth Century* (London and Toronto, 1963), pp. 287 ff. Lister was the only medical peer in the nineteenth century.

29. See: S. M. Lipset and R. Bendix, *Social Mobility in Industrial Society* (Berkeley and Los Angeles, 1967), p. 39.

30. All of the above was compiled from *Munk's Roll*. See also: [J. Vaughan-Hughes], *Seventy Years of Life in the Victorian Era* (London, 1893), p. 2; and C. J. B. Williams, *Memoirs of Life and Work* (London, 1884), p. 5.

31. *Plarr's Lives*, s.v. His eldest son first studied law; see: T. Holmes, *Sir Benjamin Collins Brodie* (London, 1897), pp. 76 ff.

32. *Plarr's Lives*, s.v. Also see the family of Victor Horsley in *Plarr's Lives* and in S. Paget, *Sir Victor Horsley* (London, 1919). Thomas Wakley, a successful medical man in his own way, wanted his eldest son to enter the church, his second son to become a barrister, and his third son to become editor of the *Lancet*; see: S. S. Sprigge, *The Life and Times of Thomas Wakley* (London, 1899), pp. 233, 347, 485, and 488–489.

33. See *Plarr's Lives*, s.v. Sir Frederick Treves. See also: Lipset and Bendix, *Social Mobility*, pp. 60–61.

34. *Report of the Committee Appointed by the Secretary of State to Enquire into the Causes which Tend to Prevent Sufficient Eligible Candidates from Coming Forward for the Army Medical Department*, 1878–79 [C. 2200], p. 29, notes that "social status and influence" increase with "increased earnings."

35. B. Brodie, Account books, 3 vols., 1824–1860 (RCS Ms.).

36. Discussed in an article entitled "Medical Fortunes," *BMJ*, 1894, i, 91. Cf. B. Brodie, *Autobiography of the Late Sir Benjamin Brodie, Bart.* (London, 1865), pp. 115, 117, and 141.

37. B. Shillitoe, Visiting Lists, Cashbooks, Accounts, and Diaries, Wellcome Historical Medical Library, Mod. Mss. 4519 (1866) and 4534 (1881).

38. H. D. Rolleston, *The Cambridge Medical School* (Cambridge, 1932), p. 98.

39. Shillitoe, Visiting Lists, Mss. 4501–4536 passim; and *Calen-*

dar of the Grants of Probate and Letters of Administration Made in the Probate Registers of the High Court of Justice in England . . . , 1917, s.v. Buxton Shillitoe.

40. *Calendar of the Grants of Probate . . . , 1881*, s.v. Benjamin Brodie.

41. Holmes, *Sir Benjamin*, pp. 147–148. See also: *BMJ*, 1894, i, 91.

42. *Plarr's Lives*, s.v.

43. S. H. Snell, *A Doctor at Work and Play* (London, 1937), pp. 7 and 39. See also: *Plarr's Lives*, s.v. John Hammond Morgan; and A. C. Doyle, *The Stark Munro Letters* (New York, 1895), pp. 128–130, 151, 158, and 179.

44. Banks, *Prosperity and Parenthood*, pp. 103 ff., and F. Musgrove, "Middle Class Education and Employment in the Nineteenth Century," *Econ. Hist. Rev.*, 2nd ser., 12 (1959), 99 ff., discuss the problems of assessing middle-class incomes. One of the rare surviving records of general practitioners' income may be found in: [W. Martin], Untitled book of accounts, 1888 to c. 1914, RCP Library Ms., a record of his practice in Thorne, near Doncaster, Yorkshire.

45. *BMJ*, 1876, i (February 12), "Advertiser," no pagination.

46. BMA, *A Tariff of Medical Fees Recommended by the Shropshire Ethical Branch of the British Medical Association* (Shrewsbury, 1870), p. 3; and *BMJ*, 1867, ii, 554.

47. See [Martin], Book of accounts, no pagination, for examples of this form of differential fees. His accounts list the occupation or status of his patients.

48. R. Hodgkinson, *The Origins of the National Health Service* (London, 1967), pp. 84–86, 89, and 105–106; and C. B. Keetley, *The Student's and Junior Practitioner's Guide to the Medical Profession*, 2nd ed. (London, 1885), pp. 40 ff. and 95. The *BMJ* carried advertisements of openings in poor law and public health: *BMJ*, 1884, ii (July 12), "Advertiser," no pagination, carries an advertisement for a full-time medical officer at £250 per year.

49. *BMJ*, 1884, ii (July 12), "Advertiser," no pagination. Cf. Ashe, *Medical Education*, p. 107, who cites a figure of £120 per year, plus housing, in 1868. See also: S. J. Novak, "Professionalism and Bureaucracy," *J. Social History* (Summer, 1973), 452.

50. *Report of the Committee Appointed . . . to Enquire into . . . the Army Medical Department*, 1878–79, p. 20, para. 89.

51. Ibid., p. 4, para. 6; also see Appendix A, pp. 28–29.

NOTES TO PAGES 194–243

52. Ibid., pp. 48 and 49.

53. Ibid., p. 20, para. 89, and p. 49.

54. *Select Committee on Metropolitan Hospitals*, 1890, p. 227, Q. 3377–78 (Farmer); and p. 241, Q. 3699 (Corbyn). See also: p. 250, Q. 3834, and p. 252, Q. 3893 (Bhakha); p. 284, Q. 4587 (Kay); and Ashe, *Medical Education*, p. 107.

55. BMA, *Medicine in Modern Times*, p. 4. See also: *Report of the Committee Appointed . . . to Enquire into . . . the Army Medical Department*, 1878–79, p. 29.

56. *Confessions of an English Doctor* (London, 1904), pp. 28, 43, and 56.

57. *Report of Sir William Plender to the Chancellor of the Exchequer on the Result of His Investigation into Existing Conditions in Respect of Medical Attendance and Remuneration in Certain Towns*, 1912–13 [Cd. 6305], lxxviii, 679. Cardiff was to have been included, but many practitioners refused to cooperate. I am grateful to Professor Bentley Gilbert for having brought this document to my attention, and to Professor Paul Kuznets for his comments and assistance on this section.

58. Computed from: P. Deane and W. A. Cole, *British Economic Growth, 1688–1959* (Cambridge, 1964), p. 8; G. Routh, *Occupation and Pay in Great Britain, 1906–1960* (Cambridge, 1965), p. 172; and *Report of Sir William Plender*, p. 4.

59. M. Friedman and S. Kuznets, *Income from Independent Professional Practice* (New York, 1945), Chapter 4, especially pp. 100–101.

60. Doyle, *Stark Munro*, pp. 16, 57, and 58.

61. *Select Committee on Metropolitan Hospitals*, 1890, p. 227, Q. 3381 and 3578–81 (Farmer).

62. *Report of Sir William Plender*, p. 4; and W. E. Steavenson, *The Medical Act (1858) Amendment Bill and Medical Reform* (London, 1880), p. 30. BMA, *A Tariff of Medical Fees*, p. 7, recommends 1¼d. per week for clubs (5s.5d. per year). William Martin charged club fees ranging from 1s.9d. to 3s.6d. in 1888 and 1889 (Book of accounts [RCP Ms., 1888–c. 1914]). The fee schedule shown in "Everybody's Pocket Cyclopaedia" for the 1890's, cited in A. F. Andrews, *The Doctor in History, Literature, Folklore* (London, 1896), p. 18, is very close to that of the 1870's.

63. Deane and Cole, *British Economic Growth*, pp. 12–18 and Figure 7 at the end of the book.

64. Sir Henry Burdett, *The Medical Attendance of Londoners* (London, 1903), p. 9.

65. F. Semon, *The Autobiography of Sir Felix Semon* (London, 1926), p. 111; also see p. 106. Semon needed £300 a year to live as a single man in the mid-1870's (p. 101), and on this amount he could not afford a consulting room in the best medical neighborhood (p. 105).

66. Ibid., p. 113. See also: Brodie, *Autobiography*, p. 117. In A. Conan Doyle's *Stark Munro*, p. 160, a poor general practitioner is described as renting a house for £40 a year; he can only afford a "grubby-faced maid." His income would probably amount to £300 to £400 a year. Cf. Banks, *Prosperity and Parenthood*, pp. 74–82 and, on rents, pp. 57 and 165.

67. Doyle, *Stark Munro*, pp. 16, 57, and 58. Cf. J. A. Banks and O. Banks, *Feminism and Family Planning in Victorian England* (Liverpool, 1964), Chapter 5.

68. *BMJ*, 1872, ii, 170.

69. *BMJ*, 1868, i, 38; W. Dale, *The State of the Medical Profession in Great Britain* (Dublin, 1875), pp. 10–12; and T. H. Huxley, "The State and the Medical Profession," *Nineteenth Century*, 15 (February, 1884), 229.

70. *Confessions of an English Doctor* (London, 1904), p. 28.

71. BMA, *A Tariff of Medical Fees*, p. 3. See also: *BMJ*, 1872, ii, 169; and Ashe, *Medical Education*, pp. 3–4.

72. See: "Competition and Underselling," *BMJ*, 1894, i, 210, 977, and 983. The debate over club practice reflects the fear of practitioners that refusing contract practice would send patients to other practitioners, to the chemist, or to charities. See also: *BMJ*, 1867, ii, 10 and 594; *BMJ*, 1868, i, 38; Huxley, "The State," p. 229; Dale, *The Medical Profession*, p. 13; H. C. Burdett, *The Medical Attendance of Londoners* (London, 1903), p. 9; and Ashe, *Medical Education*, pp. 108 and 112.

73. Carter, *Doctors*, p. 153; and *Select Committee on Metropolitan Hospitals*, 1890, p. 284, Q. 4587 (Kay).

74. S. D. Clippingdale, "Some Considerations of the Life and Work of the General Practitioner," *West London Medical Journal*, 4 (1899), 10; Hodgkinson, *National Health Service*, p. 75; and BMA, *A Tariff of Medical Fees*, p. 4n.

75. Ashe, *Medical Education*, p. 153; and R. Saundby, *Medical Ethics* (Bristol, 1902), p. 41.

76. Huxley, "The State," p. 229. Cf. J. Rogers, *Reminiscences of a Workhouse Medical Officer* (London, 1889), p. xii; *The Family Doctor. A*

Monthly Journal of Hygiene, 3:2 (1883), no pagination; Burdett, *Medical Attendance*, p. 13; and *BMJ*, 1868, i, 38, and 1857, i, 557. See also: J. Chapman, *The Medical Institutions of the United Kingdom* (London, 1870), pp. 21 and 22; and P. Eade, *The Autobiography of Sir Peter Eade* (London, 1916), p. 34.

77. *BMJ*, 1872, ii, 170; cf. p. 169 and the article, "A Large Fee and Its Use," *BMJ*, 1894, i, 210. See also: Ashe, *Medical Education*, p. 108.

78. *BMJ*, 1872, ii, 170.

79. Idem.

80. BMA, *A Tariff of Medical Fees*, p. 3. See also: *BMJ*, 1877, ii, 941, and 1878, i, 112.

81. *BMJ*, 1886, i, 1196.

82. *Select Committee on Metropolitan Hospitals*, 1890, p. 269, Q. 4232 (Bennett).

83. *Low's Handbook of Charities*, 1890, pp. vi–vii. Cf. Abel-Smith, *The Hospitals*, pp. 104 ff. and 116 ff.

84. *Select Committee on Metropolitan Hospitals*, 1890, p. 54, Q. 763 (Holmes); p. 87, Q. 1316–17 (Bousfield); and p. 513, Q. 8861 (Nixon).

85. *BMJ*, 1889, ii, 287. Cf. Abel-Smith, *The Hospitals*, pp. 117–118.

86. Burdett, *Medical Attendance*, p. 9.

87. Ibid., pp. 12–13. Cf. Carter, *Doctors*, p. 157. The general practitioners discussed this at great length before the Select Committee on Metropolitan Hospitals. See, e.g., 1890, p. 245, Q. 3777–78 (Browne).

88. *BMJ*, 1886, ii, 89. Quoted in Abel-Smith, *The Hospitals*, p. 115. Cf. *BMJ*, 1878, i, 197.

89. *BMJ*, 1872, ii, 169 and 170; and 1894, i, 210.

90. Steavenson, *Medical Act*, p. 6. Cf. RCS, *Minutes*, November 10, 1881, p. 26.

91. RCS, *Annual Report on the Affairs of the Royal College of Surgeons of England by the President [Sir James Paget], 1875–76*, (London, 1876), p. 14.

92. Steavenson, *Medical Act*, pp. 9–10.

93. Abel-Smith, *The Hospitals*, pp. 114 ff.; and Vaughan, *Doctors' Commons*, p. 53.

94. *BMJ*, 1886, ii, 1190, quoted in Abel-Smith, *The Hospitals*, pp. 115–116. See also: "Does the General Medical Council Represent the Medical Profession?" *Medical Press and Circular*, January 28, 1880. [In Sir John Simon's Papers, RCS Library Ms.]

95. *BMJ*, 1884, ii, 546–547.

96. *BMJ*, 1857, i, 259 (emphasis in the original). Cf. Dale, *The Medical Profession*, pp. 10–11; Atlay, *Sir Henry Wentworth Acland*, p. 337; Berdoe, *St. Bernard's*, pp. 180–182; and Brodie, *Autobiography*, p. 25.

97. De Styrap, *The Young Practitioner*, p. viii; and *BMJ*, 1878, i, 197.

98. Vaughan, *Doctors' Commons*, pp. 53–54 and 106.

99. Ibid., pp. 50–51.

100. RCP, Annals, XXXI (July 7, 1875), 196; and (July 19, 1875), 216. A summary of the College's past actions appears in: RCP, Annals, XXXI (December 20, 1875), 247–249.

101. G. Makins, *Autobiography* (RCS Ms., n.d.), p. 95. See also: *BMJ*, 1876, i, 181.

102. RCS, *Minutes*, 6 August 1885, p. 15; 24 November 1885, p. 71; 14 January 1886, pp. 89–90; and 13 May 1886, p. 114.

103. Ibid., 14 November 1878, 600–603. See also: 11 December 1884, p. 152; 19 December 1884, pp. 157 ff.; 8 January 1885, pp. 174–175; 9 April 1885, pp. 189 ff.; 17 November 1885, pp. 50–53; and 8 April 1886, pp. 107–109. Failing College Council action, the Members and Fellows decided to petition Parliament and the Crown (ibid., 12 November 1885, pp. 47–48).

104. Ibid., 21 February 1889, p. 255.

105. Ibid., p. 256. Also see p. 255.

106. G. Burrows, *Address of the President of the Royal College of Physicians . . . 1875* (London, 1875), p. 4.

107. Ibid., p. 5.

108. RCP, Annals, XXVIII (April 10, 1865), 367; (April 21, 1865), 371; and (June 6, 1865), 373 ff.

109. Ibid. (June 26, 1865), 388.

110. T. Watson, *Dr. Watson's Address, . . . Royal College of Physicians* (London, n.d.), p. 2.

111. Idem.

112. For just a few examples, see: RCP, Annals, XXVIII (March

21, 1865), 164–165; XXIX (January 3, 1866), 23–24; (June 15, 1866), 55–57; (July 18, 1866), 80–83; and (December 14, 1868), 317.

113. Ibid., XXXIII (April 3, 1882), 101; and (July 27, 1882), 148–150.

114. Ibid. (July 27, 1882), 151.

115. Ibid., XXX (April 11, 1870), 76–77. See also: XXXIII (November 22, 1883), 307–309, and (January 31, 1884), 340, regarding the College's action on the new problem of malpractice suits—which of course concerned consultants as well as G.P.'s.

116. Ibid., XXX (August 11, 1869), 32.

117. Burrows, *Address*, p. 14.

118. Charles Newman discusses the problem of the Conjoint Boards briefly, in *Medical Education*, pp. 232–233 and 297–299. See A. M. Cooke, *A History of the Royal College of Physicians of London* (Oxford, 1972), III, 850–861, for a fuller account.

119. The Minutes of the Royal College of Surgeons contain the fullest account of all the negotiations from 1865 to 1886. RCS, *Annual Report . . . 1875–76*, p. 8, provides a good summary of early negotiations.

120. C. R. B. Barrett, *The History of the Society of Apothecaries of London* (London, 1905), pp. 251–252; and N. G. Horner, *The Growth of the General Practitioner of Medicine in England* (London, 1922), p. 24.

121. J. Simon, *On the Claim, Asserted by the Royal College of Physicians, that the College of Itself . . . Can Grant Such Letters-Testimonial . . .* (London, 1892), pp. 17 and 19–20; Horner, *General Practitioner*, pp. 24 ff.; and Barrett, *Apothecaries*, pp. 251 ff. See also: W. Rivington, *The Medical Profession* (Dublin, 1879), pp. 61–62.

122. RCS, *Minutes*, 6 August 1885, p. 15; 24 November 1885, p. 71; 14 January 1886, pp. 89–90; 13 May 1886, p. 114; 10 June 1886, pp. 123–124; and 16 December 1886, pp. 190–198.

123. Cooke, *A History*, III, 931–971. For studies of the University of London, see: University of London, *The Historical Record (1836–1912)* (London, 1912); T. L. Humberstone, *University Reform in London* (London, 1925); and W. H. Allchin, *An Account of the Reconstruction of the University of London*, 3 Parts (London, 1905–1912). By 1938, one-half of all medical students obtained university degrees; see: R. M. Walker, *Medical Education in Britain* (London, 1965), p. 22.

124. Cooke, *A History*, III, 971.

125. Walker, *Medical Education*, p. 22.

Chapter VI

1. This and other material on Abercrombie's career are drawn from a letter from Robert Abercrombie to the Council of the Royal College of Surgeons, dated November 9, 1865, and recorded in: Royal College of Surgeons, *Minutes*, XI (9 November 1865), 254–255.

2. The *Times* (London), August 4, 1865, p. 11; August 5, 1865, p. 11; and August 9, 1865, p. 10.

3. RCS, *Minutes*, XI (9 November 1865), 252–253.

4. The *Times*, August 4, 1865, p. 11.

5. RCS, *Minutes*, XI (10 August 1865), 239–240; and XI (9 November 1865), 252–253.

6. Idem.

7. R. Abercrombie, *A Popular Treatise* . . . (London, 1864), pp. v, vi, vii, and 40–41. Cf. W. Rivington, *The Medical Profession* (Dublin, 1879), pp. 95–96.

8. The *Times*, February 11, 1873, p. 12.

9. Idem. For another of Lobb's advertisements, see: the *Times*, November 5, 1872, p. 10.

10. A. La'Mert, *Self-Preservation*, 47th ed. (London, 1852), p. 56.

11. B. Abel-Smith, *The Hospitals, 1800–1948* (London, 1964), p. 22. Cf. H. R. Haweis, *Sir Morrell Mackenzie, Physician and Operator* (London, 1893), pp. 49 and 57. Mackenzie was assistant physician at the London Hospital and apparently left that post after establishing the Throat Hospital. The conditions under which he left are not explained by his biographers.

12. Theodor Billroth, *The Medical Sciences in the German Universities* (New York, 1924), pp. 33 ff. and 85–89; Haweis, *Mackenzie*, pp. 48, 49, 59, 60*n*; and F. Semon, *The Autobiography of Sir Felix Semon* (London, 1926), pp. 60, 80–89 passim, and 102–103.

13. Haweis, *Mackenzie*, p. 58. Cf. E. O. Jewesbury, *The Royal Northern Hospital, 1856–1956* (London, 1956), p. 10.

14. Haweis, *Mackenzie*, p. 58.

15. R. S. Stevenson, *Morrell Mackenzie* (London, 1946), p. 48. See also: *BMJ*, 1857, i, 1, where it is argued that ophthalmology owed none of its advances to oculists or to doctors in special hospitals.

16. RCS, *Minutes*, XI (9 November 1865), 252–253; and XII (13 March 1873), 143. For a hint of a similar motive, see: RCS, *Minutes*, 8 July 1886, p. 136.

17. M. Mackenzie, "Specialism in Medicine," *Fortnightly Review*, 37, n.s. (1885), 773.

18. R. Kershaw, *Special Hospitals* (London, 1909), p. 26; cf. p. 25. Kershaw was the lay Secretary to the Board of the Central London Throat, Nose, and Ear Hospital. C. B. Keetley, *The Student's and Junior Practitioner's Guide to the Medical Profession*, 2nd ed. (London, 1885), p. 47, notes that specialists were known to have "a very keen eye to the main chance." Sometimes specialism was thought of as the logical pursuit for the man with ambition but without financial resources; see: W. Jenner, Presidential Addresses to the Royal College of Physicians, 1882–1888, vol. 2 (RCP Ms., 1887), irregular pagination (regarding the career of Alfred Wiltshire).

19. Mackenzie, "Specialism," p. 779. See also: *Select Committee on Metropolitan Hospitals*, 1890, p. 36, Q. 366 (Steele).

20. Jewesbury, *Royal Northern Hospital*, p. 7; also see pp. 1–3.

21. Ibid., pp. 2 and 9–13.

22. F. Davenant, *What Shall My Son Be?* (London, 1870), p. 7. See also: B. Brodie, *Autobiography of the Late Sir Benjamin Brodie, Bart.* (London, 1865), p. 87.

23. For examples, see: J. Bland-Sutton, *The Story of a Surgeon* (London, 1930), p. 68 (*re* Lawson Tait); J. Beddoe, *Memories of Eighty Years* (Bristol, 1910), pp. 173–174 (*re* William Budd); J. A. Shepherd, *Spencer Wells* (Edinburgh and London, 1965), pp. 117 and 120; S. T. Taylor, *The Diary of a Medical Student . . . 1860–64*, p. 2 (*re* Lionel S. Beale); *Munk's Roll*, III, s.v. Thomas Addison, and IV, s.v. H. M. Hughes; and J. Crichton-Browne, *Victorian Jottings* (London, 1926), p. 85. Cf. Noel Annan's "intellectual aristocracy" who, secure in their status, shunned current fashions and the "philistinism of the new rich" (N. G. Annan, "The Intellectual Aristocracy," in *Studies in Social History*, ed. J. H. Plumb [London, 1955], pp. 247–250 and 252–253).

24. *BMJ*, 1872, ii, 169, suggests that mental disorders were more common among medical men than in other social groups. Cf. R. Roose, *The Wear and Tear of London Life* (London, 1886), pp. 18–19 and 25. For cases of undiagnosed illness among socially mobile medical men, see: Z. Cope, *The Versatile Victorian* (London, 1951), p. 45; and *Plarr's Lives*, s.v. Caleb Rose, Alfred John Wall, A. E. Durham, and Henry Burford Norman. For literature on the psychology of social mobility, see: E. H. Powell, "Occupation, Status, and Suicide," *Am. Soc. Rev.*, 23 (1958), 131–139; A. B. Hollingshead, R. Ellis, and E. Kirby, "Social Mobility and Mental Illness," *Am. Soc. Rev.*, 19

(1954), 577–584; W. Breed, "Occupational Mobility and Suicide among White Males," *Am. Soc. Rev.*, 28 (1963), 179–188; and R. J. Kleiner and S. Parker, "Goal Striving, Social Status, and Mental Disorder," *Am. Soc. Rev.*, 28 (1963), 189–203.

25. A. Feiling, *A History of the Maida Vale Hospital for Nervous Diseases* (London, 1958), pp. 4 and 7.

26. C. Morson, ed., *St. Peter's Hospital for Stone, 1860–1960* (Edinburgh and London, 1960), pp. 16–18. Both Todd and Statham suffered unidentified ill health. For other cases of specialists with "difficult" personalities, see: B. Russell, ed., *St. John's Hospital for Diseases of the Skin, 1863–1963* (Edinburgh and London, 1963), pp. 5, 10, and 27; E. T. Collins, *History and Traditions of the Moorfields Eye Hospital* (London, 1929), p. 4; Haweis, *Mackenzie*, p. 47; and Stevenson, *Morrell Mackenzie*, p. 26. Cf. Rivington, *The Medical Profession*, p. 771.

27. Mackenzie, "Specialism," p. 775.

28. G. MacDonald, *The Sanity of William Blake* (London, 1908), p. 7.

29. RCP, *By-Laws of 1862*, Chapter XXIII, Section x, reprinted in A. M. Cooke, *A History of the Royal College of Physicians of London* (Oxford, 1972), III, 1174; and RCS, *Bye-Laws . . . 1860*, XVI.2, p. 14.

30. RCS, *Minutes*, XI (11 February 1869), 532.

31. The *Times*, February 11, 1873, p. 12. On galvanic treatments, see also: R. B. Carter, *Doctors and Their Work* (London, 1903), pp. 227–228. For a discussion of the treatment of venereal disease in the nineteenth century, see: A. Comfort, *The Anxiety Makers* (London, 1967).

32. RCS, *Minutes*, XII (13 March 1873), 142–143 (letter from Lobb). Cf. the *Times*, February 11, 1873, p. 12.

33. RCS, *Minutes*, XII (19 June 1873), 168–169.

34. Ibid., XII (2 January 1873), 132.

35. RCP, Annals, XXXI (June 9, 1873), 25–27; cf. ibid., XXXIII (March 1, 1881), 8, and (December 27, 1881), 75–76. See also: RCS, *Minutes*, 8 December 1887, pp. 59–60.

36. Taylor, *Diary, 1860–64*, p. 16.

37. RCS, *Minutes*, XI (8 January 1863), 7; and RCS, *Minutes*, 14 June 1888, pp. 139–140. See also: F. B. Courtenay, *On Spermatorrhoea and the Professional Fallacies and Popular Delusions which Prevail in Relation to Its Nature, Consequences, and Treatment*, 11th ed. (London, 1878), p. 4.

38. W. A. Coote, *A Romance of Philanthropy* (London, 1916), pp. 18, 102, and 104. See also: ibid., p. 101, passim; and RCS, *Minutes*, 13 December 1888, pp. 218–219. Regarding legislation on indecent advertisements, see: RCS, *Minutes*, 8 December 1887, pp. 58–59; *An Act to Suppress Indecent Advertisements*, 1889, 52 and 53 Vict. c. 18; and 337 Parliamentary Debates, 3rd series, 1354.

39. Coote, *A Romance*, pp. 14 and 108.

40. RCS, *Minutes*, 14 February 1884, p. 48. See also: ibid., 13 December 1883, p. 32; and 10 January 1884, p. 42.

41. RCP, *By-laws of 1862*, Chapter XXIII, Paragraphs V and VIII, reprinted in Cooke, *A History*, III, 1173–74. Prosecutions for violation were relatively rare; for one example, see: RCP, Annals, XXX (July 28, 1869), 24–25.

42. G. Clark, *A History of the Royal College of Physicians of London* (Oxford, 1966), I, 32–34; *Lancet*, July 2, 1887, ii, 25; and RCP, *Regulations . . .* , Section 12, Paragraph I, reprinted in Cooke, *A History*, III, 1184.

43. RCP, Annals, XXXI (October 26, 1876), 339–341; and XXXII (January 12, 1881), 341.

44. Ibid., XXXIII (January 31, 1884), 339; and XXXIV (February 26, 1884), 4. For other cases, see: Cooke, *A History*, III, 902–904. The most famous case is that of Sir Morrell Mackenzie's publication of *The Fatal Illness of Frederick the Noble* (1888); see: Cooke, *A History*, III, 904–905; and R. Saundby, *Medical Ethics* (London, 1907), p. 27.

45. Abercrombie, *Popular Treatise*, pp. v and vi.

46. The *Times*, February 11, 1873, p. 12.

47. La'Mert, *Self-Preservation*, pp. 13 and 56; also pp. 18, 29, and 38.

48. E. Jameson, *The Natural History of Quackery* (London, 1961), p. 15; and Z. Cope, ed., *Sidelights on the History of Medicine* (London, 1957), p. 21. For other studies of quackery, see: S. H. Holbrook, *The Golden Age of Quackery* (New York, 1959); C. J. S. Thompson, *The Quacks of Old London* (London, 1928); and two early works: *Exposures of Quackery*, by the Editor of "Health News" (London, [1896?]); and G. Everitt, *Doctors and Doctors* (London, 1888). The best is probably: B. Inglis, *Fringe Medicine* (London, 1964).

49. Abercrombie, *Popular Treatise*, pp. viii, 42, and 50; cf. pp. v and vi.

50. RCS, *Minutes*, 11 March 1880, pp. 11–12. The cases dis-

cussed here are drawn from the RCS records, which are more complete than those of the RCP. Some cases arose in the Physicians College, but little information appears in the Annals. For a sketch, see: Cooke, *A History*, III, 902 and 904–909.

51. RCS, *Minutes*, 11 June 1885, p. 207; 3 July 1885, p. 216; 6 August 1885, p. 18; 5 October 1885, pp. 24 and 26; 10 June 1886, p. 126; 24 June 1886, p. 131; 8 July 1886, p. 136; and 5 August 1886, pp. 149–150.

52. Ibid., 11 June 1885, p. 206; and 3 July 1885, p. 216.

53. J. L. Berlant sees the issue of trade in the context of the conflict between legal privilege and laissez faire (*Profession and Monopoly* [Berkeley and Los Angeles, 1975], p. 149).

54. Kershaw, *Special Hospitals*, p. 25. N. Parry and J. Parry, *The Rise of the Medical Profession* (London, 1976), p. 140, also see specialism as entrepreneurial behavior, but do not elaborate.

55. Clark, *A History*, I, 163.

56. Jameson, *Quackery*, Chapters 3 and 4; and E. H. Ackerknecht, *A Short History of Medicine* (New York, 1955), p. 182.

57. G. Rosen, *The Specialization of Medicine* (New York, 1944), focusses on the specialty of ophthalmology in America. It is the best study of the social context of specialism, to date. See also: Ackerknecht, *Short History*, Chapter 17 passim.

58. Abel-Smith, *The Hospitals*, pp. 22 ff.; J. Woodward, *To Do the Sick No Harm* (London and Boston, 1974), Chapter 7; and R. Hunter and I. Macalpine, *Psychiatry for the Poor* (London, 1974), pp. 13–19.

59. A. Sorsby, *The Royal Eye Hospital, 1857–1957* (London, 1957), p. 4; and *Select Committee on Metropolitan Hospitals*, 1890, p. 17, Q. 141 (Montefiore); p. 51, Q. 699 (Holmes); and pp. 71–72, Q. 1072 and 1092–93 (Hardy).

60. Billroth, *Medical Sciences*, pp. 32 ff.; E. H. Ackerknecht, *Medicine at the Paris Hospital, 1794–1848* (Baltimore, 1967), pp. 163–164; and Ackerknecht, *Short History*, pp. 181 ff. Sir Felix Semon describes the tension he felt as a German-trained medical man practicing in the anti-specialist environment of London hospitals (*Autobiography*, pp. 80–102 and 115).

61. Mackenzie, "Specialism," p. 776.

62. T. Higgins, *Great Ormond Street Hospital for Children, 1852–1952* (London, 1952), pp. 7 and 10.

63. Russell, *St. John's Hospital*, pp. 2–3; and *Lancet 1864*, ii, 530. Historically, skin and venereal disease practice have been re-

lated; see: Ackerknecht, *Short History*, p. 186. For other instances of medical initiative in special hospital foundations, see: Sorsby, *Royal Eye Hospital*, p. 5; Haweis, *Mackenzie*, pp. 57–58; Feiling, *Maida Vale Hospital*, pp. v and 1; and St. Mark's Hospital for Fistula, London, *Collected Papers of St. Mark's Hospital . . . 1835–1935* (London, 1935), pp. 1–2. Richard Kershaw assumes that special hospitals were the creations of medical men (*Special Hospitals*, p. 25).

64. Haweis, *Mackenzie*, pp. 58 ff. See also: Kershaw, *Special Hospitals*, p. 25; St. Mark's Hospital, *Collected Papers*, p. 1; and Rivington, *The Medical Profession*, p. 771.

65. Russell, *St. John's Hospital*, passim.

66. Morson, *St. Peter's Hospital*, pp. 3–4, 8, and 18–19.

67. Haweis, *Mackenzie*, pp. 58 ff.

68. Jewesbury, *Royal Northern Hospital*, p. 13.

69. Higgins, *Hospital for Children*, p. 10.

70. G. M. Holmes, *National Hospital, Queen Square, 1860–1948* (London, 1954), p. 10.

71. Jewesbury, *Royal Northern Hospital*, p. 22. See also: Sorsby, *Royal Eye Hospital*, p. 6; and Morson, *St. Peter's Hospital*, p. 60. *The London and Provincial Medical Directory* listed the patrons of each hospital.

72. Hospital for Diseases of the Throat and Chest, London, *Statement by the Medical Council to the Committee of Management . . .* [London, 1886], p. 15. This ideal did not always work out in practice; see: Haweis, *Mackenzie*, pp. 65 ff.; and Russell, *St. John's Hospital*, pp. 27 ff.

73. Reprinted in: *Mr. Punch among the Doctors*, p. 25.

74. Quoted in: R. Pound, *Harley Street* (London, 1967), p. 10. See also: Ackerknecht, *Short History*, p. 182.

75. See, e.g., statistics in: Higgins, *Hospital for Children*, p. 30; and Russell, *St. John's Hospital*, passim. *Low's Handbook to the Charities of London* (London, various years), published information on the income of special hospitals.

76. Russell, *St. John's Hospital*, p. 27.

77. Feiling, *Maida Vale Hospital*, pp. 1, 4, and 5.

78. *BMJ*, 22 October 1864, quoted in Russell, *St. John's Hospital*, p. 33.

79. Sorsby, *Royal Eye Hospital*, p. 10.

80. Haweis, *Mackenzie*, pp. 65 ff., 83, and 85; and Stevenson, *Morrell Mackenzie*, pp. 47–48.

81. Eliot Freidson is suggestive here (*Profession of Medicine* [New York, 1970], pp. 162 and 194–200).

82. Collins, *Moorfields Eye Hospital*, p. 161.

83. Russell, *St. John's Hospital*, pp. 45–46.

84. W. R. Lefanu, *British Periodicals of Medicine* (Baltimore, 1938), items 234 and 268.

85. J. M. M. Kerr et al., eds., *Historical Review of British Obstetrics and Gynaecology, 1800–1950* (Edinburgh and London, 1954), p. 312.

86. Lefanu, *British Periodicals*, items 326, 380, 445, 474, and 540.

87. Sorsby, *Royal Eye Hospital*, p. 10.

88. Ibid., p. 3.

89. *London and Provincial Medical Directory*, 1861.

90. *Low's Handbook*, 1890.

91. Russell, *St. John's Hospital*, pp. 33–35.

92. *Plarr's Lives*, s.v.

93. Quoted in Sorsby, *Royal Eye Hospital*, p. 4 (from the *Lancet*). The *BMJ* in 1873 called special hospitals "mischievous excrescences on our system of hospital charity" (quoted in Morson, *St. Peter's Hospital*, p. 7).

94. Quoted in Sorsby, *Royal Eye Hospital*, p. 4.

95. Stevenson, *Morrell Mackenzie*, pp. 47–48.

96. Mackenzie, "Specialism," p. 777.

97. *Select Committee on Metropolitan Hospitals*, 1890, p. 250, Q. 3834.

98. Ibid., p. 221, Q. 3280. See also: p. 235, Q. 3608–09 (Corbyn); and p. 284, Q. 4587 (Kay).

99. *The General Practitioner*, I (January 6, 1900), 6.

100. Idem.

101. Idem. Other general practitioners suggested making general practice a specialty; see, e.g., S. D. Clippingdale, "Some Considerations of the Life and Work of the General Practitioner," *West London Medical Journal*, 4 (1899), 1.

102. Quoted in Pound, *Harley Street*, p. 11.

103. Letter dated July 16, 1860, from Sir Benjamin Brodie to the Members of the Deputation Appointed by the Representatives of the Medical Staffs of General Hospitals, in: RCS, Circulars and letters from well-known surgeons relating to Special Hospitals, 1860. Brodie's letter was printed and distributed nationally.

104. Sorsby, *Royal Eye Hospital*, p. 4. See also: Ackerknecht, *Short*

History, p. 181; letter dated 28 June 1860, E. H. Sieveking to John Erichsen, in: RCS, Circulars and letters; and *The General Practitioner*, 1 (January 6, 1900), 6.

105. RCP, Annals, XXXIII (December 27, 1881), 75–76; and RCS, *Minutes*, X (10 December 1862), 651. A. M. Cooke indicates that free choice of medical theories was stipulated in the Medical Act of 1858 (*A History*, III, 908).

106. "Special Hospitals," a printed circular, in: RCS, Circulars and letters. The signed and returned circulars, together with many letters, are on file at the RCS Library. The circular was published in the *BMJ*, 1860, ii, 582. See also: Committee Minutes, October 19, 1860, no pagination, and letter dated August 10, 1860, from John Erichsen and W. H. Flower (printed), in: RCS, Circulars and letters, 1860.

107. "Special Hospitals," in: RCS, Circulars and letters, 1860.

108. Idem.

109. Letter dated June 26, 1860, from W. Basham to John Erichsen, in: RCS, Circulars and letters. See also: Letter dated July 16, from E. H. Greenhow to J. Erichsen; and letter dated July 2, 1860, from Bernard Holt to J. Erichsen. Also see: *Select Committee on Metropolitan Hospitals*, 1890, p. 253, Q. 3937 (Bhakha).

110. "Special Hospitals," in: RCS, Circulars and letters.

111. Idem.

112. Idem.

113. Letter dated June 28, 1860, from E. H. Sieveking to J. Erichsen, in: RCS, Circulars and letters.

114. This disapproval may have had some effect; see: *My Doctors*, "By a Patient" (London, 1891), pp. 7–8; J. L. Hammond and B. Hammond, *Lord Shaftesbury*, 4th ed. (London, 1936), p. 204*n*; Keetley, *Guide*, pp. 34–35, 47, 87, and 94; and *Lancet*, ii (1864), 497–498. See also: Freidson, *Profession of Medicine*, pp. 193–198.

115. Semon, *Autobiography*, p. 102.

116. Morson, *St. Peter's Hospital*, p. 21.

117. Ibid., p. 42.

118. *Munk's Roll*, IV, s.v.

119. D. Power and H. J. Waring, *A Short History of St. Bartholomew's Hospital, 1123–1923* (London, 1923), p. 50; G. Whitteridge and V. Stokes, *A Brief History of the Hospital of Saint Bartholomew* (London, 1961), pp. 45 and 46; E. M. McInnes, *St. Thomas' Hospital* (Lon-

don, 1963), pp. 135 and 147; and H. C. Cameron, *Mr. Guy's Hospital, 1726–1948* (London, 1954), pp. 116, 190–191, and 358–361.

120. *Select Committee on Metropolitan Hospitals*, 1890, p. 32, Q. 288 (Steele), and p. 50, Q. 696 (Holmes).

121. McInnes, *St. Thomas' Hospital*, p. 147; and Semon, *Autobiography*, pp. 82–84, 106–107, and 114–116. Later awarded a knighthood and the FRCP, Semon had studied with Traube in Heidelberg and considered Rudolph Virchow his "paternal friend" (*Autobiography*, pp. 41–42 and 62).

122. McInnes, *St. Thomas' Hospital*, p. 147.

123. Cameron, *Mr. Guy's Hospital*, pp. 3, 117, 191, 358–362, and 418.

124. Kerr et al., *Historical Review*, pp. 332–333.

125. Cooke, *A History*, III, 885–889.

126. Semon, *Autobiography*, p. 81. See also: Ackerknecht, *Short History*, p. 144; G. Geison, "Social and Institutional Factors in the Stagnancy of English Physiology, 1840–1870," *Bulletin of the History of Medicine*, 46:1 (1972), 30–58; and R. D. French, *Antivivisection and Medical Science in Victorian Society* (Princeton, N.J., 1975), pp. 328 ff.

127. T. Underhill, *On Hospitals and Medical Education* (Birmingham, [1870]), p. 26. See also: Carter, *Doctors*, p. 287. For an excellent discussion of early nineteenth-century medical ethics, see: I. Waddington, "The Development of Medical Ethics—A Sociological Analysis," *Medical History*, 19:1 (1975), 36–51.

128. Saundby, *Medical Ethics*, pp. 4–5.

129. Carter, *Doctors*, p. 252.

Conclusion

1. T. Hardy, *The Woodlanders* (London, 1958), Chapter XVII.

2. B. Gilbert, *The Evolution of National Insurance in Great Britain* (London, 1966), pp. 411–412 and 440.

3. R. D. French, *Antivivisection and Medical Science in Victorian Society* (Princeton, N.J., 1975), p. 329 and note 93.

4. T. Underhill, *On Hospitals and Medical Education* (Birmingham, [1870]), p. 27.

5. G. B. Shaw, "Preface on Doctors," *The Doctor's Dilemma* (New York, 1942), p. v.

6. H. Perkin, *The Origins of Modern English Society, 1780–1880* (London and Toronto, 1969), p. x.

Bibliography

1. Official Documents

GOVERNMENT

The General Council of Medical Education and Registration of the United Kingdom. *The Medical Register: Pursuant to an Act Passed in the XXI and XXII Victoria, Cap. xc, To Regulate the Qualifications of Practitioners in Medicine and Surgery, 1859* [etc.]. London: General Council of Medical Education and Registration of the United Kingdom, 1859, etc. [After 1885, published by H.M.S.O.]

————. *Minutes of the General Medical Council, of its Executive and Dental Committees, and of its Branch Councils, for 1859* [etc.] London: Spottiswoode, 1859, etc.

Parliament. *Parliamentary Debates*.

————. *Sessional Papers*.

Select Committee on Medical Education, Schools of Anatomy, 1828 (568), vii.

Select Committee on Medical Education, 1834 (602-I, II, and III), Parts I-III, xiii.

32nd Report of the Charity Commissioners, Pt. VI, 1840 [219], xix.

Report of the Committee Appointed by the Secretary of State to Enquire into the Causes which Tend to Prevent Sufficient Eligible Candidates from Coming Forward for the Army Medical Department, 1878–79 [C. 2200], xliv, 257.

Report from the Select Committee of the House of Lords on Metropolitan Hospitals, &c.; with the Proceedings of the Committee, Minutes of Evidence, Appendix, and Index, 1890 (392), xvi; *2nd Report*, 1890–91 (457), xiii; *3rd Report*, 1892, Sess. 1 (321), xiii.

Report of Sir William Plender to the Chancellor of the Exchequer on the Result of his Investigation into Existing Conditions in Respect of

Medical Attendance and Remuneration in Certain Towns, 1912–13 [Cd. 6305], lxxviii, 679.

Prerogative Court of Canterbury, Principal Registry of the Family Division (formerly Principal Probate Registry).

———. *Calendar of the Grants of Probate and Letters of Administration made in the Probate Registers of the High Court of Justice in England.* Hastings: H.M.S.O., various years.

Privy Council. *Report as to the Practice of Medicine and Surgery by Unqualified Persons in the United Kingdom.* Presented to Both Houses of Parliament by Command of His Majesty. London: H.M.S.O., 1910.

ROYAL COLLEGE OF PHYSICIANS OF LONDON

[Alderson, Sir James]. *Address* [Presidential Address to the RCP, 1870]. [RCP Library]

Annals of the College, 1857–1890. Vols. XXV–XXXVI. RCP Mss.

Burrows, Sir George. *Address of the President of the Royal College of Physicians to the Fellows, at the Annual General Meeting, 22nd March, 1875.* London: Harrison & Sons, for the College, 1875.

A Catalogue of the Fellows, Candidates, and Licentiates of the Royal College of Physicians. London: For the College, 1830–1871. [Subsequently publ. as: *A List . . .* ,q.v.]

The Charter, Bye-Laws, and Regulations of the Royal College of Physicians of London and the Acts of Parliament Especially Relating Thereto. London: Harrison & Sons, for the College, 1892.

Jenner, Sir William. Presidential Addresses to the Royal College of Physicians, 1882–1888. 2 vols. [RCP Ms.]

A List of the Fellows, Members, Extra-Licentiates, and Licentiates of the Royal College of Physicians of London. London: For the College, 1871–1890. [See also: *A Catalogue. . . .*]

Lives of the Fellows of the Royal College of Physicians, 1826–1925. G. H. Brown, comp. London: Royal College of Physicians, 1955. [*Munk's Roll*, IV.]

Payne, Joseph Frank. *History of the College Club of the Royal College of Physicians of London.* London: For the Club, 1909.

The Roll of the Royal College of Physicians of London. 2nd ed., comp. William Munk. 3 vols. London: Royal College of Physicians, 1878 [*Munk's Roll*, I–III.—Continued as *Lives of the Fellows . . . 1826–1925*, q. v.]

[Watson, Sir Thomas]. *Dr. Watson's Address, March 26th, 1866. Royal College of Physicians* [Presidential Address]. London: T. Richards, for the College, n.d. [RCP Library]

ROYAL COLLEGE OF PHYSICIANS OF EDINBURGH

Royal College of Physicians of Edinburgh. *Historical Sketch and Laws of the Royal College of Physicians from its Institution to December, 1865*. Edinburgh: For the College, 1867.

ROYAL COLLEGE OF SURGEONS OF ENGLAND

Annual Report on the Affairs of the Royal College of Surgeons of England, 1875–76. By the President [Sir James Paget]. London: Taylor and Francis, for the College, 1876.

Bye-Laws of the Royal College of Surgeons of England. London: For the College, [1860].

Calendar of the Royal College of Surgeons of England. London: Taylor & Francis, for the College, 1865, etc. [Previously published as *List . . .* , q.v.]

Circulars and letters from well-known surgeons relating to Special Hospitals. Secretary of Committee, W. H. Flower. RCS Mss., 1860.

A Few Words on the Fellowship, with a Suggestion Concerning the Present Crisis, Addressed to the President and Council of the Royal College of Surgeons of England by an Old Member of the College. London: Churchill, 1845.

Finch, Sir Ernest. *History of the College Council Club, 1869–1958*. London: For the Club, 1960.

List of the Fellows, Members, Licentiates in Midwifery, and Persons Who Have Received the Certificate of Qualification in Dental Surgery of the Royal College of Surgeons of England. London: For the College, 1857–1864. [Subsequently published as *Calendar . . .* , q. v.]

List of Officers, &c. of the Royal College of Surgeons of England, 1800–1895. London: Taylor & Francis, for the College, 1896.

Lives of the Fellows of the Royal College of Surgeons of England, 1930–1951. By Sir D'Arcy Power and W. R. Lefanu. London: By the College, 1953. [Cited here as *Plarr's Lives*, III.]

Minutes of Council. Vols. X–XII, 1854–1879. RCS Mss. [Continued as *Minutes of Council*, 1880, etc. London: For the College, 1880, etc.]

Plarr's Lives of the Fellows of the Royal College of Surgeons of England. Rev. by Sir D'Arcy Power, with W. G. Spencer and G. E. Gask. 2 vols. Bristol: John Wright & Sons, for the College, 1930. [Continued as *Lives of the Fellows . . . 1930–1951*, q.v.]

SOCIETY OF APOTHECARIES OF LONDON

An Address by the Society of Apothecaries to the General Practitioners of England and Wales on the Provisions of the Bill "For the Better Regula-

tion of Medical Practice Throughout the United Kingdom," and Their Probable Influence on the Position and Prospects of That Branch of the Medical Profession. London: Samuel Highley, 1844.

Apprenticeship contract of Richard Hughes, bound to Henry Reynolds, November 4, 1851 [Guildhall Ms.].

Court Minute Books. Vols. 10–12, 1817–1858 [Guildhall Ms. 8200/11–13]. [Continued as Minutes of the Court . . . , q.v.]

Friendly Medical Society. Minute Books, 1775–1844, 1875–1917. 5 vols. [Guildhall Ms. 8278].

Minutes of the Court of Assistants, 1859–1890 [Society of Apothecaries Mss.].

HOSPITALS AND MEDICAL SCHOOLS

Hospital for Diseases of the Throat and Chest, London. *Statement by the Medical Council to the Committee of Management on the Differences that Have Lately Arisen between These Two Bodies.* [London, 1886].

Lock Hospital and Asylum, and Male Hospital. Minutes of the Weekly Board, 1862–73 [RCS Ms.].

St. Bartholomew's Hospital. Administration. Minutes of the Board of Governors.

———. Medical Council. Correspondence.

———. Medical Council. Minutes of the Medical Council.

———. Medical School. Copies of entries in the Journals concerning the Medical School, 1842–1851 ["Collegiate Committee"].

———. Medical School. Number of Students, 1851–1904.

———. Medical School. Regulations, Medical College Hall.

St. Thomas's Hospital. General Court Minute Books [Greater London Record Office].

———. Minute Books of the Grand Committee [GLRO].

———. *Rules and Orders for the Government of St. Thomas's Hospital.* [GLRO]

———. *A List of Governors of St. Thomas's Hospital in Southwark*, various years.

———. Miscellanea associated with St. Thomas's Hospital [GLRO].

———. [Papers relating to St. Thomas's Hospital 1863–98]. [RCS Library]

———. Medical School. *Prospectus for the Year Commencing October 1st, 1898.* London: W. P. Griffith, [1898].

2. *Other Manuscript and Printed Primary Sources*

Abercrombie, Robert. *A Popular Treatise on the Anatomy, Physiology, Pathology, and New Treatment of Specific Diseases of the Genital Organs in Males.* London: Job Caudwell, 1864.

Allbutt, Sir Thomas Clifford. "Medicine in the 19th Century." *Bull. of the Johns Hopkins Hospital*, 9 (1898), 277–285. [Reprinted with explanatory notes by A. M. Chesney, in *J. Med. Educ.*, 31 (1956), 460–468.]

———. *The Need for a Liberal Education in Medicine.* London: n.p., 1889.

———. *On Professional Education. With Special Reference to Medicine. An Address Delivered at King's College, London, on October 3, 1905.* London: Macmillan, 1906.

Arnold, Matthew. *Essays in Criticism*, 2nd ser., in: *Works of Matthew Arnold*, IV. London: Macmillan, 1903.

Ashe, Isaac. *Medical Education and Medical Interests. Being the Essay to Which Was Awarded the Carmichael Prize of £100 by the Council of the Royal College of Surgeons, Ireland, 1868.* Dublin: Fannin, 1868.

Ashurst, Frederick. *Memoirs of a Young Surgeon.* London: Digby Long & Co., 1898.

Barker, Sir Herbert A. *Leaves from My Life.* London: Hutchinson, 1927.

Beddoe, John. *Memories of Eighty Years.* Bristol: Arrowsmith, 1910.

Belcher, [Robert] Henry. *Degrees and "Degrees." Or, Traffic in Theological, Medical and Other "Diplomas" Exposed.* London: Hardwicke, 1872.

Berdoe, Edward [pseud. Scalpel Aesculapius]. *St. Bernard's. The Romance of a Medical Student.* London: Swan Sonnenschein, Lowrey & Co., 1887.

British Medical Association. *Medicine in Modern Times; or, Discourses Delivered at a Meeting of the British Medical Association at Oxford by Dr. Stokes, Dr. Acland, Professor Rolleston, Rev. Prof. Haughton, and Dr. Gull, August 5–7, 1868.* London: Macmillan, 1869.

———. *A Tariff of Medical Fees Recommended by the Shropshire Ethical Branch of the British Medical Association* [Prepared by Jukes De Styrap]. Shrewsbury: Privately printed, 1870.

The British Medical Journal: Being the Journal of the BMA. [*BMJ*]

Brodie, Sir Benjamin. Account books, 1824–1860. 3 vols. [RCS Ms.]

———. *Autobiography of the Late Sir Benjamin Brodie, Bart.* London: Longman, Green, Longman, Roberts & Green, 1865.

———. *Introductory Discourse on Duties and Conduct of Medical Students and Practitioners. Addressed to the Students of the Medical School of St. George's Hospital, October 2, 1843.* London: Longman, Brown, Green, & Longman, 1843.

Browne, Sir James Crichton-. *Victorian Jottings. From an Old Commonplace Book.* London: Etchells & MacDonald, 1926.

Burdett, Sir Henry Charles. *Hospitals and Asylums of the World: Their*

Origin, History, Construction, Administration, Management, and Legislation. 4 vols. London: Churchill, 1891–93.

————. *The Medical Attendance of Londoners. An Economical System of Medical Relief Freed from Existing Abuse. A Speech....* London: Scientific Press, 1903.

Carter, Robert Brudenell. *Doctors and Their Work; or, Medicine, Quackery, and Disease*. London: Smith, Elder & Co., 1903.

Chapman, John. *The Medical Institutions of the United Kingdom: A History Exemplifying the Evils of Over-Legislation* [reprinted from the *Medical Mirror*, n.s., nos. 7–13, 1869–70]. London: Churchill, 1870.

Churchill's Medical Directory. See: *The London and Provincial Medical Directory*.

Clippingdale, Samuel Dodd. Medical Court-Roll. Physicians and Surgeons and Some Apothecaries, Who Have Attended the Sovereigns of England, from William I to George V, with a Medical Note on Harold. 2 vols. [typescript] 1922 [RCS Ms.].

————. "Some Considerations of the Life and Work of the General Practitioner" [Presidential Address, West London Med. Soc.]. *West London Medical Journal*, 4 (1899), 1–12.

[Cobbe, F. P.]. *The Medical Profession and its Morality*. [Reprinted, with additions, from *The Modern Review*, April, 1881.] London: Pewtress & Co., 1886.

Collins, Wilkie. *The Moonstone. A Romance*. London: Thos. Nelson, n.d.

Confessions of an English Doctor. [Anon.] London: George Routledge & Sons, 1904.

Corfe, George. *The Apothecary, Ancient and Modern, of the Society, London, Blackfriars*. London: Elliot Stock, 1885.

Counsell, Herbert Edward. *37 The Broad. The Memoirs of an Oxford Doctor*. London: Robert Hale, 1943.

Courtenay, Francis Burdett. *On Spermatorrhoea and The Professional Fallacies and Popular Delusions Which Prevail in Relation to Its Nature, Consequences, and Treatment*. London: H. Baillière, 1878.

Cronin, A. J. *Adventures in Two Worlds*. Boston: Little, Brown, 1952.

Cullingworth, Charles J. *On the Importance of Personal Character in the Profession of Medicine. An Address Delivered at the Opening of the Winter Session of the Medical Department of the Yorkshire College, Leeds. October 3, 1898*. London: Henry J. Glaisher, 1898.

Dale, William. *The State of the Medical Profession in Great Britain. Being the Successful Carmichael Prize Essay in 1873....* Dublin: J. Atkinson & Co., 1875.

Davenant, Francis. *What Shall My Son Be? Hints to Parents on the Choice of a Profession or Trade; and Counsels to Young Men on Their Entrance into Active Life*. London: S. W. Partridge, 1870.

De la Ramée, Marie Louise—see: Ouida.

De Styrap, Jukes. *The Young Practitioner: With Practical Hints and Instructive Suggestions . . . for His Guidance on Entering into Private Practice. . . .* London: H. K. Lewis, 1890.

Dickens, Charles. *Bleak House*. London: Dent, 1966.

Doran, Alban Henry Griffiths. *Life Memories*. [Typescript with ms. additions], 1923. [RCS Library]

Doyle, Arthur Conan. *Memories and Adventures*. Boston: Little, Brown, 1924.

————. *The Stark Munro Letters. Being a Series of Twelve Letters Written by J. Stark Munro, M.B., to His Friend and Former Fellow-Student, Herbert Swanborough, of Lowell, Massachusetts, during the Years 1881–1884*. New York: Appleton, 1895.

Eade, Sir Peter. *The Autobiography of Sir Peter Eade, With Selections from His Diary*. S. H. Long, ed. London: Jarrold & Sons, 1916.

Eliot, George. *Middlemarch. A Study of Provincial Life*. London: Oxford University Press, 1947.

Evans, George W. *Health, Life, and the Laws of God; A Pure Mind in a Pure Body is Health. . . . The Antiseptic Treatment*. Reading: n.p., 1870.

Everitt, G. *Doctors and Doctors: Some Curious Chapters in Medical History and Quackery*. London: Sonnenschein & Co., 1888.

Exposures of Quackery: Being a Series of Articles upon, and Analyses of, Various Patent Medicines. By the Editor of "Health News." 2 vols. London: Savoy Press, n. d. [1896?].

The Family Doctor. A Monthly Journal of Hygiene.

Farquharson, Rt. Hon. Robert. *In and Out of Parliament*. London: Williams and Norgate, 1911.

Gamgee, Sampson. *Medical Reform: The Present Crisis*. London: n.p., 1870. [In: Sir John Simon's Papers, File Box "Medical Profession: Bills, etc., " RCS Ms.]

Gant, Frederick J. *Auto-Biography*. London: Baillière, Tindall & Cox, 1905.

The General Practitioner [official journal of the Incorporated Medical Practitioners' Association, London].

Glenn, Robert G. *A Manual of the Laws Affecting Medical Men*. London: Churchill, 1871.

Griffin, Richard. *The Grievances of the Poor Law Medical Officers, Elucidated in a Letter to the Members of the Legislature, and a Commentary on the Proposed Act of Parliament.* . . . London: Simpkin, Marshall, 1858.

Gull, William W. "On the Nursing Crisis at Guy's Hospital" (No. I). *Nineteenth Century*, 7 (May, 1880), 884–891.

Habershon, S. O. "On the Nursing Crisis at Guy's Hospital" (No. II). *Nineteenth Century*, 7 (May, 1880), 892–901.

Haight, Gordon. *George Eliot and John Chapman, With Chapman's Diaries.* New Haven: Yale University Press, 1940.

Hardy, Thomas. *The Woodlanders.* London: Macmillan, 1969.

Henery, A. F. *Cure Yourself! A Textbook of Practical and Effective Instruction.* . . . London: By the author, 1863.

Henriques, Alfred G. "On the Nursing Crisis at Guy's Hospital" (No. III, concl.). *Nineteenth Century*, 7 (May, 1880), 902–904.

[Hughes, James Vaughan-]. *Seventy Years of Life in the Victorian Era. Embracing a Travelling Record.* . . . By "A Physician." London: T. Fisher Unwin, 1893.

Huxley, T. H. "The State and the Medical Profession." *Nineteenth Century*, 15 (February, 1884), 228–238.

Jones, Henry Bence-. *An Autobiography, 1813–1873.* London: Privately printed, 1929.

Keetley, Charles Bell. *The Student's and Junior Practitioner's Guide to the Medical Profession.* 2nd ed. Ed. by the Author and Robert Wharry. London: Baillière, Tindall, & Cox, 1885.

Kershaw, Richard. *Special Hospitals: Their Origins, Development and Relationship to Medical Education: Their Economic Aspects and Relative Freedom from Abuse.* London: George Pulman, 1909.

La'Mert, Samuel. *Self-Preservation: A Medical Treatise on the Secret Infirmities and Disorders of the Generative Organs, Resulting from Solitary Habits, Youthful Excess, or Infection; With Practical Observations on The Premature Failure of Sexual Power.* 47th ed. London: Published by the Author, 1852.

The Lancet. A Journal of British and Foreign Medicine, Physiology, Surgery, Chemistry, Criticism, Literature, and News [London].

The London and Provincial Medical Directory. London: Churchill, various years.

Lonsdale, Margaret. "Doctors and Nurses" (No. III, concl.). *Nineteenth Century*, 7 (June, 1880), 1105–08.

———. "The Present Crisis at Guy's Hospital." *Nineteenth Century*, 7 (April, 1880), 677–684.

Low's Handbook to the Charities of London. Giving the Objects, Date of Formation, Office, Income, Expenditure . . . of Over a Thousand Charitable Institutions. London: Sampson Low, Marston, Searle &

Rivington, various years. [Also published earlier under various titles, as, e.g., *The Charities of London in 1861*, and *Low's One Shilling Guide to the Charities of London*.]

MacDonald, Greville Matheson. *Reminiscences of a Specialist*. London: George Allen & Unwin, 1932.

———. *The Sanity of William Blake*. London: Fifield, 1908.

Mackenzie, Morrell. "Specialism in Medicine." *Fortnightly Review*, n.s., 37 (June 1, 1885), 772–787.

Makins, Sir George. *Autobiography* [RCS Ms., n.d.].

[Martin, William]. Untitled. Book of accounts, 1888 to c. 1914. [RCP Ms.]

Medical & Surgical Association of the Borough of Marylebone. *A Manifesto by the Medical and Surgical Association of the Borough of Marylebone*. 2nd ed. London: Churchill, 1884.

Medical Institutions of London. [Reprinted from the *BMJ*, June–July, 1895.] London: At the Office of the BMA, 1895.

Memoirs of the Life of a Country Surgeon. [Anon.] London: Reeve Bros., 1845.

Moxon, Walter. "Miss Lonsdale on Guy's Hospital." *Contemporary Review*, 37 (May, 1880), 872–892 and 1063.

Muggeridge, H. H. *Treatise on Recent and Old Ulcerated Wounds of the Legs, the Opprbrium* (sic) *of Hospitals*. N.p., n.d.

Munk's Roll: See Section 1, under Royal College of Physicians of London.

My Doctors. [Anon.] "By a Patient." London: Skeffington & Son, 1891.

Ouida [Marie Louise de la Ramée]. *The New Priesthood*. London: E. W. Allen, 1893.

Paget, Sir James. "The Advantages of Medical Societies" [an address to the Abernethian Society—RCS Ms., n.d.].

———. *Memoirs and Letters of Sir James Paget*. Stephen Paget, ed. London: Longmans, Green, & Co., 1901.

———. *Memoirs of Sir James Paget* [RCS Ms., n.d.].

———. "What Becomes of Medical Students." *St. Bartholomew's Hospital Reports* (1869). Reprinted in: *Selected Essays and Addresses*. London: Longmans, Green, & Co., 1902.

Plarr's Lives: See Section 1, under Royal College of Surgeons of England.

Power, Sir D'Arcy. *The Evolution of the Surgeon in London. The Mid-Sessional Address Delivered at the Abernethian Society, January 11th, 1912* [reprinted from *St. Bartholomew's Hospital Journal*, February, 1912]. London: Adlard & Son, Bartholomew Press, 1912.

Punch [London].

Punch. *Mr. Punch among the Doctors.* London: Methuen, 1933.

Quain, Richard. *Observations on Medical Education. Being the Introductory Lecture in the Faculty of Medicine of University College, London, for the Session 1864–65. With Additions.* London: Walton & Maberly, 1865.

Rainow, G. K. [pseud.] *"G.P."* London and Glasgow: Blackie & Son, 1939.

Rivington, Walter. *The Medical Profession: Being the Essay to Which Was Awarded the First Carmichael Prize . . . by the Council of the Royal College of Surgeons, Ireland, 1879.* Dublin: Fannin & Co., 1879.

Rogers, Joseph. *Reminiscences of a Workhouse Medical Officer.* J. E. Thorold Rogers, ed. London: T. Fisher Unwin, 1889.

Roose, [E. C.] Robson. *The Wear and Tear of London Life. Rest and Repair in London Life. Health Resorts and Their Uses* [Reprinted from *The Fortnightly Review*]. London: Chapman & Hall, 1886.

Salter, John Henry. *Dr. Salter of Tolleshunt D'Arcy in the County of Essex, Medical Man, Freemason, Sportsman, Sporting-dog Breeder and Horticulturalist. His Diary and Reminiscences from the Year 1849 to the Year 1932.* J. O. Thompson, comp. London: John Lane, 1933.

Saundby, Robert. *Medical Ethics: A Guide to Professional Conduct.* Bristol: J. Wright, 1902.

Sayers, Dorothy. *Whose Body?* New York: Harper & Row, 1923.

Semon, Sir Felix. *The Autobiography of Sir Felix Semon.* Henry C. Semon and Thomas A. McIntyre, eds. London: Jarrolds, 1926.

Sharkey, Seymour J. "Doctors and Nurses" (No. II). *Nineteenth Century,* 7 (June, 1880), 1097–1104.

Shaw, George Bernard. *The Doctor's Dilemma. With a Preface on Doctors.* New York: Dodd, Mead, 1942.

Sheen, A. *The Workhouse and Its Medical Officer.* Cardiff: n.p., , 1875.

Shillitoe, Buxton. Visiting Lists, Cashbooks, Accounts, and Diaries. [Wellcome Historical Medical Library, Mod. Mss. 4501–4536.]

Simon, Sir John. *On the Claim, Asserted by the Royal College of Physicians, that the College of Itself, Apart from Any Other Examining Authority, Can Grant Such Letters-Testimonial or Licenses in Medicine, Surgery and Midwifery, As Shall Be Valid Diplomas of Qualification in All Those Branches, under Sections 2 and 3 of the Medical Act, 1886.* London: n.p., March, 1892. [RCS Library, with ms. annotations by John Simon.]

———. *Personal Recollections of Sir John Simon, KCB.* London: Privately printed, 1894. [RCS Lib., with ms. corrections by John Simon.]

Snell, Sidney H. *A Doctor at Work and Play*. London: John Bale, Sons, & Curnow, 1937.

South, John Flint. *Memorials of the Craft of Surgery*. D'Arcy Power, ed. London: Cassell, 1886.

Sprigge, S. Squire. *Physic and Fiction*. London: Hodder and Stoughton, 1921.

Steavenson, W. E. *The Medical Act (1858) Amendment Bill and Medical Reform. A Paper Read before the Abernethian Society at St. Bartholomew's Hospital on Thursday, January 29th, 1880*. London: Baillière, Tindall, and Cox, 1880.

Stevens, John. *Man-midwifery Exposed*. London: n.p., [c. 1866].

Sturges, Octavius. "Doctors and Nurses" (No. 1). *Nineteenth Century*, 7 (June, 1880), 1089–1096.

Sutton, Sir John Bland-. *The Story of a Surgeon*. With a preamble by Rudyard Kipling. London: Methuen, 1930.

Talley, W. *He, or Man-Midwifery, and the Results; or, Medical Men in the Criminal Courts*. London: Job Caudwell, 1863.

Taylor, Shephard Thomas. *The Diary of a Medical Student during the Mid-Victorian Period, 1860–64*. Norwich: Jarrold & Sons, 1927.

———. *Diary of a Norwich Hospital Medical Student, 1858–1860*. Norwich: Jarrold & Sons, 1930.

Thackeray, William Makepeace. *The History of Pendennis. His Fortunes and Misfortunes, His Friends and His Greatest Enemy*. New York: Scribners, 1917.

Thomson, Henry Byerley. *The Choice of a Profession. A Concise Account and Comparative Review of the English Professions*. London: Chapman & Hall, 1857.

The *Times* [London].

Trollope, Anthony. *Barchester Towers*. Oxford: University Press, 1929.

Turner, Sir George Robertson. *Unorthodox Reminiscences*. London: John Murray, 1931.

Twining, Louisa. *Recollections of Workhouse Visiting and Management during Twenty-five Years*. London: n.p., 1880.

Underhill, Thomas. *On Hospitals and Medical Education, Being the Inaugural Address Delivered at the Fifteenth Annual Meeting of the Birmingham and Midlands Counties' Branch of the British Medical Association, Held June 17th, 1870*. Birmingham: Cornish Bros., [1870].

Williams, Charles James Blasius. *Memoirs of Life and Work*. London: Smith, Elder & Co., 1884.

Winslow, Forbes. *Physic and Physicians: A Medical Sketch Book, Exhibiting the Public and Private Life of the Most Celebrated Medical Men of Former Days. With Memoirs of Eminent Living London Physicians and Surgeons*. 2 vols. London: Longman, Orme, Brown & Co., 1839.

3. *Secondary Literature: Medical Profession, Medicine, and Science*

Ackerknecht, Erwin H. *Medicine at the Paris Hospital, 1794–1849*. Baltimore: Johns Hopkins University Press, 1967.

———. *A Short History of Medicine*. New York: Ronald Press, 1955.

Andrews, A. F. *The Doctor in History, Literature, Folk-Lore*. London: Hull, Andrews and Co., 1896.

Atlay, J. B. *Sir Henry Wentworth Acland, Bart., KCB, FRS, Regius Professor of Medicine in the University of Oxford. A Memoir*. London: Smith Elder & Co., 1903.

Ayers, Gwendolyn. *England's First State Hospitals and the Metropolitan Asylums Board, 1867–1930*. London: Wellcome Institute of the History of Medicine, 1971.

Barrett, Charles Raymond Booth. *The History of the Society of Apothecaries of London*. London: Elliot Stock, 1905.

Bell, Enid Moberly. *The Story of Hospital Almoners. The Birth of a Profession*. London: Faber & Faber, 1961.

Berlant, Jeffrey L. *Profession and Monopoly. A Study of Medicine in the United States and Great Britain*. Berkeley, Los Angeles, and London: University of California Press, 1975.

Billroth, Theodor. *The Medical Sciences in the German Universities. A Study in the History of Civilization*. New York: Macmillan, 1924.

Brand, Jeanne L. *Doctors and the State: The British Medical Profession and Government Action in Public Health, 1870–1912*. Baltimore: Johns Hopkins University Press, 1965.

Brockbank, E. M. *The Foundation of Provincial Medical Education in England, and of the Manchester School in Particular*. Manchester: Manchester University Press, 1936.

Brook, Charles Wortham. *Battling Surgeon*. Glasgow: Strickland, 1945.

Cameron, H. C. *Mr. Guy's Hospital, 1726–1948*. London, New York, and Toronto: Longmans, Green, 1954.

Clark, Sir George. "The History of the Medical Profession: Aims and Methods." *Medical History*, 10:3 (1966), 213–220.

———. *A History of the Royal College of Physicians of London*. 2 vols. Oxford: University Press, 1966.

Collins, E. T. *The History and Traditions of the Moorfields Eye Hospital*. London: H. K. Lewis, 1929.

Comfort, Alex. *The Anxiety Makers*. London: Nelson, 1967.

Cooke, Alexander M. "The College and Europe" [The Langdon-Brown Lecture, delivered at the Royal College of Physicians, Oct., 1968]. *J. Roy. Coll. Phys. London*, 4:2 (1970), 97–113.

———. *A History of the Royal College of Physicians of London*. Vol. III. Oxford: Clarendon Press, for the College, 1972.

Coombe, Russell. *Medico-Political History of the British Medical Association*. London: n.p., 1921.

Cope, Sir [Vincent] Zachary. *History of St. Mary's Hospital Medical School*. London: Heinemann, 1964.

———. *The Royal College of Surgeons of England. A History*. London: Anthony Blond, 1959.

———, ed. *Sidelights on the History of Medicine*. London: Butterworth, 1957.

———. *The Versatile Victorian. Being the Life of Sir Henry Thompson, Bt., 1820–1904*. London: Harvey and Blythe, 1951.

Copeman, W. S. C. *The Worshipful Society of Apothecaries of London. A History, 1617–1967*. Oxford: Pergamon Press, 1967.

Crawford, Dirom Grey. *History of the Indian Medical Service, 1600–1913*. 2 vols. London: Thacker, 1914.

Dainton, Courtney. *The Story of England's Hospitals*. London: Museum Press, 1961.

Darwin, Charles. *The Life and Letters of Charles Darwin. Including an Autobiographical Chapter*. Francis Darwin, ed. 2 vols. New York: Basic Books, 1959.

Davidson, Maurice. *The Royal Society of Medicine. The Realization of an Ideal (1805–1955)*. Written at the request of the President and Council. London: The Royal Society of Medicine, 1955.

———, and F. G. Rouvray. *The Brompton Hospital for Diseases of the Chest*. London: Lloyd-Luke, 1954.

Davies, J. Langdon-. *Westminster Hospital. Two Centuries of Voluntary Service, 1719–1948*. London: John Murray, 1952.

Donnison, Jean. *Midwives and Medical Men. A History of Inter-Professional Rivalries and Women's Rights*. New York: Schocken, 1977.

Eckstein, Harry H. *Pressure Group Politics: The Case of the British Medical Association*. Stanford: Stanford University Press, 1960.

Feiling, Anthony. *A History of the Maida Vale Hospital for Nervous Dis-*

eases. London: Published for the Board of Governors of the Hospital by Butterworth, 1958.

Figlio, Karl. "The Historiography of Scientific Medicine: An Invitation to the Human Sciences." *Comp. Stud. Soc. and Hist.*, 19:3 (July, 1977).

Finer, S. E. *Life and Times of Edwin Chadwick*. London: Methuen, 1952.

French, Richard D. *Antivivisection and Medical Science in Victorian Society*. Princeton, N.J.: Princeton University Press, 1975.

Geison, Gerald. "Social and Institutional Factors in the Stagnancy of English Physiology, 1840–1870." *Bulletin of the History of Medicine*, 46:1 (1972), 30–58.

Gordon-Taylor, Sir George. *Sir Charles Bell. His Life and Times*. Edinburgh: Livingstone, 1958.

Haller, John S. "Bachelor's Disease: Etiology, Pathology, and Treatment of Spermatorrhea in the Nineteenth Century." *New York State Journal of Medicine*, 73 (1973), 2076–82.

Haweis, H. R. *Sir Morrell Mackenzie. Physician and Operator. A Memoir, Compiled and Edited from Private Papers and Personal Reminiscences*. 2nd ed. London: W. H. Allen, 1894.

Higgins, Thomas T. *Great Ormond Street Hospital for Children, 1852–1952*. London: Odhams Press, for the Hospital, 1952.

Hodgkinson, Ruth G. *The Origins of the National Health Service. The Medical Services of the New Poor Law, 1834–1871*. London: Wellcome Historical Medical Library, 1967.

Holbrook, Stewart H. *The Golden Age of Quackery*. New York: Macmillan, 1959.

Holloway, S. W. F. "The Apothecaries' Act of 1815: A Reinterpretation." 2 parts. *Medical History*, 10:2 (1966), 107–129; and 10:3 (1966), 221–236.

———. "Medical Education in England, 1830–1858: A Sociological Analysis." *History*, 49 (1964), 299–324.

Holmes, Sir Gordon M. *The National Hospital, Queen Square, 1860–1948*. London: E. & S. Livingstone, 1954.

Holmes, Timothy. *Sir Benjamin Collins Brodie*. London: T. F. Unwin, 1897. [Masters of Medicine, ed. E. A. Hart.]

Horner, Norman Gerald. *The Growth of the General Practitioner of Medicine in England*. London: Printed for the author by Bridge & Co., 1922.

Hunter, Richard, and Ida Macalpine. *Psychiatry for the Poor. 1851 Colney Hatch Asylum—Friern Hospital 1973*. London: Dawsons of Pall Mall, 1974.

Hunter, William. *Historical Account of Charing Cross Hospital and Medical School (University of London) . . . with . . . Some Account of the Origin of the Other Hospitals and Schools in London*. London: John Murray, 1914.

Inglis, Brian. *Fringe Medicine*. London: Faber & Faber, 1964.

Ives, A. G. L. *British Hospitals*. London: Collins, 1948.

Jameson, Eric. *The Natural History of Quackery*. London: Michael Joseph, 1961.

Jewesbury, Eric C. O. *The Royal Northern Hospital, 1856–1956. The Story of a Hundred Years' Work in North London*. London: H. K. Lewis, 1956.

Jewson, N. D. "Medical Knowledge and the Patronage System in Eighteenth-Century England." *Sociology*, 8:3 (1974), 369–385.

Kerr, J. M. M., et al., eds. *Historical Review of British Obstetrics and Gynaecology, 1800–1950*. Edinburgh and London: Livingstone, 1954.

King, Lester S. "Medical Philosophy, 1836–1844." In *Medicine, Science, and Culture. Historical Essays in Honor of Owsei Temkin*, ed. Lloyd G. Stevenson and Robert P. Multhauf. Baltimore: Johns Hopkins University Press, 1968, pp. 143–159.

————. *The Medical World of the Eighteenth Century*. Chicago: University of Chicago Press, 1958.

Laffin, John. *Surgeons in the Field*. London: Dent, 1970.

Lambert, Royston. *Sir John Simon and English Social Administration, 1816–1904*. London: MacGibbon & Kee, 1963.

Lankford, Nelson D. "Status, Bureaucracy, and Professionalism: The Surgeon in the British Army, 1860–1914." Ph.D. dissertation, Indiana University, 1976.

Lefanu, W. R. *British Periodicals of Medicine. A Chronological List* [reprinted from *Bull. Institute Hist. Med.*, 5:8 (1937), 5:9 (1937), and 6:6 (1938)]. Baltimore: Johns Hopkins University Press, 1938.

Little, Ernest M., comp. *History of the British Medical Association, 1832–1932*. London: BMA, [1932].

Lloyd, C., and J. L. S. Coulter. *Medicine and the Navy, 1200–1900*. Vol. 3, ed. John J. Keevil. Edinburgh and London: Livingstone, 1963.

MacIlwain, George. *Memoirs of John Abernethy, FRS*. New York: Harper, 1853.

McInnes, E. M. *St. Thomas' Hospital*. London: George Allen & Unwin, 1963.

McKeown, Thomas. "A Sociological Approach to the History of Medicine" [Inaugural Lecture, Society for the Social History of

Medicine, London, May 8th, 1970]. *Medical History*, 14:4 (1970), 342–351.

McLeod, Roy M. "The Anatomy of State Medicine: Concept and Application." In *Medicine and Science in the 1860's*, ed. F. N. L. Poynter. [Proceedings of the 6th British Congress on the History of Medicine, University of Sussex, 6–9 September, 1967.— Pub. of the Wellcome Institute of the History of Medicine, n.s., Vol. 16.] London: Wellcome Institute of the History of Medicine, 1968, pp. 199–228.

———. "The Frustration of State Medicine, 1880–1899." *Medical History*, 11 (1967), 15–40.

McMenemey, W. H. *The Life and Times of Sir Charles Hastings, Founder of the British Medical Association*. Edinburgh and London: Livingstone, 1959.

MacNalty, Sir Arthur Salusbury. *The History of State Medicine in England. Being the Fitzpatrick Lectures of the Royal College of Physicians of London for the Years 1946 and 1947*. London: Royal Institute of Public Health and Hygiene, 1948.

Matthews, Leslie G. *History of Pharmacy in Britain*. Edinburgh and London: Livingstone, 1962.

———. *The Royal Apothecaries* [Publications of the Wellcome Historical Medical Library. Gen. Ed., F. N. L. Poynter, n.s., Vol. XIII]. London: Wellcome Historical Medical Library, 1967.

Merrington, W. R. *University College Hospital and Its Medical School: A History*. London: Heinemann, 1976.

Minney, R. J. *The Two Pillars of Charing Cross. The Story of a Famous Hospital*. London: Cassell, 1967.

Moore, Sir Norman. *History of St. Bartholomew's Hospital*. 2 vols. London: C. Arthur Pearson, 1918.

———, and Stephen Paget. *The Royal Medical and Chirurgical Society of London. Centenary, 1805–1905*. Aberdeen: University Press, 1905.

Morris, E. W. *A History of The London Hospital*. 2nd ed. London: Edward Arnold, 1910.

Morson, Clifford, ed. *St. Peter's Hospital for Stone, 1860–1960*. Edinburgh and London: Livingstone, 1960.

National Hospital, Queen Square. *Queen Square and the National Hospital, 1860–1960*. London: E. Arnold, 1960.

Newman, Charles. *The Evolution of Medical Education in the Nineteenth Century*. London: Oxford University Press, 1957.

Novak, Steven J. "Professionalism and Bureaucracy: English Doctors and the Victorian Public Health Administration." *Journal of Social History* (Summer, 1973), 440–462.

Oppert, Franz. *Hospitals, Infirmaries and Dispensaries: Their Construction, Interior Arrangement, and Management, etc*. London: Churchill, 1867.

Paget, Stephen. *Sir Victor Horsley. A Study of His Life and Work*. London: Constable, 1919.

Parry, Noel, and Jose Parry. *The Rise of the Medical Profession. A Study of Collective Social Mobility*. London: Croom Helm, 1976.

Peachey, George C. *History of St. George's Hospital*. Pt. 1–6. London: John Bale, Sons, & Co., 1910–1914.

Pound, Reginald. *Harley Street*. London: Michael Joseph, 1967.

Power, Sir D'Arcy, ed. *British Medical Societies*. London: The Medical Press and Circular, 1939.

———, and H. J. Waring. *A Short History of St. Bartholomew's Hospital, 1123–1923*. London: For the Hospital, 1923.

Poynter, Frederick Noel Lawrence, ed. *The Evolution of Hospitals in Britain*. London: Pitman, 1964.

———, ed. *The Evolution of Medical Education in Britain*. London: Pitman, 1966.

———, ed. *The Evolution of Medical Practice in Great Britain* [Papers read at the First British Congress on the History of Medicine and Pharmacy]. London: Pitman, 1961.

Puschmann, Theodor. *A History of Medical Education from The Most Remote to the Most Recent Times*. Trans. and ed. E. H. Hare. London: Lewis, 1891.

Robb-Smith, A. H. T. *A Short History of the Radcliffe Infirmary*. Oxford: Church Army Press, for the United Oxford Hospitals, 1970.

Rolleston, Sir Humphry Davy. *The Cambridge Medical School. A Biographical History*. Cambridge: University Press, 1932.

———. *The Rt. Hon. Sir Thomas Clifford Allbutt, KCB. A Memoir*. London: Macmillan, 1929.

Rook, Arthur, ed. *Cambridge and its Contribution to Medicine* [Proceedings of the 7th British Congress on the History of Medicine, University of Cambridge, 10–13 September, 1969]. London: Wellcome Institute of the History of Medicine, 1971.

Rosen, George. *The Specialization of Medicine, with Particular Reference to Ophthalmology* [Columbia University Ph.D. thesis]. New York: Froben Press, 1944.

Royal Cancer Hospital, Fulham Road, London. *A Short History of the Royal Cancer Hospital. Prepared for the Centenary, 1951*. London: n.p., [1951].

Russell, Brian, ed. *St. John's Hospital for Diseases of the Skin, 1863–1963*. Edinburgh and London: Livingstone, 1963.

St. Mark's Hospital for Fistula, London. *Collected Papers of St. Mark's*

Hospital, London, Including a History of the Hospital. Centenary Volume, 1835–1935. Comp. by the Medical Committee. London: H. K. Lewis, 1935.

Shepherd, John A. *Spencer Wells. The Life and Work of a Victorian Surgeon.* Edinburgh and London: Livingstone, 1965.

Sherrington, Edwina Chadwick. "Thomas Wakley and Reform: 1832–62." D.Phil. thesis, Oxford University, 1973.

Shryock, Richard H. *The Development of Modern Medicine. An Interpretation of the Social and Scientific Factors Involved.* London: Gollancz, 1948.

Smith, Brian Abel-. *A History of the Nursing Profession in Great Britain.* New York: Springer, 1960.

————. *The Hospitals, 1800–1948. A Study in Social Administration in England and Wales.* London: Heinemann, 1964.

Smith, Cecil Woodham-. *Florence Nightingale, 1820–1910.* London: Constable, 1950.

Sorsby, Arnold. *The Royal Eye Hospital, 1857–1957.* London: Royal Eye Hospital, 1957.

Sprigge, S. Squire. *The Life and Times of Thomas Wakley, Founder and First Editor of the "Lancet," Member of Parliament for Finsbury, and Coroner for West Middlesex.* London: Longmans, Green, & Co., 1899.

Stephen, G. N. *The British Medical Association and the Medical Profession.* London: 1914.

Stevens, Rosemary. *Medical Practice in Modern England. The Impact of Specialization and State Medicine.* New Haven and London: Yale University Press, 1966.

Stevenson, R. Scott. *Morrell Mackenzie. The Story of a Victorian Tragedy.* London: Heinemann, 1946.

Thompson, C. J. S. *The Quacks of Old London.* London: Brentano's, 1928.

Turner, Frank M. "Rainfall, Plagues, and the Prince of Wales: A Chapter in the Conflict of Religion and Science." *Journal of British Studies,* 13:2 (1974), 46–65.

Vaughan, Paul. *Doctors' Commons. A Short History of the British Medical Association.* London: Heinemann, 1959.

Waddington, Ivan. "The Development of Medical Ethics—A Sociological Analysis." *Medical History,* 19:1 (1975), 36–51.

————. "The Role of the Hospital in the Development of Modern Medicine: A Sociological Analysis." *Sociology,* 7:2 (1973), 211–225.

————. "The Struggle to Reform the Royal College of Physicians,

1767–1771: A Sociological Analysis." *Medical History*, 17:2 (1973), 107–126.

Walker, R. Milnes. *Medical Education in Britain* [The Rock Carling Fellowship, 1965]. London: Nuffield Prov. Hospitals Trust, 1965.

Wall, Cecil. *A History of the Worshipful Society of Apothecaries of London*. Vol. 1, 1617–1815 [no further vols. published]. Abstracted & arr. by H. C. Cameron; rev., annotated, and ed. by E. Ashworth Underwood [Wellcome Historical Medical Museum Publication, n.s., no. 8]. London: Oxford University Press, 1963.

——. *The London Apothecaries, Their Society and Hall*. London: For the Apothecaries Hall, 1932.

Whitteridge, Gweneth, and Veronica Stokes. *A Brief History of the Hospital of Saint Bartholomew*. London: The Governors of the Hospital of St. Bartholomew, 1961.

Wilks, Samuel, and G. T. Bettany. *A Biographical History of Guy's Hospital*. London: Ward and Lock, 1892.

Wilson, T. G. *Victorian Doctor. Being the Life of Sir William Wilde*. New York: Fischer, 1946.

Woodward, John. *To Do the Sick No Harm. A Study of the British Voluntary Hospital System to 1875*. London and Boston: Routledge & Kegan Paul, 1974 [International Library of Social Policy, ed. Kathleen Jones].

Young, James Harvey. *The Toadstool Millionaires. A Social History of Patent Medicines in America before Federal Regulation*. Princeton, N.J.: Princeton University Press, 1961.

4. Other Secondary Literature (selected)

Allchin, Sir William Henry. *An Account of the Reconstruction of the University of London*. 3 parts. London: Lewis, 1905–1912.

Annan, Noel G. "The Intellectual Aristocracy." In *Studies in Social History: A Tribute to G. M. Trevelyan*, ed. J. H. Plumb. London: Longmans, 1955, pp. 243–287.

Bamford, T. W. *The Rise of the Public Schools. A Study of Boys' Public Boarding Schools in England and Wales from 1837 to the Present Day*. London: Nelson, 1967.

Banks, J. A. *Prosperity and Parenthood: A Study of Family Planning among the Victorian Middle Classes*. London: Routledge & Kegan Paul, 1954.

——, and Olive Banks. *Feminism and Family Planning in Victorian England*. Liverpool: University Press, 1964.

Bellot, H. Hale. *University College London, 1826–1926*. London: University of London Press, 1929.

Black, C. E. *The Dynamics of Modernization. A Study in Comparative History*. New York: Harper and Row, 1966.

Breed, Warren. "Occupational Mobility and Suicide among White Males." *Am. Soc. Rev.*, 28 (1963), 179–188.

Burn, W. L. *The Age of Equipoise. A Study of the Mid-Victorian Generation*. New York: Norton, 1964.

Campbell, J. K. *Honour, Family, and Patronage. A Study of Institutions and Moral Values in a Greek Mountain Community*. Oxford: Clarendon Press, 1964.

Carr, John Dickson. *The Life of Sir Arthur Conan Doyle*. New York: Harper, 1949.

Cecil, Lady Gwendolyn. *Life of Robert Marquis of Salisbury*. 4 vols. London: Hodder and Stoughton, 1921–32.

Cominos, Peter J. "Late Victorian Sexual Respectability and the Social System" (Parts I and II). *International Review of Social History*, 8 (1963), 18–48, 216–250.

Coote, W. A. *A Romance of Philanthropy. Being a Record of the . . . Work of the National Vigilance Association*. Asst. ed. A. Baker. London: National Vigilance Association, 1916.

Curtis, Stanley J. *The History of Education in Great Britain*. 7th ed. London: University Tutorial Press, 1967.

Dahrendorf, Ralf. *Class and Class Conflict in Industrial Society*. Stanford: Stanford University Press, 1959.

Deane, Phyllis, and W. A. Cole. *British Economic Growth, 1688–1959. Trends and Structure* [University of Cambridge Department of Applied Economics, Monograph 8]. Cambridge: University Press, 1964.

Dictionary of National Biography [*DNB*].

Freidson, Eliot. "The Organization of Medical Practice." In *Handbook of Medical Sociology*, ed. Howard E. Freeman, Sol Levine, and Leo G. Reeder. Englewood Cliffs, N.J.: Prentice-Hall, 1963, pp. 299–319.

———. *Professional Dominance: The Social Structure of Medical Care*. New York: Atherton Press, 1970.

———. *Profession of Medicine. A Study of the Sociology of Applied Knowledge*. New York: Dodd, Mead, 1970.

Friedman, Milton, and Simon Kuznets. *Income from Independent Professional Practice*. New York: National Bureau of Economic Research, 1945.

Gilbert, Bentley. *The Evolution of National Insurance in Great Britain. The Origins of the Welfare State*. London: Michael Joseph, 1966.

Hall, Oswald. "The Stages of a Medical Career." *Am. J. Soc.*, 53:5 (1948), 327–336.

Hammond, J. L., and Barbara Hammond. *Lord Shaftesbury*. 4th ed. London: Longmans, Green, 1936.

Harrison, Brian. *Drink and the Victorians: The Temperance Question in England, 1815–1872*. London: Faber & Faber, 1971.

Hollingshead, A. B., Robert Ellis, and E. Kirby. "Social Mobility and Mental Illness." *Am. Soc. Rev.*, 19 (1954), 577–584.

Humberstone, T. L. *University Reform in London*. London: Unwin, 1926.

Hunt, Edward H. *Regional Wage Variations in Britain, 1850–1914*. Oxford: Clarendon Press, 1973.

Jones, Kathleen. *A History of the Mental Health Services*. London and Boston: Routledge & Kegan Paul, 1972.

Kleiner, Robert J., and Seymour Parker. "Goal-Striving, Social Status, and Mental Disorder: A Research Review." *Am. Soc. Rev.*, 28:2 (1963), 189–203.

Kuhn, Thomas S. *The Structure of Scientific Revolutions*. 2nd ed. [International Encyclopedia of Unified Science, Vol. II, no. 2, ed. Otto Neurath]. Chicago: University of Chicago Press, 1970.

Lipset, Seymour M., and Reinhard Bendix. *Social Mobility in Industrial Society* [Pub. of the Institute of Industrial Relations, University of California]. Berkeley and Los Angeles: University of California Press, 1967.

Longford, Elizabeth (Countess of). *Victoria R. I.* London: Weidenfeld and Nicolson, 1964.

McCormack, Thelma H. "The Druggist's Dilemma: Problems of a Marginal Occupation." *Am. J. Soc.*, 61:4 (1956), 308–315.

Marder, Arthur. *From the Dreadnought to Scapa Flow. The Royal Navy in the Fisher Era, 1904–1919*. 5 vols. London: Oxford University Press, 1961–1972.

Marshall, Thomas H. *Class, Citizenship, and Social Development. Essays by T. H. Marshall*, ed. S. M. Lipset. Garden City, N.Y.: Doubleday, 1964.

Merton, Robert K. "The Institutional Imperatives of Science." In *Sociology of Science. Selected readings*, ed. Barry Barnes. Harmondsworth: Penguin, 1972 [Penguin Modern Sociology Readings, ed. Tom Burns].

Millerson, Geoffrey. *The Qualifying Associations. A Study in Professionalization*. London: Routledge & Kegan Paul, 1964.

Morgan, D. H. J. "The Social and Educational Background of Anglican Bishops—Continuities and Changes." *Brit. J. Soc.*, 20:3 (1969), 295–310.

Mousnier, Roland. *Les Hierarchies Sociales de 1450 à nos jours*. Paris: Presses Universitaires de France, 1969.

Musgrove, Frank. "Middle Class Education and Employment in the Nineteenth Century." *Econ. Hist. Rev.*, 2nd ser., 12 (1959), 99–111.

Namier, Sir Lewis. *The Structure of Politics at the Accession of George III*. 2nd ed. London: Macmillan, 1965.

Otley, C. B. "Social Origins of British Army Officers." *Soc. Rev.*, 18:2 (1970), 213–240.

Owen, David. *English Philanthropy, 1660–1960*. Cambridge, Mass.: Belknap Press, 1964.

Parry-Jones, William. *The Trade in Lunacy. A Study of Private Madhouses in England in the Eighteenth and Nineteenth Centuries*. London: Routledge & Kegan Paul, 1972.

Parsons, Talcott. *The Social System*. Glencoe, Ill.: Free Press, 1958.

Perkin, Harold. *The Origins of Modern English Society, 1780–1880*. London: Routledge & Kegan Paul, 1969.

Pitt-Rivers, J. A. *The People of the Sierra*. London: Weidenfeld and Nicolson, 1954.

Powell, Elwin H. "Occupation, Status and Suicide." *Am. Soc. Rev.*, 23 (1958), 131–139,

Reader, W. J. *Professional Men. The Rise of the Professional Classes in Nineteenth-Century England*. London: Weidenfeld and Nicolson, 1966.

Roberts, David. *Victorian Origins of the British Welfare State* [Yale Historical Publications Miscellanea: 73]. New Haven: Yale University Press, 1960.

Rothblatt, Sheldon. *The Revolution of the Dons. Cambridge and Society in Victorian England*. New York: Basic Books, 1968.

Routh, Guy. *Occupation and Pay in Great Britain, 1906–1960*. Cambridge: University Press, 1965.

Saunders, A. M. Carr-, and P. A. Wilson. *The Professions*. Oxford: University Press, 1933. Reprinted: London: Cass, 1964.

Thackray, Arnold. "Natural Knowledge in Cultural Context: The Manchester Model." *American Historical Review*, 79:3 (1974), 672–709.

Thomas, Keith. *Religion and the Decline of Magic. Studies in Popular Beliefs in Sixteenth- and Seventeenth-Century England*. London: Weidenfeld and Nicolson, 1971.

Thompson, F. M. L. *English Landed Society in the Nineteenth Century*. London: Routledge & Kegan Paul, 1963.

Turner, Ralph. "Acceptance of Irregular Mobility in Britain and the United States." *Sociometry*, 29:4 (1966), 334–352.

——. "Modes of Social Ascent through Education: Sponsored and Contest Mobility." In *Education, Economics and Society*, ed. Neil Smelser and Seymour M. Lipset. New York: Free Press, 1961, pp. 121–139.

University of London. *The Historical Record (1836–1912). Being a Supplement to the Calendar*. London: University of London Press, 1912.

Weber, Max. *From Max Weber: Essays in Sociology*. H. H. Gerth and C. Wright Mills, eds. and trans. New York: Oxford University Press, 1958.

Weinberg, Ian. *English Public Schools: The Sociology of Elite Education*. New York: Atherton, 1967.

Wilkinson, Rupert. *Gentlemanly Power. British Leadership and the Public School Tradition. A Comparative Study in the Making of Rulers*. London and New York: Oxford University Press, 1964.

Index

Abercrombie, Robert, 244–246, 247, 248, 253, 256
Abernethy, John, 120, 146
Accoucheurs, 260. *See also* Midwifery; Obstetrics
Acland, Henry Wentworth, 58–59, 333
Acland, T. D., 333, 336
Adams, J. E., 333
Adams, John, 77
Addison, Thomas, 146, 148, 352
Admiralty, 237
Advertising, 96, 127–128, 248, 252
  of patent medicines, 257
  Royal College regulations on, 252–253
  and trade, 134, 253, 280
Ager, Joseph, 329
Airedale, 1st Lord, 201
Alabone, Edwin W., 257
Aldersgate School of Medicine, 77
Alderson, James, 315, 334
Allbutt, Thomas, 207
Althaus, Julius, 251, 265
Ambition, 163, 246
  education and, 54, 80, 83, 158–159
  personality and, 250–251
  specialism and, 249
Anatomy, 15, 161

in medical curriculum, 60, 61, 62 (Table 4), 80–81
  morbid, 61, 62, (Table 4), 63
Anatomy schools, private, 15, 64–65, 72
Andrews, John Goldwyer, 323
Annan, Noel, 148
Antisepsis, 229
Antivivisectionists, 196
Apothecaries, hospital, 159, 160, 160n
Apothecaries, Society of, 5–6, 11, 12, 19, 20, 32n, 35, 37n, 204, 204n
  and Conjoint Board Examinations, 191–192, 241
  cost of apprenticeships in, 69–70, 70 (Table 6)
  and drug trade, 94, 226n
  family connections in, 41, 42
  income of, 192n
  License of (LSA), 10, 60–63, 62 (Table 4), 85
  social origins of apprentices at, 197, 198 (Table 9), 199n, 291–293
  wealth of officers of, 207–209, 208 (Table 11)
Apothecaries' Act of 1815, 11, 17, 21–22, 28
Apprenticeship, 10, 11, 14, 60, 64, 65, 71

cost of, 69–71, 70 (Table 6)
decline of, 15, 16, 65, 71
family and, 41–42, 70 (Table 6), 76–77
and hospital appointments, 77, 147, 152n, 165, 165n
See also Pupillage
Aristocracy: family ties of, with medical profession, 197, 198 (Table 9), 201–204, 202–203 (Table 10); hospital patronage by, 13, 264; medical attendance to, 85, 120–121, 154–155; professional men in, 204
Army Medical Department, 214. See also Military medical services
Army officers, social origins of, 199–200
Army Surgeons, Association of, 23
Arnold, Matthew, 342
Arts examinations, 56–57, 80. See also Degrees, arts; Education, general
Ashburner, John 328
Ashe, Isaac, 131
Associated Faculty, 20
Association of Apothecaries and Surgeon-Apothecaries, 20
Association of Army Surgeons, 23
Association of General Practitioners, 231
Association of Officers of Hospitals for the Insane, 23, 267
Australia, 126
Authority, medical 3–4, 112, 123–124, 132, 134, 283–284, 286
and government, 116, 237
in hospitals, 141, 180, 182–183
and knowledge, 183, 185, 187–188, 281–282
and medical education, 164, 173
and nurses, 180–183
over patients, 14
and religion, 180
and secret remedies, 258
Autonomy, professional, 38, 39, 90, 175–6, 180, 189
and income, 117, 215
in public employment, 112–114, 125
vs. trade practices, 258–259
See also Authority; Dependence, medical; Lay values
Avebury, 1st Lord, 201
Aveling, J. H., 129

Babington, Benjamin Guy, 148, 149
Babington, William, 148
Back, William, 328 (66)
Bacot family, 105
Badham, Charles, 320, 328, 329
Baillie, Matthew, 155
Bain, Andrew, 329
Baker, Alfred, 312
Balliol College (Oxford), 45, 88
Banks, J. A., 221, 221n, 222
Barber-Surgeons' Company, 8
Barendt, Frank, 312
Barker, Edgar, 312, 315
Barnes, J. W., 315, 317
Barnes, John, 312
Barnes, Samuel, 312
Barnes family, 315
Baronets: in medical profession, 202–203 (Table 10), 204; physicians' family connections with, 201–204, 202–203 (Table 10)
Barter, C. S., 317
Bartlet, Alexander H., 312
Bates, William, 312
Beale, Lionel S., 312
Beaman, George, 317

Beard, Francis, 317
Beck, Marcus, 310, 316, 333
Beddoe, John, 45, 48, 106
Bell, Charles, 152, 156–157
Bellot, Thomas, 310
Bellot, W. H., 316
Belgium, 64n
Benfield, Thomas Warburton, 107–108
Bennett, James Risdon, 325
Berry, James, 166
Best, Alexander, 312
Bhakha, S. D., 273
Bickersteth, Edward R., 312
Bickersteth family, 106, 315
Bills, medical, 225, 225n, 226
Billing, Archibald, 306, 328
Biology, 60
Birkett, John, 77
Birmingham Infirmary, 120
Birth order and medical careers, 205–206
Bishop, John, 317
Bishop, Thomas, 307
Blantyre, 10th Lord, 201
Blewitt, Byron, 254
Boards of governors. *See* Hospitals, governance of
Bodington, George F., 312, 315
Botany, 61, 62 (Table 4), 81, 161
Bowlby, Anthony, 323
Boyd, James S. N., 108, 316
Bree, Robert, 319, 329
Bright, Richard, 148, 149, 328
Briscoe, John, 307, 327
Bristol, 3, 66
Bristol Infirmary, 106
British Journal of Dermatology, 267
British Medical Association (old), 23
British Medical Association, 27, 134, 232, 232n
and fees, 224–225, 227, 237
and general education of

medical men, 56, 232
and general practitioners' interests, 232–233
and medical corporations, 231–232, 237, 240
and Parliament, 232–233
and public employment, 117
and social status of profession, 56, 232
See also Provincial Medical and Surgical Association
British Medical Journal: practices for sale advertised in, 99, 209–210; prizes announced in, 84; scientific articles in, 232
Brodie, Benjamin, 329
on education, 55, 59
family of, 151, 206
income and wealth of, 207, 208
on independence, 156
influence of, 146, 150
on medical careers, 46, 48
on specialism, 273–274
Brodsham, J. Mill, 265
Brooke, Charles, 307, 327
Brown, Isaac B., 323
Brown, Robert C., 310
Bryant, Thomas, 310
Buchanan, A., 317
Budd, William, 52, 352
Bullar family, 315
Bulley family, 315
Buncombe, Charles H., 317
Burd family, 315
Bureaucratic practice, 110, 112. *See also* General practice, salaried
Burrows, George, 166, 192, 237, 240
Burt, Margaret E., 180, 183, 186
Businessmen, sons of, in medical profession, 198 (Table 9), 205
Butlin, H. T., 159

Cambridge, University of, 66, 147, 206
  and diploma in public health, 279
  and FRCP, 7–8, 57 (Table 5), 153–154
  social origins of students of, 197–199
Callaway, Thomas, 146, 326
Callaway, Thomas, Jr., 326
Career choice, medical, 40–48
Carrick, Andrew, 24, 25
Carter, R. B. 266, 281
Casualty department (hospital), 175
Ceeley, J. H., 316 (59)
Challinor, Henry, 321
Chambers, Thomas King, 148
Chambers, William F., 155
Chapman, John, 128
Charing Cross Hospital, 13, 142 (Table 8)
  Medical School, 65, 75
Charity, medical 12, 13–14, 13n
  and contract practice, 114
  lay control of, 116
  medical education in conflict with, 174–176
  and practitioners' incomes, 215, 228–229
  and specialism, 264–265
Charity Commissioners, 143, 145, 148, 149–150
Cheadle, W. B., 320, 336
Chemistry, 60, 61, 62 (Table 4)
Chevass family, 315
Cheyne, Watson, 334
Children, hospitals for, 261, 262–263 (Table 15)
Childs, George Borlase, 120n
Church, William Selby, 334
Church of England: bishops, social origins and connections of, 200, 204; clergy, connections of, with medical profession, 198 (Table 9), 204–205.

206, 291 (App. B); M. D. Lambeth, 35; nursing sisterhood of, 180
Church of England Purity Society, 254
Clapton, Edward, 333
Clark, Andrew, 323, 336
Clark, Frederick LeGros, 334
Clark, James, 106, 274
Clarke, Horatio, 321
Clarkson, Thomas, 257
Classical education: of medical men, 10, 57, 75; and status, 8–9, 38–39, 56; See also Education, general; Liberal education
Churchill, J. & A. (publishers), 252–253
Clergy, Anglican. See Church of England
Clergy, dissenting, in medical profession, 198 (Table 9)
Clifton, Nathaniel Henry, 104–105
Cline, Henry, 144, 311, 326
Cline, Henry, Jr., 41, 326
Clinical clerks, 84–85, 159
Clinical practice, 14, 15, 64, 66, 68
Clubs, sick. See Contract practice
Coate family, 315
Cock, Edward, 76, 146, 147, 311
Colby family, 315
Colleagueship, 157, 188–189
College of General Practitioners, proposed, 32
Competition, medical, 29, 37, 100, 126, 228n, 229, 246
  in consulting careers, 137, 162, 170
  and fees, 210, 225
  among general practitioners, 100, 115, 116, 117–118, 126, 133
  between G.P.'s and consultants, 227–228, 229

and overcrowding of profession, 238–239
and status, 196, 225
and trade practices, 252, 258
Conjoint Board Examinations, 191–192, 240–241
Connections: in consulting careers, 121, 155; and general practice, 95, 96–97, 98, 104, 109, 111–112; and hospital posts, 14, 87, 121, 142 (Table 8); and medical education, 76, 77, 78, 79, 88; and social status, 195; *See also* Family; Friendship; Nepotism; Patronage
Conquest, John, 328
Consultants, 16, 28, 154–155
career patterns of, 137, 161–162
conflicts among, 188
income and fees of, 155, 207–209, 212–213 (Table 13), 221
and general practitioners, 18, 227–230, 230n
in hospital governance, 140–141, 174–175, 176–178, 176n, 180, 186–188
numbers of, 137, 296–297 (App. D)
and nurses, 181
personal traits of, 156, 250–251
and specialism, 260, 273–276, 279
wealth of, 207–209, 208 (Table 11)
See also Physicians, Royal College of; Royal Colleges; Surgeons, Royal College of
Contract practice, 114–116, 117, 127, 225
income from 115, 116n, 117
Cooke, Alexander, 242
Cooke, Thomas, 167

Cooper, Alfred, 312, 323
Cooper, Astley, 85, 144, 148, 149, 311
family of, 41, 76, 147, 151
income of, 207
influence of, 146, 150
Cooper, Bransby, 41, 146, 147, 149
Cooper, William, 151
Coote, Holmes, 165n, 167
Corporations, medical, 5–6, 31, 241
and general practitioners, 16–19, 20n, 25, 30, 31
incomes of, 192n
list of, 289 (App. A)
and medical education, 63
and Provincial Medical and Surgical Association, 24–25
and reform, 12, 20, 21, 30, 31–33, 36–37
wealth of leaders, of, 207–209, 208 (Table 11)
See also Apothecaries, Society of; Physicians, Royal College of; Royal Colleges; Surgeons, Royal College of;
Coulson, Walter John, 120n
Coulson, William, 119, 120n
Counsell, H. E., 44, 88, 127–128, 319
Cowper, W. F., 34
Crabb, Alfred, 317
Craft and medical profession, 8, 9, 10, 49, 196
Craven, Robert, 105
Cripps, W. H., 166
Criticism of medical colleagues, 252, 255–256, 258
Cross, William, 120n
Crowfoot, W. H., 319
Crowfoot family, 105
Cumberland Infirmary, 121, 127
Curling, Thomas Blizard, 77, 310, 326
Curnow, John, 322

Curriculum, medical, 66, 71, 191
   changes in, 60–64, 62 (Table 4)
Currie, E. H., 188
Cutler, Edward, 165n, 323, 326

Dalby, William, 120n
Dale, William, 55, 170, 171
Dalrymple, Archibald, 315, 316
Darwin, Robert Waring, 129
Davies, Herbert, 311
Davies, John, 321
Davies-Colley, John, 166
Davis, David, 328
Davy, T. G., 58
De la Ramée, Marie Louise (Ouida), 196, 282n
de Morgan, Campbell, 78
De Styrap, Jukes, 43, 48
Degrees, arts, 57–58, 59
   numbers of, among Royal College Fellows, 50 (Table 1), 51 (Table 2), 58
Degrees, foreign, 64n
Degrees, medical, 64n, 67 (Table 5), 130, 131, 242
   numbers of, among Royal College Fellows, 50 (Table 1), 51 (Table 2)
Demonstrators, 160, 162
Dennison, Richard, 328
Dent, C. T., 334
Dentistry, 268 (Table 16), 278, 279
Dependence, lay, on medical men, 281–282, 285–286
Dependence, medical, 4, 91, 122, 128, 196
   Brodie and Bell on, 156–157
   of consultants, 138, 150
   in military medicine, 125
   in poor law practice, 112
Dermatology, 261
   hospitals, 262–263 (Table 15), 265
   and medical education, 269

periodicals, 267, 270–271 (Table 17)
societies, 266, 268 (Table 16)
   in voluntary hospitals, 278
Diagnosis, changes in, 14
Dickinson, William Howship, 166, 333
Dispensary for Diseases and Ulceration of the Legs, 267, 269
Disputes among medical men, 157, 255–256
Division of labor in medicine, 12
Dr. Kahn's Museum, 253–254
Doctor-patient ratios, 218, 220, 220n, 221
"Doctor" (title), 17n, 233–234, 233n, 234n
Dodd, H. W., 312
Donkin, Horatio Bryan, 255–256
Dossiers, professional, 121, 122–124
Down, J. L. H. Langdon-, 310
Doyle, Arthur Conan, 44, 109, 109n, 129.
   Stark Munro Letters, 93–98, 109n, 219
Dressers, 84–85, 159, 164n
Druggists, 20n, 239–240
Drugs: and consultants' practice, 7, 10, 225, 225n; and entrepreneurship, 246; and general practice, 11, 99, 128, 133–134, 225–226; laws re prescription of, 239–240; and medical authority, 239–240; and medical income, 210, 211 (Table 12), 212–213 (Table 13), 217 (Table 14), 223; profit-sharing in sale of, 255; in poor law practice, 111, 113; and Society of Apothecaries, 11, 226n
Du Pasquier, C. F., 119
Dublin, 3

Duckworth, Dyce, 334
Duka, 319
Duffin, A. B., 315, 333
Duffin, E. W., 315
Duncan, W. A., 312
Durham, A. E., 352

Eade, Peter, 52
Earle, Henry, 144, 206n, 326
East India Company, 124
Eastes, Thomas, 311
Eastlin, John B., 316
Edinburgh, 3, 153
Education, general, 49–57,
    59–60
  of consultants, 50 (Table 1),
    51 (Table 2)
  economic factors in, 59
  of general practitioners, 52,
    59
  prizes for, 75
  in university, 57–59, 153–154,
    206
  See also Classical education;
    Degrees, arts; Liberal Educa-
    tion; Public schools
Education, medical, 9–10, 60–85
  economic factors in, 42–43,
    43n, 66, 68–76, 72–75, 74
    (Table 7), 86, 224n
  family and, 41–42, 41n, 42n,
    45
  G.P.'s role in, 65
  versus hospital charity, 174–
    196
  and hospital governance, 178
  as private enterprise, 15
  and professional socialization,
    15, 88
  provincial, 65, 66, 72, 73–75,
    74 (Table 7)
  scholarships for, 75
  and scientific developments,
    14–15
  Select Committee on, 153, 156
  social aspects of, 79

and specialism, 86–87, 272,
    275–276, 278–279
  and staff appointments,
    141–142, 169
  as technical education, 60,
    196
  See also Apprenticeship; Cur-
    riculum; Medical schools;
    Universities
Efficacy of medical practice, 4,
    130
Electricity, medical, 247, 252
Elliotson, John, 140
Ellis, W. A., 235
Erichsen, John, 276
Emigration, 126
Employment, medical. See Gen-
    eral practice, salaried
Entrepreneurship in medical
    careers, 244–282
  See also Secret remedies;
    Specialism; Trade
Epsom School, 195
Equipment, medical, 74 (Table
    7), 93
Estates. See Medical Profession,
    social structure of
Ethics, medical, 280. See also
    Etiquette, medical; Unprofes-
    sional conduct
Ethnicity and practice, 109–110
Etiquette, medical, 96. See also
    Ethics, medical; Unprofes-
    sional conduct
Examinations, qualifying, 74
    (Table 7), 81, 85
Expertise, medical, 36, 38, 141,
    280–281, 286–287. See also
    Merit; Skill; Science

Falconer, R. W., 306
Family, 52, 148
  and choice of medical career,
    41–42, 43–45
  and general practice, 104–
    110, 120

and hospital posts, 87, 143–144, 147–148, 165–166
and medical education, 42n, 66, 70, 75–80
succession in professions, 198, 200
See also Connections; Friendship; Nepotism; Patronage
Farmer, Cottenham, 273
Farnell, H. D., 108
Favoritism, 144–145, 149, 150, 169, 188
Fees, medical, 58, 95, 116n, 218–219, 218n, 227
consultant-G. P. conflict over, 227-228
in contract practice, 115, 117
and income, 210
schedules of, 210, 211 (Table 12), 212–213 (Table 13), 219
Fenwick, Samuel, 173, 316
Fergusson, William, 158–159
Fever: cases and general hospitals, 174, 260; hospitals, 13, 262–263 (Table 15)
Fildes, Luke,131
Forensic medicine, 62 (Table 4), 63
Forster, John Cooper, 167, 311, 334
Forster, Thomas, 146
Fox, Edward Long, 106
Fox, Herbert, 321
Fox, Tilbury, 265
Frampton, Algernon, 148, 328
France, 64n, 247–248, 250, 260
Freidson, Eliot, 3n
Friedman, Milton, 218, 222n, 224n
Friendship, 88, 103
doctor-patient relationship as, 131–132
and general practice, 98, 109
and hospital posts, 85, 143–145, 165–166
and medical education, 66, 70, 76–77, 78, 79
See also Connections; Family; Nepotism; Patronage
Furner, Edmund J., 312

Gee, Samuel, 335
General Medical Council, 35, 38, 68, 74 (Table 7), 231
disciplinary action by, 259
and general practitioners, 230, 233, 235n
and professional unity, 36, 191
role of, in education of medical men, 35, 56, 61, 80
survey of medical students, 86
General Pharmaceutical Association of Great Britain, 19, 20n
General practice, 7, 84, 87, 133, 140
building a, 92–93, 94–97, 126–131, 255
choice of location for, 92–93, 100, 104–110
and competition, 92, 100, 102, 133–134
connections and, 95, 96–97, 98
drugs supplied in, 99, 226
economic factors in, 91–95, 97, 98, 103, 124, 126, 132
emergence of, 17–18, 22–23, 28–29
ethnicity and, 109–110
failure in, 126
family and, 91, 104–110
fees for, 211 (Table 12), 212–213 (Table 13)
income in, 97, 99, 111, 209–224
in London, 98
marriage as avenue to, 107–108

partnership in, 102–103
personal traits and, 97, 101, 104, 106–107, 108, 128–130
provincial, 93
purchase of, 98–104, 209–210
and religion, 109–110, 109n, 128
salaried, 43, 110–118, 124–125
skill in, 107, 130
General Practitioner, The, 273
General practitioners, 16, 26, 27, 32, 33, 52, 112, 222, 233
BMA support of, 117
college of, proposed, 23, 32
and consultants, 16, 226–231
as friend, 131–132
and hospitals, 160, 229
licensing of, 37n, 85–86, 191, 241
and medical corporations, 16–17, 21–25, 27, 237–240
organizations of, 23, 27, 231
representation of, in professional governance, 31–33, 31n, 33n, 35, 233, 235, 235n
role of, in medical education, 16, 65, 71
sons of, in medical careers, 205–206
and specialists, 272–273
status of, 22–23, 33, 37, 195, 240–242
trade practices of, 133–134, 255
and university medical degrees, 242
Genito-urinary diseases, 261, 262–263 (Table 15), 278
Gentleman, 135, 194
education of, 55, 56, 154, 196
and medical income, 92, 206, 221, 224
professional ideal of, 130, 195, 196, 251

sons of, recruited into medical profession, 75, 76, 79, 197
Germany, 64n, 87, 247–248, 260
Glasgow, 3
Glynn, T. R., 316
Godlee, Rickman, 310, 333
Golden Square Hospital for Throat Diseases, 261, 266
Golding-Bird, Cuthbert, 333
Goodsall, David, 305
Government, 33, 214, 239–240, 241
medical employment, 110–114, 126
and status of the profession, 112, 134
and Royal Colleges, 236, 237–238
Gower, Charles, 328, 329
Gowers, William R., 335
Graham, James, 31–33
Grainger, Richard, 149
Grammar Schools, 50 (Table 1), 51 (Table 2), 52
Great Ormond Street Hospital for Children, 261
Green, J. H., 310, 326
Green, Thomas H., 323
Greenhow, E. H., 315
Greenhow, H. M., 315
Greenwich Hospital, 87, 121
Griffith, Thomas, 105
Grocers' Company, 11
Grosvenor Street School of Anatomy and Medicine, 72
Gull, William Withey, 136, 255, 319, 333
on medical authority, 183
on nursing, 180, 182
patronage in career of, 146, 148
on specialism, 264, 273
Guy's Hospital, 12, 138, 143
Cooper influence at, 146–147
crisis at, 180–187

Medical School, 44, 65, 88, 123
posts at, 159, 160
special departments at, 278
staff, 77, 142 (Table 8), 144, 148, 149, 165n, 166, 167, 168
treasurer of, 145–147
Gwynn, S. B., 315
Gynecology, 129
departments in voluntary hospitals, 278
diplomas in, 279
periodicals, 270–271 (Table 17)

Habershon, Samuel, 183, 184
Harley, John, 334
Haldane, 1st Lord, 201
Hale-White, William, 173
Halford, Henry, 153
Hall, Marshall, 316
Hardy, Thomas, 283
Harrison, Benjamin, 145
Harrison, Benjamin, Jr., 145–147
Hastings, Charles, 24, 26, 48
Haward, F. Robertson, 254
Hawes, Benjamin, 30
Hawkins, Caesar H., 147, 148, 165n, 310, 326
Heath, Charles J., 334
Heath, George Y., 305
Herman, G. E., 109
Hewett, P. G., 326, 333
Hey, Samuel, 316
Hey family, 105
Hill, Matthew Berkeley, 310
Hodgkin, Thomas, 144, 146, 149
Hodgson, Joseph, 120
Holland, Henry, 155, 274, 307, 320
Holmes, Timothy, 57, 326
Holthouse, Edwin, 335
Horsley, Victor, 43, 344
Hospitals, 12–16
appointments system in, 121–122, 141–145, 142 (Table 8), 144–150, 161, 165, 168–172, 186–188
boards of governors of, 13, 139, 143
casualty departments of, 175
and charity, 12, 13, 228–229
family influence in, 87, 143–144, 147–151, 165–166, 168–169
and G.P.s' incomes, 214–215, 228–229
governance of, 13, 63, 138–141, 144–145, 175–178, 183–188
income of, 13, 138
junior posts in, 87, 123, 141, 160–165
lay-medical relations in, 174–186
and medical education, 15, 60–61, 62 (Table 4), 63–65, 74 (Table 7), 152n, 157–158, 190
organization of, 295 (App. C)
patients in, 13, 13n, 138, 139–140, 145, 157–158, 168, 174–176, 260
pay wards in, 229, 229n
physicians and, 142, 147–148, 152
retirement policies of, 248
Select Committee on Metropolitan, 175, 214–215, 272–273
senior staff of, 77, 87–88, 127, 137, 142–145, 162–163, 189–190, 296–297 (App. D)
special wards in, 174, 178, 277–278, 296–297 (App. D)
student posts in, 84–85, 159–163
treasurers' role in, 143, 145, 157, 184, 187
See also Charity Commissioners; Consultants; Nursing:

394

Special hospitals; Entries for individual hospitals
Hovell, Dennis, 77
Hudson, C. E. L. B., 312
Hughes, James Vaughan, 55–56
Hughes, H. M., 325
Hume, Thomas, 329
Hunter, John, 10, 10n
Hurlock, Joseph, 328
Hussey, E. L., 307, 327
Hypogastria, 245n, 247
  See also Venereal disease

Income, medical, 207–224, 217 (Table 14), 249, 273
  and cost of living, 222, 223–224
  distribution of, 215–221
  efforts to improve, 224–229
  examples of, 97, 99, 100, 115, 116, 155, 159
  and expenses, 214, 217 (Table 14), 223–224
  and hospitals, 228–229, 266
  in London, 221–222, 222n
  and professional autonomy, 215, 222
  salaried, 118, 126, 211, 214
  and social status, 215, 222–224
Indian Army Medical Service, 124, 125
  See also Military medical services
Ireland, 35, 50, 51, 86n, 125

Jacobson, W. H. A., 333
Jeaffreson, Henry, 328
Jenner, William, 47–48, 48n, 173
Jessop, W. H. H., 312
Johnson, E. C., 319
Johnson, George, 255
Johnson, John, 321
Johnstone, James, 315
Jones, Henry Bence, 261, 264
Jones, Sydney, 333, 335

Jordan, R. J., 254
Journal of Mental Science, 267
Jowett, Benjamin, 88
Julius, F. C., 316

Keate, Robert, 107, 326
Keetley, Charles Bell, 43, 78–79, 83, 92, 171, 336
Keser, Jean Samuel, 109
Kerrison, Robert M., 328
Key, Charles Aston, 41, 146, 147, 148, 334
Kiernan, Francis, 327
King's College Hospital and Medical School, 13, 45, 65, 68, 142 (Table 8), 162, 242n
Knight, Charles, 321
Knights: in medical profession, 202–203 (Table 10), 204, 266; physicians' family connections with, 201–204, 202–203 (Table 10)
Kuznets, Simon, 218, 222n, 224n

La'Mert, Abraham, 247, 256
Laboratory studies in medical curriculum, 61, 62 (Table 4)
Laffan, Joseph, 343
Lancet, The, 26, 84, 117
Landed classes, sons of, in medical profession, 197, 198 (Table 9)
Lane, James E., 77, 312, 333
Lane, J. R., 311
Lane, Samuel, A., 77, 326
Langstaff, George, 120
Laryngology: departments in general hospitals, 278; hospitals for, 261, 262–263 (Table 15), 266; periodicals re, 270–271 (Table 17); societies for, 268 (Table 16)
Latham, Peter Mere, 144, 147–148, 201, 206n, 308, 328
Laurence, 1st Lord, 201
Lawrence, J. Z., 266, 267

Lawrence, John, 106, 312
Lawrence, William, 120, 326, 334
Lay society: authority of, in medical affairs, 189, 255, 258–259; attitudes of, to medical profession, 38, 39, 90, 91, 113, 117, 195–196; exclusion of, from medical sphere, 253, 280–282, 285; power of, in medical institutions, 13, 138, 184–185, 264–265; power of, over medical men, 111–114, 116, 118, 125, 140–141, 156–157; reliance of, on medical authority, 122, 188; values of, in medical life, 59, 60, 76, 123, 128, 153–154, 232, 280–281
Leach, D.J., 316
Legal profession, sons of, in medical profession, 198 (Table 9), 204–205, 291 (App. B)
Legislation. See Apothecaries' Act of 1815; Medical Act of 1858; Medical Act Amendment Act, 1886
Leicester Infirmary, 107
Leicester Provident Dispensary, 116
Ley, Hugh, 328
Liberal education, 55–56, 196 See also Classical education; Public schools
Licensing bodies (medical). See Corporations, medical; and Entries for individual corporations
Lister, Joseph, 204, 310
Little, Louis S., 311, 333
Liveing, Robert, 323
Liverpool, 3, 66
Liverpool Infirmary, 106, 123
Lloyd, E. A., 326
Lobb, Harry, 247, 248, 252–253, 256

Lock Hospital (London), 119, 120n
Locock, Charles, 322, 329, 337
London, University of, 66–68, 67 (Table 5), 120, 242
London Anatomical Museum, 254
London Dermatological Society, 266
London Hospital, 12, 121, 142 (Table 8), 148, 188
    Medical School, 65, 77, 177
London Medical Gazette, 43
London School of Anatomy, 15
Lonsdale, Margaret, 181, 182
Lowe, Mr. (museum proprietor), 254
Lubbock, Montague, 201
Lucas, William, Jr., 146, 149, 151, 168
Lukes, C. P., 312

MacCormac, William, 85
Maccullock, John, 328
MacDonald, Greville, 251
McGill, Arthur F., 311
Mackenzie, Morrell, 248, 261, 266, 272, 276, 278, 351, 354
Macmichael, William, 153, 154, 319, 329
Macmurdo, G., 165n
Macnamara, C. N., 321
McWhinnie, A. M., 327
Mahomed, Frederick Akbar, 167–168
Maida Vale Hospital for Nervous Diseases, 251, 265
Makins, George, 52, 65–66, 78, 85, 87, 121
Mallett, George, 312
Malpractice, 254, 350
Mantell, G. A., 119
Markham, W.O., 272
Marriage, 92, 107–108, 162, 222, 201–204
Marriott, C. H., 315

Marsh, Frederick H., 307
Marshall, T. H., 6
Martin, J. M., 109
Martin, William, 115, 127, 132
Masonic lodges, 82
Materia medica, 62 (Table 4), 81, 161
Maternity: hospitals, 87, 267, 268 (Table 16); patients, 140, 260; *See also* Midwifery; Obstetrics
Maton, William, 120, 155, 328
Maunder, Charles F., 310
Maurice, J. B., 315
Mayo, Thomas, 274, 315
Medical Act Amendment Act (1886), 3, 31n, 233, 235n
Medical Act of 1858, 2, 30, 34–37, 37n, 231, 240
Medical Defence Association, 230
Medical Jurisprudence, 161
Medical Officers of Health, 211, 214
    Association of, 117
    See also Public health
Medical profession. *See* Profession, medical
Medical Register. See Registration
Medical schools, 65, 88, 121, 157–158, 163, 173, 246, 249, 295 (App. C)
    choice of, 77–80
    collegiate residences in, 81, 161
    competition in, 82–84
    enrollments in, 66, 238–239, 238n
    fees at, 69, 71, 72, 74 (Table 7)
    fiscal arrangements in, 71, 158, 163–164
    governance of, 63, 156, 161, 177–178
    and hospitals, 15, 158, 177–179, 190
    junior posts in, 160–164
    prizes in, 83–84, 159, 172
    provincial, 72, 73–75, 74 (Table 7)
    scholarships in, 75
    societies in, 268 (Table 16)
    students in, 40, 64, 76, 81–82, 85–86, 158–159, 171
    teachers in, 76, 80, 121, 161, 171, 190, 229
    and University of London, 242, 242n
    See also Curriculum; Education, medical; Universities
Medicine, principles and practice of, 60, 62 (Table 4), 63, 81, 161
Medico-Psychological Association, 267, 269n
Mental illness. *See* Nervous diseases; Psychological medicine
Merchant Taylor's School, 49
Merit, 118, 170n, 171–172
    in hospital appointments, 141–145, 150, 152, 164n, 170–172
    See also Expertise; Science; Skill; Talent
Meryon, Edward, 265
Metropolitan Asylums Board, 110
Metropolitan Society of General Practitioners in Medicine and Surgery, 23
Middlemore, Richard, 120
Middlesex Hospital, 12–13, 142 (Table 8), 152, 167
    Medical School, 65, 66, 75, 78
Midwifery, 62 (Table 4), 63, 99n, 100, 260
    fees for, 99, 209, 211 (Table 12), 212–213 (Table 13)
Military Medical practice, 85, 124–125, 125n, 211, 214, 237, 270–271 (Table 17)
    See also Individual services and societies

Milton, John Laws, 261, 265
Moore, James, 119
Moorfields Club, 266
Moreton, James E., 316
Morgan, D. H. J., 200, 204
Morgan, John Hammond, 77, 146, 345
Morgan, Thomas C., 230
Morton, Thomas, 326, 333
Moxon, Walter, 184
Munro, Henry, 315
"Munro, Stark," 93–98, 219, 222
Museums, medical, for laymen, 245, 253, 254

Nairne, Robert, 328
Namier, Lewis, 98
Neale, Adam, 327
National Association of General Practitioners, 23
National Hospital, Queen Square, 264
National Insurance Act 1911, 116n, 216, 226n, 284
National Vigilance Association, 254
Naval Surgeons, Society of, 23
Navy medical services, 124, 237
Nedham, John, 107
Nepotism, 143, 144, 147–50, 151, 169–171, 206
See also Connections; Family; Friendship; Patronage
Nervous diseases: hospitals for, 262–263 (Table 15), 264, 265; periodicals re, 270–271 (Table 17); societies re, 268 (Table 16); See also Psychological medicine
Neurology, 278
Nevison, Charles D., 329
Newman, William, 319
Nicholson, Simon, 319
Nightingale, Florence, 179
Noble, Daniel, 306
Norman, George, 105

Norman, Henry Burford, 352
Nottingham, John, 123
Nunn, Thomas William, 78, 276
Nursing (hospital), 179–183
Nussey, John, 119

Obstetrical Society, 279
Obstetrics: diploma in, 279; in general practice, 87, 99–100, 99n; in medical education, 161, 174, 269, 278; See also Maternity; Midwifery
Oculists, 260
Ogle, Cyril, 333
Ogle, John W., 333
Ophthalmic Review, 267
Ophthalmic Society of the United Kingdom, 266
Ophthalmology, 260, 269
diploma in, 279
hospitals for, 13, 262–263 (Table 15), 264, 266
periodicals of, 267, 270–271 (Table 17)
societies re, 266, 268 (Table 16)
Ord, William, 315
Ormerod, J. A., 166, 333
Otley, C. B., 199–200
Otology, 278
Ouida. See De la Ramée, Marie Louise
Owen, E. B., 311, 312
Oxbridge, 8n, 68, 81, 82, 190
and FRCP, 152, 153–154
and London hospitals, 147
and medical education, 14, 15, 66, 68, 69n, 142, 153
and University of London, 242
See also Cambridge, University of; Oxford, University of
Oxford (city of), 88
Oxford, University of, 57, 58, 66, 147, 148, 206
and FRCP, 7–8, 67 (Table 5), 153–154

Page, Harry, 335
Page, William B., 85, 121, 127
Page, William E., 328
Paget, George E., 328
Paget, James, 133n, 159, 230, 323, 332
Paget, Stephen, 163, 206n, 335
Paget, Thomas, 235n
Paris, John Ayrton, 120, 155, 329
Parkes, Edmund A ., 333
Parliament, 34, 36, 153–154, 216–218
  and BMA, 232
  and hospitals, 143, 148, 186, 187, 214–215
Partnership in medical practice, 102, 118–119
Patent medicines, 90, 247, 254, 256–259
  See also Quackery; Secret remedies; Unlicensed practioners; Unprofessional conduct
Patients, 14, 134, 154, 189, 222n, 247
  class of, and medical income, 100, 132, 209, 210, 211 (Table 12)
  competition for, 102, 228, 228n, 272
  criteria of, in selection of practitioner, 101, 104, 106–107, 109–110, 128–131
  and drug dispensing, 113, 226
  middle-class, 99, 127
  recruitment of, 94–97, 119, 128, 253
  upper class, 136, 156, 173, 221
  women, 129–130
  working-class, 114–116, 127
  See also Doctor-patient ratios; Hospitals; Special hospitals
Patronage, 156–157, 170n
  lay, 4, 14, 143, 150
  professional, 84–85, 118–124, 154–155, 163–165, 166–168,
178, 191
  See also Connections; Friend-ship; Family; Nepotism
Pavy, Frederick, 255
Pearse, T. F., 312
Pemberton, Oliver, 310
Percival, William, 315
Periodicals, medical, 84, 172, 267, 270–271 (Table 17), 298 (App. E)
Personal traits and medical careers, 8, 91, 128–130, 250–251
Pettigrew, William, 315
Physicians, 8, 8n, 84, 237
  hospital, 147–148, 152, 161–162
  house, 84
Physicians, Royal College of, 5–9, 19, 20, 257, 279
  and general practitioners, 22, 237–240
  income of, 192n
  and lay society, 154, 240
  licentiates of, 7, 37n, 62 (Table 4), 85–86, 233–234, 240
  members of, 240n
  officers of, 151–152, 190–191, 190n, 207–209, 208 (Table 11), 209n
  and provincial practitioners, 7, 67
  and trade, 225n, 255
  and universities, 7–8, 67, 152, 153–154
  and unprofessional behavior, 252, 253, 255–256
  See also Physicians, Royal College of, Fellowship; Royal Colleges
Physicians, Royal College of, Fellowship, 6–7, 67
  age at, 137n, 152, 152n
  criteria for, 152–153, 156, 173
  and education, 49, 50 (Table 1), 52n, 53–55, 54 (Table 3),

58, 66–67, 67 (Table 5)
and family, 41, 201–206,
202–203 (Table 10)
and hospitals, 151–152
and social origins, 197, 198
(Table 9), 291–293 (App. B)
Physics, 60
Physiology, 60, 61, 62 (Table 4),
81
Pick, Thomas Pickering, 334
Pitman, H. A., 320
Playfair, 1st Lord, 201
Playfair, William, 201
Plender, William, 216–219, 217
(Table 14)
Poland, John, 335
Pollock, G. D., 326
Poor Law Medical Officers: As-
sociation of, 23, 117–118, 240;
incomes of, 211, 214; practice
of, 110–114, 115, 134
Postgate, John 52
Powell, Richard Douglas, 144,
334
Power, D'Arcy, 166
Power, Henry, 166
Power, James Joseph, 122
Power, W. H. 315
Price, Charles, 328
Priestley, William Overend, 334
Profession, definition of, 37, 37n
Profession, medical, 8n, 90, 135
aristocratic connections of,
201–204, 202–203 (Table 10)
birth order and careers in,
205–206
choice of career in, 40–48
conflict in, 189, 226–231
overcrowding in, 116, 238–
239, 246, 249
social origins of, 197, 198
(Table 9), 199–201, 291–293
(App. B)
social status of, 3–4, 56, 112,
131, 194–197, 200–201, 206,
215, 226, 251, 253–255, 258

social structure of, 5–6, 12,
15, 16, 18, 19, 20, 22, 28–30,
36–37, 63, 71, 236, 241, 243,
246, 249, 283–285, 287
solidarity of, 117, 118, 228n,
231, 255, 258
unity of, 6, 15, 28, 37–38, 68,
71–72, 189–190, 231
Professional conduct, 188–190,
255
See also Medical ethics; Medical etiquette; Unprofessional
conduct
Professions other than medicine,
170, 197–200, 198 (Table 9),
204–205, 206
Profit and medical practice,
131–133, 196, 245, 247, 248–
251, 258
See also Trade
Provident dispensaries, 110, 115
Provincial Medical and Surgical
Association, 24–25, 26, 27
See also British Medical Association
Provincial practice, 3, 54 (Table
3), 54n, 93–98, 207
and family connection, 106,
108
and medical associations,
23–24, 27
and Royal Colleges, 7, 19–20,
67, 235n
Psychological medicine, 23,
262–263 (Table 15), 267, 268
(Table 16), 269, 269n, 270–
271 (Table 17), 278, 279
See also Nervous diseases
Public health, 110–114, 117, 134,
270–271 (Table 17), 279
See also Medical Officers of
Health
Public schools, 56, 57, 136, 206
medical men at, 49, 50 (Table
1), 51 (Table 2), 52, 53–55, 54
(Table 3)

See also Classical education;
Education, general; Liberal
education
Publication, medical, 172
  for lay readers, 247, 258
  and professional status, 153,
  246
Punch, 61n, 264
Pupillage, 42, 42n, 65
  See also Apprenticeship

Quackery, 5, 244n, 247, 254
  definition of, 257–258, 257n,
  258n
  general practitioners, competition from, 26, 37, 38
Quain, Jones, 77, 120
Quain, Richard, 77, 310, 327
Qualifications, medical, 33,
  35–36, 85–86, 130, 240–242
Queens' College Birmingham,
  72n

Ramage, Francis, 122
Ransome family, 105
Rawes, William, 312
Rayner, Hugh, 58
Redfern, Peter, 319
Reform, medical, 12, 19–25, 26,
  30–37
Registrar (hospital), 160
Registration, medical, 30, 33,
  34n, 35
  in *Medical Register*, 85, 258
Religion in medical life, 109–110,
  109n, 128, 144
Rendle, Richard, 321
Rentoul, Robert, 229
Research, medical, 196, 247–248
Residents (hospital), 160
Reynolds, J. R., 316
Richardson, Benjamin, 265
Ringer, Sydney, 167, 173
Rivington, Walter, 77, 333
Robertson, James, 321
Robinson, Benjamin, 328

Robinson, H. B., 312
Rogers, Joseph, 111
Rogers-Harrison, Charles H.,
  319
Roget, Peter Mark, 320, 329
Rose, Caleb, 352
Rose, H. J., 108
Rose, William, Jr., 44, 323
Rothblatt, Sheldon, 197–199
Roughton, Edmund, 334
Routh, Guy, 215–216, 219
Royal College of Medicine, 242
Royal Colleges, 12, 33, 35, 83,
  122, 241
  disciplinary action by, 259
  fees of Fellows of, 212–213
  (Table 13)
  and general practitioners, 26,
  117, 192, 230, 233, 240, 255
  and government, 188, 236,
  237–239
  and hospitals, 16, 190
  and lay society, 150–154, 240
  and M.D. degree, 241–242
  and secret remedies, 257–258
  and specialism, 277, 277n,
  279
  See also Corporations, medical; Physicians, Royal College
  of; Surgeons, Royal College
  of
Royal family, medical attendants
  of, 146, 155, 204, 266
Royal London Eye Hospital,
  264, 266
Royal (formerly Great) Northern Hospital, 264
Royal Universal Dispensary for
  Children, 261
Ruddall, James T., 321

St. Bartholomew's Hospital, 12,
  65, 120, 138, 146, 147–148,
  159, 167, 174–175, 206
  family connections at, 41, 144,
  166

governors of, 143
Medical Council of, 177, 187
Medical School, 65, 81, 177, 238, 238n
staff of, 141–142, 142 (Table 8), 162, 165n, 187
students of, 107, 133n
St. George's Hospital, 12, 57, 146
Medical School, 77
staff of, 142 (Table 8), 147, 148, 162, 165n, 166
St. John's Hospital for Diseases of the Eyes, Legs, and Breasts, 267
St. John's Hospital for Diseases of the Skin, 261, 265, 266, 269
St. Mary's Hospital and Medical School, 13, 65, 77, 142 (Table 8), 177
St. Paul's School, 49
St. Peter's Hospital for Stone, 261, 265, 274, 276–277
St. Saviour's Hospital, 269
St. Thomas's Hospital, 12, 41, 45, 85, 138, 149, 162, 179–180, 278
governors of, 140, 143
Medical School, 65, 66, 75, 76, 78, 178
staff of, 77, 142 (Table 8), 143, 144, 165n, 168–169
Sanderson, John, 201
Saunders, Edwin, 319
Saunders, Henry W., 321
Savory, Borradaile, 206
Savory, William Scovell, 206, 334
Science, 14, 57, 60, 66, 232
and careers in medicine, 41, 44–48
and lay values, 232, 282n, 283
and medical authority, 3–4, 183, 286
and specialism, 247–248, 267
as source of status, 171n, 172–173, 226
and Royal Colleges, 10, 10n,

152–153, 154
See also Expertise; Merit; Skill; Talent
Scotland, 35, 50 (Table 1), 51 (Table 2), 67 (Table 5), 86n, 125, 190
Scott, John, 121, 149, 328
Secret infirmities, 247, 256
See also Venereal disease
Secret remedies, 248, 252, 256–259
See also Patent medicines; Quackery
Secretary of State for War, 237–238
Select Committee on Medical Education, 153, 156
Select Committee on Metropolitan Hospitals, 175, 214–215, 272–273
Semon, Felix, 109, 222, 276, 278, 310 (74), 355 (60), 359 (121)
Seniority, 141, 142, 169
Seymour, Edward J., 329
Shaw, Alexander, 326
Shaw, G. B., 285–286
Shaw, George, 316
Shearman, William, 328
Shepherd, A. B., 334
Shillitoe, Buxton, 109, 119, 207–208, 315
Shillitoe, Richard Rickman, 316
Sick clubs. See Contract practice
Simmons, Richard, 328, 329
Skey, F. C., 326
Sibley, S. W., 235
Sieveking, E. H., 276
Simon, John, 34, 34n, 45–46, 162, 165n
Sims, Francis M. B., 316
Skill, 122–123, 127, 128, 130, 155
in hospital appointments, 141, 148–149, 166–168
See also Expertise; Merit; Science; Talent
Smith, Eustace, 319

Smith, Thomas, Heckstall, 43
Snell, S. H., 44–45, 45n, 101, 209
Social Mobility, 2, 204, 250–251
Socialization, 15, 44, 65, 71–72, 82, 88
Societies, medical, 18–20, 134–135, 172, 225, 268 (Table 16)
  in London, 20–21, 23, 27
  and medical corporations, 18, 18n, 19, 23
  provincial, 19–20, 24–25
  student, 81–82
  specialist, 23, 266–267, 268 (Table 16)
  See also Entries for individual societies
Society for the Suppression of Vice, 254
Society of Collegiate Physicians, 19
Society of Naval Surgeons, 23
Solly, Samuel, 77
Somerville, William, 343
South, John Flint, 149, 179, 274, 326
Southey, Herbert Henry, 329
Southey, Reginald, 47, 156, 333
Special hospitals, 248, 249, 261, 266, 267, 269
  economic factors in, 261, 264–265
  and general hospitals, 260, 265–266, 274–276
  lay support for, 264–265
  numbers of, 261, 262–263 (Table 15)
  patients in, 264–265
  profession's response to, 272–277
  See also Specialism
Specialism, 86–87, 247–248, 259
  consultants' opposition to, 273–277
  general practitioners' objections to, 272–273
  and medical education, 62

(Table 4), 190n, 269, 272, 277–279, 296–297 (App. D)
  motives for, 246, 248–251
  periodicals devoted to, 267, 270–271 (Table 17)
  and science, 247–248, 260, 267, 273–274
  societies devoted to, 266–267, 268 (Table 16)
Spermatorrhea, 244, 244n, 261
  See also Venereal disease
Sports, 82, 97, 128
Sprigge, S. Squire, 83, 84
Standard of living, 93–94, 95, 223–224
Stanley, Edward, 326
Statham, Sherard Freeman, 250, 264
Steele, W. C., 235
Stephens, James, 316
Stevenson, W. E., 219
Stewart, Alexander Patrick, 201
Stokes, William, 56, 194
Stone, William Henry, 45, 335
Strand Museum, 245, 253
Students, medical. See Medical schools
Surgeons, 9–10, 20
  hospitals, 142 (Table 8), 147, 161–162
  house, 84
  ship's 126
Surgeons, Royal College of, 5, 9–10, 26–27, 57
  Association of Fellows of, 234–235
  Association of Members of, 234–236
  conflict in, 235–236
  Council of, 10, 150–151, 151n, 234–236
  disciplinary action by, 246, 252–253, 254, 257
  family connections in, 42, 151
  and general practitioners, 16–17, 22, 31n, 85, 234–235,

234n
and hospitals, 142 (Table 8), 150–151, 190n
income of, 192n
Membership of, 10, 17, 60, 62 (Table 4), 63, 63n, 85
officers of, 9, 59, 59n, 207–209, 208 (Table 11), 209n
and professional conduct, 245–246, 252–253, 254
and specialism, 269, 279
See also Royal Colleges; Surgeons, Royal College of, Fellowship
Surgeons, Royal College of, Fellowship, 9, 10, 124–125, 130
age at, 137n
and education, 49–54, 51 (Table 2), 57, 58, 59, 59n, 67–68
and family, 41, 105–106, 108–109
and social origins, 197, 198 (Table 9), 291–294 (App. B)
Surgeons' Association, 19
Surgery: practice of, 7, 9, 10; principles and practice of, 62 (Table 4), 63, 81, 161
Sussex County Hospital, 106
Sutherland, Alexander J., 326
Sutherland's "Rheumaticon" Manufacturing Co., 254
Sutton, H. G., 336
Sutton, John Bland-, 43, 45, 78, 167
Symonds, J. A., 315
Sympson, Thomas, 315

Tait, Lawson, 352
Talent, 79, 80, 165, 167–169, 171
See also Expertise; Merit; Science; Skill
Tattersall, James, 328
Tatum, Thomas, 151, 326
Taylor, Frederick, 173

Taylor, Shephard Thomas, 82, 158–159, 253–254
Teachers, medical. *See* Medical schools
Teale, T. R., 315
Textbooks, medical, 172
Thomas, Honoratus L., 108, 311
Thompson, Henry, 320, 323
Thomson, Alexander Thom, 316
Thomson, H. B., 47, 55
Thomson, Hale, 140, 144, 147, 149–150
Thorburn, William, 311
Thorpe, Robert, 105
Thudichum, J. L., W., 277
Times (London), 184, 187, 252
Todd, Armstrong, 251
Tomes, Charles Sissmore, 311
Trade, 7, 11, 12, 128, 258
and competition, 225, 255
and general practice, 38, 113, 133–134
medical affiliation with, 253–255
and professional status, 8, 49, 131, 196, 225–226, 253, 280
secret remedies and, 256–259
Tradesmen, sons of, in medical profession, 198 (Table 9), 205, 293 (App. B)
Travers, Benjamin, Jr., 311
Treasurer (hospital). *See* Hospitals
Treves, Frederick, 335, 344
Trinity College, Dublin, 8n, 279
Trollope, Anthony, 194
Tropical medicine, 270–271 (Table 17), 279
Tuke, Daniel Hack, 109
Turner, George, 57, 195
Turner, William, 319, 335
Turton, James, 312, 316
Tutors, medical, 74 (Table 7)
Tweedie, Alexander, 47–48, 48n
Tyrell, Frederick, 41, 327

Universities, 5, 7, 35
  and conjoint examinations,
  241
  and general education of
  medical men, 57–59
  and medical education, 50
  (Table 1), 51 (Table 2), 60–61,
  67 (Table 5), 290–291 (App.
  A)
  See also Education, general;
  Education, medical; Entries
  for individual universities
University College Hospital, 13,
  140, 142, 167, 242n, 250
  Medical School, 65, 68, 176–
  177
Unprofessional conduct, 245–
  246, 252–253, 254, 255–256,
  256–259
  See also Ethics, medical;
  Etiquette, medical
Unqualified practitioners, 29,
  30–32, 32n, 36, 90, 231, 233,
  260
  See also Quackery

Vaux, Bowyer, 105
Venereal disease, 244, 244n,
  245, 245n, 247, 252, 266
  and hospitals, 140, 260,
  262–263 (Table 15), 266
  periodicals re, 270–271 (Table 17)
Vinrace, F. C., 312
Vienna, 86

Wadham, Frederick, 321
Wadham, William, 311
Wagstaffe, William Warwick, 75
Wainewright, Benjamin, 323
Wakley, Thomas, 24, 25–28,
  120, 227, 344
  and medical reform, 26–27,
  30, 33, 34–35
  and nepotism, 150, 169–170

Wall, Alfred John, 352
Walton, H. Haynes, 333
Warburton, Henry, 30
Waring, Edward J., 321
Warren, Pelham, 156
Waterlow, Sidney, 187
"Watston, Dr.," 125
Watson, Thomas, 47, 189, 237–
  238, 307, 334
Webb, William, 305
Weber, Frederic, 322
Weber, Hermann, 173, 323
Weber, Max, 6
Wells, J. A. Spencer, 209
Wells, John S., 323
Wells, Thomas Spencer, 320
  (109), 321
West, Charles, 261, 264
West Kent Infirmary and Dis-
  pensary, 122
Westminster Hospital, 12, 140,
  155, 182, 187
  governors of, 143, 144
  Medical School, 65, 62, 177
  staff of, 142 (Table 8), 147,
  149
Wheeler, Thomas Rivington,
  307, 311, 315
White, Anthony, 168
Whitelock, R. H., 312
Whitfield, Richard Gullett, 179
Whittle, E. G., 312
Wigg, Thomas, Jr., 321
Wilkinson, John S., 321
Wilks, Samuel, 173, 316
Willan Society, 266
Willett, Alfred, 166, 333
Williams, Caleb, 109
Williams, Charles J. B., 52, 53,
  315
Williams, D. J., 321
Williams, Robert, 328
Willis, William, 316
Wilson, J. A., 320, 329, 333
Wilson, James H., 329

Wilson, William James Erasmus, 120, 265, 269
Windmill Street School of Anatomy, 15
Winkfield, Alfred, 307, 327
Women
  diseases of, in medical curriculum, 62 (Table 4), 63
  hospitals for, 262–263 (Table 15)
  in medical profession, 2, 108n, 268 (Table 16)
  in nursing, 179, 183
  as patients, 92, 129–130, 131, 174
  as wives of medical men, 107–108
  See also Gynecology; Maternity; Midwifery; Obstetrics
Woods, George, 312
Woolf, Abraham, 109
Wormald, Thomas, 165n, 326
Wrench, E. M., 320

Yeats, G. D., 320, 329
Yeo, I. B., 322, 323
Young, John, 257
Young, Thomas, 328, 329